MRCPCH
MasterCourse
Volume ❶

Commissioning Editors: Ellen Green, Timothy Horne and Pauline Graham
Development Editor: Janice Urquhart
Project Manager: Gail Wright/Emma Riley
Senior Designer: Sarah Russell
Illustration Manager: Merlyn Harvey
Illustrator: Cactus

MRCPCH
MasterCourse
Volume 1

Editor in Chief

Malcolm Levene
MD FRCPCH FRCP FMedSc

Professor of Paediatrics and Child Health,
University of Leeds,
Leeds General Infirmary,
Leeds, UK

Foreword by

Professor Sir David Hall
FRCPCH FRCP FRCP(Edin)

Emeritus Professor of Community Paediatrics,
University of Sheffield;
President of the Royal College of Paediatrics and Child Health
2000–2003

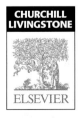

EDINBURGH LONDON NEW YORK OXFORD PHILADELPHIA ST LOUIS SYDNEY TORONTO 2007

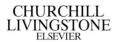

An imprint of Elsevier Limited

© 2007, Royal College of Paediatrics and Child Health

The right of Malcolm Levene to be identified as editor of this work has been asserted by him in accordance with the Copyright, Designs and Patents Act 1988

First published 2007
  Reprinted 2008 (twice), 2009, 2010

ISBN: 978-0-443-10142-7

British Library Cataloguing in Publication Data
A catalogue record for this book is available from the British Library

Library of Congress Cataloging in Publication Data
A catalog record for this book is available from the Library of Congress

Notice
Knowledge and best practice in this field are constantly changing. As new research and experience broaden our knowledge, changes in practice, treatment and drug therapy may become necessary or appropriate. Readers are advised to check the most current information provided (i) on procedures featured or (ii) by the manufacturer of each product to be administered, to verify the recommended dose or formula, the method and duration of administration, and contraindications. It is the responsibility of the practitioner, relying on their own experience and knowledge of the patient, to make diagnoses, to determine dosages and the best treatment for each individual patient, and to take all appropriate safety precautions. To the fullest extent of the law, neither the Publisher nor the Editors assume any liability for any injury and/or damage to persons or property arising out of or related to any use of the material contained in this book.

The Publisher

ELSEVIER   your source for books,
journals and multimedia
in the health sciences
www.elsevierhealth.com

Working together to grow
libraries in developing countries

www.elsevier.com | www.bookaid.org | www.sabre.org

ELSEVIER   BOOK AID International   Sabre Foundation

The
publisher's
policy is to use
**paper manufactured
from sustainable forests**

Printed in China

Foreword

Reflecting on their work to establish the structure of DNA, Watson and Crick remarked that 'they knew it would be beautiful'. And so it was — I still remember my biology master reading us their classic letter to *Nature* and explaining the implications of this awe-inspiring discovery, just a few years after it was published. But no-one then could possibly have predicted the progress that would follow in genetics, linking over the next half century with molecular and cell biology and neuroscience, nor the ways in which medicine, and paediatrics in particular, would benefit. Advances in technology have kept pace with biology — ultrasound, CT scanning, magnetic resonance imaging and endoscopic surgery were unheard of when my generation of paediatricians began their training. But some of the most important advances did not need technological genius — just careful listening, acute observation and an open mind. Just a few years after Watson and Crick published their findings, Kempe told a disbelieving medical profession and public that some parents batter their children, sometimes with fatal consequences. We have learned slowly and often reluctantly the full extent of cruelty to children and still find this distressing topic among the hardest aspects of looking after children, whether in general practice or as a paediatrician.

Developments in other areas of the medical sciences have been less dramatic but equally important. Epidemiology and public health have come of age — studies of disease patterns in populations remind us to think of the whole community and to question the way we provide medical care. Continuing advances in the methodology of clinical trials have delivered spectacular improvements in survival for children with conditions like cystic fibrosis and leukaemia. Evidence-based medicine and critical analysis of the literature, backed up by increasingly sophisticated statistics, have revolutionized our attitudes to all aspects of diagnosis and management — the wisdom received from those distinguished older colleagues who taught us when we were junior paediatricians is no longer taken as gospel.

Medical ethics and consumer involvement have had a major influence on the quality and safety of research — in particular, we have learned how to involve children and young people in decisions that affect them or their peers. Issues arising from paediatric and neonatal intensive care, and the nutritional support of profoundly disabled children, present our discipline with sometimes agonizing dilemmas for which we have to seek help from parents, colleagues, and sometimes the Courts.

The picture is less encouraging in the social sciences. We now know far more about the ways in which inadequate nutrition, poverty, bad parenting and soulless communities interact to produce child abuse, educational failure, crime and mental illness. Currently, 10–20% of UK children and young people have mental health problems that are intrusive and cause distress to themselves and their families. These problems are no less common in children who also have organic disease, and unravelling the relative contributions of each to the child's symptomatology is often very difficult. In resource-poor countries around the world, civil unrest, war and extreme poverty combined with the HIV-AIDS epidemic,

TB and malaria have devastating effects on children. Children die from treatable diseases and injuries and often lack even basic symptom relief such as analgesia. Sadly, so far most of these socially determined ills have proved equally resistant to the efforts of professional services and of politicians.

My generation has been privileged to observe and participate in what must be the most exciting period of change in the whole history of medicine. But we also recognize that the explosion of knowledge over the last half century presents enormous challenges to young doctors embarking on a career in paediatrics. The body of scientific knowledge underpinning clinical medicine is now so vast that no-one can hope to acquire a comprehensive knowledge of every topic, yet without some familiarity with the basic biological and social sciences we cannot hope to offer our patients the highest possible standards of care, nor can tomorrow's paediatricians play their full part in the further advances to come.

In many countries, membership by examination of a UK Royal College was, and still is, a highly regarded qualification. Nevertheless, when the British Paediatric Association became a Royal College in 1996, we were aware that the examination system was in urgent need of an overhaul. Candidates needed guidance on how they should apportion their study time between the scientific foundations of paediatrics and the body of clinical knowledge. The exam system encouraged candidates to focus on the complexities of paediatrics and neglect the common problems seen in primary care settings, particularly preventive care, atypical growth and development, and emotional and behavioural problems.

In order to address these problems, the College decided that a new approach to preparation for the Membership examination was needed. After reviewing the experience of other Royal Colleges, we invited Professor Malcolm Levene to lead the development of a project, which we designated 'MasterCourse', that would amalgamate the biological and social sciences with essential clinical practice in a way that would be relevant to any doctor practising paediatrics, whether in primary care or as a hospital general or specialist paediatrician. We wanted something that was not a traditional textbook — there are plenty of those around already, yet they are by their nature out of date almost before they are published, and easy access to the medical and scientific literature over the Internet simplifies searches for the latest information on practically any topic. The aim was rather to create a more interactive product that would make full use of various modes of learning. The result far exceeds my original expectations — Professor Levene and his team in partnership with Elsevier have done a wonderful job, producing a study guide that will smooth the path to Membership and raise the standard of paediatric practice across the country. But those who buy this MasterCourse will need to guard it well, for I have a sneaking suspicion that their seniors will find it a valuable way of keeping up with their trainees!

The project was conceived to meet the needs of UK trainee paediatricians — but my contacts with colleagues in other EU countries and my own experience in Southern Africa have taught me that the fundamentals of our discipline are much the same whether you work in Bristol, Budapest or Blantyre and whether you are working for the UK exams or some other system of assessment. I hope that Professor Levene's work will be of benefit to young doctors studying paediatrics in many parts of the world.

Professor Sir David Hall
Sheffield, 16th January 2007

Preface

MasterCourse is a comprehensive teaching package developed for paediatricians in training to prepare them for admission to the British Royal College of Paediatrics and Child Health by examination. These examinations are taken by young paediatricians after 2–3 years of training at SHO level and are constructed by the College to test aspects of knowledge and skills. The package has also been developed for doctors who do not intend to be full-time paediatricians but whose career aim is in the field of family medicine or with a primary care interest in Child Health. Volume 1 of the package is aimed at primary care paediatrics and Volume 2 at secondary care (hospital-based) paediatrics. Career paediatricians should know the principles in Volume 1 as well as those in Volume 2.

MasterCourse has had a long gestation since the original concept by Professor David Hall, when President of the College, who identified a proportion of paediatric trainees who were presenting to their membership examinations with a poor level of basic science knowledge intended to underpin the practice of Paediatrics and Child Health. It was suggested that a teaching package be developed to incorporate the basic science of Paediatrics together with the clinical science in a single package to help candidates pass their Membership examinations. Hence MasterCourse was conceived. Since then we have seen publication of the College competencies document as well as changes in the structure of the MRCPCH examination. The MasterCourse teaching package has been developed to take account of these changes.

To support the written material an accompanying DVD is provided to give visual and auditory data to supplement the text. This can be played on many desktop or laptop computers or on a stand-alone digital DVD player. A major component of the MasterCourse package is the supporting website, which purchase of the package entitles you to access for 3 years. The website will allow MasterCourse to grow and meet the needs of the trainees between published editions of the books. The website will provide additional data to complement the written material and give links to detailed information as well as useful websites. We will also commission new articles for the website on a regular basis to provide an overview on controversial or rapidly changing areas within our specialty. Finally the website provides extensive self-assessment material to gauge your progress in learning and also to practise for the various parts of the Membership examinations.

In producing the MasterCourse package I am grateful for the great support of three successive Presidents of the College who have seen the project through some rocky times. These include David Hall, Alan Craft and Patricia Hamilton. I am also indebted to Elsevier for their foresight in supporting the project and in particular Martin Delahunty, Ellen Green and Janice Urquhart. Finally a project of this size and complexity would not have been possible without the considerable efforts of the many authors and in particular my co-editors, who have given many hours to help to prepare the finished product. I wish to record my gratitude to the Module editors, Jonathan Darling, Mary Rudolf, Mitch Blair,

Henry Halliday, Martin Ward-Platt and Mike Hall, the DVD editor Andy Spencer and the website editors Ian Spillman and Colin Melville.

Malcolm Levene
Editor in Chief
May 2006

How to use this book

Thank you for purchasing MasterCourse. It has been written to provide you with information and skills that you will require to pass your Membership examination. We hope that as well as passing your examinations, you will adopt a style of working through this package which will stay with you for lifelong learning.

Written material

The written material is contained in two volumes. Volume 1 is directed towards the tool-kit of skills and knowledge that you will require to become proficient in the care of children, both in the community and in hospital. Volume 2 contains material relevant to career paediatricians and those working mainly in a hospital setting. It is essential that aspiring career paediatricians see Volumes 1 and 2 as equally important to pass the College examinations.

Children rarely present with a diagnosis but much more commonly present with a symptom or abnormal sign. The clinical material is initially presented as a 'Problem-orientated topic' abbreviated to 'POT' in both volumes. Each POT contains a short clinical vignette followed by a number of questions. We recommend that you read the POT and think about the answers to each of the questions before reading on. This will allow you to gauge your level of knowledge and understanding at an early stage of your learning. At the end of each POT the answer to each question is provided and the disorders are discussed.

DVD

A numbered DVD icon points to where supporting video clips are provided on the separate DVD to aid learning. These may illustrate a disorder, clinical sign or show a competency that you will be expected to know. These clips can also be used later to prepare for the clinical examination as they may be presented in a similar manner in the MRCPCH examination.

An index of icons describing the contents of each clip is supplied on page xi.

Website

Many paediatricians in training may want more than the core knowledge contained in the text, and the website provides valuable additional pointers as to how to obtain wider information. In many places in the books, a website icon has been placed to signpost towards additional reading. Many of these URLs are linked through the website to the source material. In addition, the website provides further reading at a higher level for those interested in reading around the subject.

The website also contains self-assessment questions similar to those presented in the various parts of the MRCPCH examination and these in turn are designed to cover the range of competencies required to pass the examination. The self-assessment can be accessed on the website by chapter title or can be presented in random format for examination practice. Details on how to access the website are available on the inside front cover. Finally, the website will provide regular updates on topics of current interest to trainee paediatricians, written by experts in the field.

We hope that you enjoy using MasterCourse and, of course, we hope you enjoy working with children in your professional life and that what you learn from the MasterCourse package provides you with life-long skills used for the benefit of children.

Good Luck.

Index of DVD clips

Module editors

Mitch Blair
MBBS BSc MSc FRCP FRCPCH FRIPH MILT
Consultant Reader in Paediatrics and Child Public Health, Imperial College (Northwick Park Campus), London, UK

Jonathan Darling
MB ChB MD FRCPCH
Senior Lecturer in Paediatrics and Child Health, St James's University Hospital, Leeds, UK

Michael A. Hall
MB ChB FRCPCH FRCP DCH
Consultant Neonatologist and Paediatrician, Honorary Senior Clinical Lecturer, University of Southampton Princess Anne Hospital and Southampton General Hospital, Southampton, UK

Henry L. Halliday
MD FRCP FRCPE
Honorary Professor of Child Health and Consultant Neonatologist, Regional Neonatal Unit, Royal Maternity Hospital, Belfast, UK

Malcolm Levene
MD FRCPCH FRCP FMedSc
Professor of Paediatrics and Child Health, University of Leeds, Leeds General Infirmary, Leeds, UK

Mary Rudolf
MB BS BSc DCH FRCPCH FAAP
Professor of Child Health and Consultant Paediatrician, University of Leeds, Leeds, UK

Martin Ward-Platt
MB ChB MD FRCP FRCPCH
Consultant Paediatrician, Newcastle upon Tyne Hospitals NHS Trust; Reader in Neonatal and Paediatric Medicine, Newcastle University, Newcastle, UK

DVD Editor

S. Andrew Spencer
BM BS BMedSci MRCP DM FRCPCH
Consultant Paediatrician, University Hospital North Staffordshire; Honorary Reader in
Neonatal Medicine, Keele University, North Staffordshire, UK

Website Editors

Ian Spillman
FRCPCH DA DCH DTM&H
Consultant Paediatrician, Macclesfield District General Hospital, UK

Colin Melville
MB ChB MMedEd FRCPCH
Senior Lecturer in Paediatrics and Consultant Paediatrician, Keele University, UK

Contributors

Julie-Clare Becher
MB ChB MD MRCPCH
Higher Specialist Trainee in Neonatology, Department of Neonatology, Simpson Centre
for Reproductive Health, Royal Infirmary of Edinburgh, Edinburgh, UK

Mark Bradbury
MB BS
Consultant Paediatric Nephrologist, Central Manchester and Manchester Children's
University Hospital, NHS Trust, Manchester, UK

Alan Cade
MB ChB DCH MRCP FRCPCH
Consultant Respiratory Paediatrician, Derriford Hospital, Plymouth, UK

Imti Choonara
MD FRCPCH
Professor in Child Health, University of Nottingham, Derbyshire Children's Hospital, UK

Angus J. Clarke
DM FRCP FRCPCH
Professor and Honorary Consultant in Clinical Genetics, Cardiff University,
University Hospital of Wales, Cardiff, UK

Sir Alan Craft
MD FRCPCH FRCP FMedSci
Professor of Child Health, University of Newcastle upon Tyne, Newcastle upon Tyne, UK

Rachel Crowther
MB BChir MSc MFPH DipLATHE
Consultant in Public Health Medicine, South East Public Health Observatory, UK

Jonathan Darling
MB ChB MD FRCPCH
Senior Lecturer in Paediatrics and Child Health, St James's University Hospital, Leeds, UK

Mark Davies
MA MB BCh MRCP
Specialist Registrar in Medical Genetics, Institute of Medical Genetics,
University Hospital of Wales, Cardiff, UK

Melanie Epstein
MBBCh MRCPCh Dip Psych
Department of Community Paediatrics, St James's University Hospital, Leeds, UK

David Evans
BM BCh MA MRCP FRCPCH
Consultant Neonatologist, Southmead Hospital, Bristol, UK

Simon Frazer
MB ChB MRCPCH
Consultant Paediatrician, Bradford Teaching Hospitals Foundation Trust, Bradford, UK

Sue Gentle
FRCPCH
Consultant Paediatrician, Ryegate Children's Centre, Sheffield Children's NHS Trust, Sheffield, UK

John Hain
MB ChB BSc MRCGP DFFP Dip Derm
General Practitioner and Approved GP Trainer for the Yorkshire Deanery, Yorkshire, UK

Richard Hain
MB BS MSc MD MRCP FRCPCH DipPalMed
Senior Lecturer/Honorary Consultant in Paediatric Palliative Medicine, Department of Child Health, Cardiff School of Medicine, University Hospital of Wales, Cardiff, UK

Valerie Harpin
FRCP FRCPCH MD
Consultant Paediatrician (Neurodisability), Ryegate Children's Centre, Sheffield Children's NHS Trust, Sheffield, UK

Delyth Howard
MB BChir MRCP MSc
Consultant Community Paediatrician, Great Ormond Street NHS Trust and Islington Primary Care Trust, London, UK

Alison Kelly
MB ChB MRCPCH
Consultant Community Paediatrics, Yorkhill Hospitals, Glasgow, UK

Nigel Kennedy
MB BS FRCP FRCPCH DCH DRCOG
General Practitioner, Aylesbury; Hospital Practitioner, Paediatrics, Stoke Mandeville Hospital, Aylesbury, UK

Malcolm Levene
MD FRCPCH FRCP FMedSc
Professor of Paediatrics and Child Health, University of Leeds, Leeds General Infirmary, Leeds, UK

Aidan MacFarlane
MB BChir FRCP FRCPCH FFPH
Independent International Consultant in Child and Adolescent Health, Oxford, UK

Neil McIntosh
DSc(Med) FRCP FRCPE FRCPCH
Professor of Child Life and Health, University of Edinburgh; Honorary Consultant
Paediatrician, Lothian University Hospitals NHS Trust, Edinburgh, UK

Colin Morgan
MD MRCP FRCPCH
Consultant Neonatologist, Liverpool Women's Hospital, Liverpool, UK

Ed Peile
MB BS EdD FRCP FRCGP FRCPCH MRCS DCH DRCOG
Professor, Associate Dean (Teaching), Head of Institute of Clinical Education,
Medical Teaching Centre, Warwick Medical School, The University of Warwick, Coventry, UK

Alison Pike
MD DCH MRCP FRCPCH
Consultant Neonatologist, Southmead Hospital, Bristol, UK

Gillian Robinson
MB ChB MRCP(Paeds) MMedSc
Consultant Paediatrician, Leeds PCT, Leeds, UK

Mary Rudolf
MB BS BSc DCH FRCPCH FAAP
Professor of Child Health and Consultant Paediatrician, University of Leeds, Leeds, UK

Arnab K. Seal
MD DCH FRCPCH
Consultant Paediatrician, Leeds General Infirmary, Leeds, UK

Neela Shabde
FRCP FRCPCH DCH DCCH
Consultant Paediatrician, Northumbria Healthcare NHS Trust,
North Tyneside General Hospital, North Shields, UK

Kathleen Skinner
MB ChB MRCP MRCPCH MPH
Specialist Registrar in Public Health, Oxford City PCT, Oxford, UK

Ragbir Thethy
MBChB MRCPI MSc
Consultant Paediatrician, St James's University Hospital, Leeds, UK

Amanda J. Thomas
MB BS DCH MMedSci MA FRCPCH
Consultant Community Paediatrician, East Leeds Primary Care Trust, Leeds, UK

Charlotte M. Wright
BMedSci BM BCH MSc MD FRCPCH FRCP
Professor of Community Child Health, Glasgow University, Yorkhill Children's Hospital,
Glasgow, UK

Linda Wolfson
RM ADM/DPSM BSc Mid
Infant Feeding Specialist, Queen Mother's Maternity Hospital, Yorkhill Hospitals,
Glasgow

List of abbreviations

AAP	American Academy of Pediatrics
ABR	auditory brainstem responses
ACE	angiotensin-converting enzyme
ACPC	Area Child Protection Committee
ADH	antidiuretic hormone
ADHD	attention deficit hyperactivity disorder
ADR	adverse drug reaction
AFP	alpha-fetoprotein
ALSG	Advanced Life Support Group
ALTE	apparent life-threatening event
AOM	acute otitis media
AP	antero-posterior
ASD	atrial septal defect
BCG	bacille Calmette–Guérin
BMA	British Medical Association
BMI	body mass index
BNF	*British National Formulary*
CCK	cholecystokinin
cDNA	complementary DNA
CGH	comparative genomic hybridization
CHT	congenital hypothyroidism
CI	confidence interval
CNS	central nervous system
CNSD	chronic non-specific diarrhoea
CPCC	Child Protection Case Conference
CRH	corticotrophin-releasing hormone
CRP	C-reactive protein
CSF	cerebrospinal fluid
CSOM	chronic suppurative otitis media
CT	computed tomography
CTG	cardiotochograph
CVS	chorionic villus sampling
CXR	chest X-ray
DCH	Diploma of Child Health
DDH	developmental dysplasia of the hip
DFES	Department for Education and Skills
DLA	Disability Living Allowance
DTaP/IPV/Hib	diphtheria, tetanus, acellular pertussis, polio and Hib
EBM	evidence-based medicine
EBV	Epstein–Barr virus

ECG	electrocardiography
ECMO	extra-corporeal membranous oxygenation
EDD	expected delivery date
EMG	electromyography
ENT	ear, nose and throat
FBC	full blood count
FII	factitious or induced illness
FIL	feedback inhibitor
FISH	fluorescent in situ hybridization
FTT	failure to thrive
FXTAS	fragile X-associated tremor/ataxia syndrome
GMC	General Medical Council
GP	general practitioner
GRF	growth hormone releasing factor
GUM	genitourinary medicine
HBV	hepatitis B vaccine
hCG	human chorionic gonadotrophin
HDN	haemolytic disease of the newborn
hGH	human growth hormone
HIV	human immunodeficiency virus
HPV	human papillomavirus
HSV	herpes simplex virus
HTA	Health Technology Assessment
ICD-10	International Statistical Classification of Diseases — 10th revision
ICF	International Classification of Functioning and Disability
ICIDH	International Classification of Impairments, Disabilities and Handicaps
IDT	infant distraction test
IGF	insulin-like growth factor
IMD	Index of Multiple Deprivation
IMPS	injury minimization and prevention
IMR	infant mortality rate
IPV	inactivated polio vaccine
IRT	immunoreactive trypsinogen
LABA	long-acting bronchodilator
LP	lumbar puncture
LRTI	lower respiratory tract infection
LSCB	Local Safeguarding Children Board
MCAD(D)	medium chain acyl CoA dehydrogenase (deficiency)
MCH	mean cell haemoglobin
MCV	mean cell volume
MELAS	mitochondrial encephalomyopathy with lactic acidosis and stroke-like episodes
MMR	measles/mumps/rubella vaccination
MRCPCH	Membership of the Royal College of Paediatrics and Child Health
mRNA	messenger RNA
MRSA	meticillin-resistant *Staphylococcus aureus*
MSH	melanocyte-stimulating hormone
MSU	midstream urine
NGT	nasogastric tube
NHS	National Health Service
NICE	National Institute for Clinical Excellence
NICU	neonatal intensive care unit
NOFTT	non-organic failure to thrive
NPA	nasopharyngeal aspirate
NPY	neuropeptide Y

NSAID	non-steroidal anti-inflammatory drug
NSF	National Service Framework
NSPCC	National Society for Prevention of Cruelty to Children
NT	nuchal translucency
OAE	oto-acoustic emissions
OFTT	organic failure to thrive
ONS	Office for National Statistics
OPCS–4	Office of Population, Censuses and Surveys' Classification of Surgical Operations and Procedures — 4th revision
OPV	oral polio vaccine
PA	pulmonary artery; postero-anterior
PAPP-A	pregnancy-associated plasma protein-A
PAS	Patient Administration System
PCR	polymerase chain reaction
PCT	Primary Care Trust
PDA	patent ductus arteriosus
PEFR	peak expiratory flow rate
PET	positron emission tomography
PHCT	primary healthcare team
PICU	paediatric intensive care unit
PKU	phenylketonuria
PWS	Prader–Willi syndrome
RAST	radioallergosorbence testing
RCPCH	Royal College of Paediatrics and Child Health
RCT	randomized controlled trial
RSV	respiratory syncytial virus
RTA	road traffic accident
SEN	special education needs
SENCO	special educational needs coordinator
SGA	small for gestational age
SHO	senior house officer
SIDS	sudden infant death syndrome
SIGN	Scottish Intercollegiate Guideline Network
SLE	systemic lupus erythematosus
SNP	single nucleotide polymorphism
SUDI	sudden unexplained death in infancy
SVT	supraventricular tachycardia
TDM	therapeutic drug monitoring
TPN	total parenteral nutrition
tRNA	transfer RNA
TSH	thyroid-stimulating hormone
UE	unconjugated oestriol
U&Es	urea and electrolytes
UNCRC	United Nations Convention on the Rights of the Child
UNHS	universal newborn hearing screening
UNICEF	United Nations Children's Fund
URTI	upper respiratory tract infection
UTI	urinary tract infection
VAPP	vaccine-associated paralytic polio
VSD	ventricular septal defect
VT	ventricular tachycardia
WHO	World Health Organization
ZIG	zoster immunoglobulin

Contents

Contents

Edited by Jonathan Darling

Normal children and child health

MODULE ONE

Alan Craft

Child health in a changing society

LEARNING OUTCOMES

By the end of this chapter you should know and understand the following principles concerning paediatrics and child health:

- The duties of a paediatrician
- The need for changes to the service in light of social, environmental, economic and disease changes
- The major causes of mortality and morbidity in childhood
- The skills required to be a good paediatric practitioner.

MODULE ONE

Introduction

Children are a nation's most important asset and their health and welfare must be safeguarded. In 2005 a report was published in England entitled 'Every Child Matters'. It emphasized the need to commit to support children in order to:

- Be healthy
- Stay safe
- Enjoy and achieve
- Make a positive contribution
- Achieve economic wellbeing.

Paediatricians play a crucial role in achieving these aims, where necessary working with other healthcare professionals, social workers and teachers.

Paediatrics is not just about the recognition and treatment of illness in babies and children. It also encompasses child health, which covers all aspects of growth and development and the prevention of disease. At the end of childhood, paediatricians must ensure a smooth transition of care to adult services, especially for those with chronic conditions.

Paediatrics and child health include every aspect of life from birth (and often before) up to adulthood. Paediatricians are usually responsible for children up to the age of 18 years, although in practice, for those in the latter years of childhood, care is shared with adolescent or adult practitioners.

Paediatrics covers everyone from a totally dependent newborn baby to a fully independent adult, and from a 24-week-gestation baby weighing less than 500 g to an obese teenager of 150 kg or more.

Every facet of paediatrics is coloured by the fact that a child is growing and developing in both a physical and an emotional sense. More than in any other aspect of medicine, the needs of the family and carers have to be considered in everything that is done.

There is increasing evidence that factors operating in fetal life, infancy and childhood are important determinants of adult health.

Paediatrics and child health are about ensuring optimum health during a critical period of life and, by so doing, putting the young adult on the road to a healthy future.

What is a paediatrician?

He or she is someone who is medically qualified and who commits himself or herself to a career of working with children. Paediatrics covers a huge spectrum of different areas so it is difficult to say that there is a typical paediatrician profile. The specialty includes everything from neonatal and paediatric intensive care, where very sick children have to be managed, rapid decisions have to be made and the outcomes are often uncertain, to areas such as neurodisability, where different skills are required to manage a chronic condition and outcomes may not be seen for many years. There is also the public health role of disease prevention and the planning and evaluation of services.

So are there any particular attributes necessary to be a paediatrician? A liking for children is obviously a prerequisite, along with an ability to communicate with children and their families.

The need for triadic consultations, e.g. taking a history from a child as well as a parent or carer, makes paediatricians unusual but not unique.

The Royal College of Paediatrics and Child Health (RCPCH) has a statement indicating the duties of a paediatrician and this gives a good summary of the very wide roles that should be played (Box 1.1).

The paediatrician must be aware of the United Nations Convention on the Rights of the Child (1989), to which virtually every country in the world has signed up. This embodies the right of every child to:
- Equality regardless of race, religion, nationality or sex
- Special protection for full physical, intellectual, moral, spiritual and social development in a healthy and normal manner
- A name and nationality
- Adequate nutrition, housing and medical services
- Special care if handicapped
- Love, understanding and protection
- Free education, play and recreation
- Priority for relief in times of disaster
- Protection against all forms of neglect, cruelty and exploitation
- Protection from any form of discrimination, and the right to be brought up in a spirit of universal brotherhood, peace and tolerance.

Paediatrics is changing

In the early part of the 20th century infection was the major cause of both morbidity and mortality. There was

---

BOX 1.1 Duties of a paediatrician

- Paediatricians should commit themselves to practise in accordance with the Objects of the College and the UN Convention on the Rights of the Child
- Paediatricians have a responsibility to safeguard the reputation of paediatrics through their personal clinical practice and through participation in continuing professional development, enabling them to maintain and enhance their knowledge, skills and competence for effective clinical practice to meet the needs of children
- Paediatricians should recognize the limitations of their skills and seek advice and support when this would be in the best interests of the child
- Paediatricians should espouse paediatric research and promote interchange between medical science and clinical practice as it affects the life and health of children
- Paediatricians should pay due regard to the domestic, sociological, environmental and genetic dimensions of the health of children
- Paediatricians, whatever their specialty interest, should understand their particular responsibilities for the holistic and life-long health of children who come under their care; each contact is an opportunity for health promotion and disease prevention
- Paediatricians should serve as clinicians to the individual child while contributing to public health medicine
- Paediatricians should be aware of current medical and political affairs affecting the lives and health of children
- Paediatricians should serve as advocates for the health needs of children locally, nationally and internationally
- Paediatricians should see themselves as ambassadors for children and for the specialty of paediatrics
- Above all, paediatricians should be courteous and compassionate in all their professional dealings with children, their parents and other carers, placing the child's best interests at the centre of all clinical considerations

---

a clear link between infection and social circumstances. Improvements in housing and the environment began the trend for improvements to the health of the population and this was accelerated by the introduction of both immunization to prevent infections and antibiotics to treat them. The first day of life is the time when children are most vulnerable but improvements in antenatal and neonatal care have done much to minimize the dangers present at this time.

There are many indicators used to monitor the health of populations and those applied to children are often a good measure of the health and health services of the total population. The key measures are:

- *Perinatal mortality*: stillbirths plus first week deaths per 1000 total births
- *Infant mortality rate (IMR)*: deaths in the first year per 1000 live births
- *Under-5 mortality*: deaths in the first 5 years of life per 1000 live births.

There has been a steady fall in all of these indicators over the last 100 years and both babies and children are now very healthy. However, this is not universal. Although economically advantaged countries have IMRs in single figures, economically less well-off countries, for example in sub-Saharan Africa, still have levels of over 200. More worrying is the fact that, for some of the least well-off countries, indicators of health are getting worse. It is also interesting to note that there can be substantial differences within individual countries according to social class and other factors; for example, in the US in 1998, the IMR for babies with white mothers was 6.0 but more than double at 14.1 for those with non-white mothers. This racial difference probably accounts for the striking variation in IMR between the state of New Hampshire, where it is 4.3, and the District of Columbia, at 13.2.

So, in spite of children getting healthier, demands for health services are increasing. The reasons for this paradox are complex. Parents are much less experienced than previously as they have usually grown up in small families with few siblings. Parental and grandparent support used to be readily available from relatives who were experienced. In addition, the 'nuclear' family is now no longer the closed unit of the past. A great deal more can be done for those who are ill and more is expected. Finally, parents are better educated but because of this they are more worried and concerned about ill health. Each year in the UK:

- 1 in 12 0–4-year-olds and 1 in 25 5–15-year-olds are admitted to hospital
- 1 in 4 children visit an accident and emergency department
- Under-5s visit a general practitioner 7 times and 5–15-year-olds 3 times.

The average length of hospital stay has declined from over 8 days 40 years ago to less than 2 days in 2005.

Causes of morbidity and mortality

These vary according to the different stages of life.

Table 1.1 Major causes of death

Stage of life	Cause of death
Stillbirth	Hypoxia/asphyxia (20%) Congenital abnormalities (7%) Prematurity (5%) Maternal causes (14%)
Neonatal death	Congenital abnormalities (25%) Prematurity (28%) Non-infectious respiratory disorders, including respiratory distress syndrome (20%) Infections (5%)
Post-neonatal deaths	Congenital abnormalities (27%) Sudden unexplained death in infancy (SUDI) (20%) Late effects of perinatal problems (17%) Infection (6%) Respiratory problems (10%)
1–4 years	Accidents Congenital abnormalities Infections
5–14 years	Malignancy Accidents Infections Congenital abnormalities

Mortality

The major causes of death in the UK are given in Table 1.1.

It is important to note that infection remains the leading cause of death in children in economically disadvantaged countries, with the human immunodeficiency virus (HIV) playing an increasingly important role.

Morbidity

General practice remains the first port of call for most children with an acute problem. The average number of consultations in the first 4 years of life is 6 per year, falling to 2.5 in the 5–14 age group. Boys are slightly more likely to consult than girls (ratio 1.1:1).

Common causes of consultation are non-infectious respiratory problems and acute infections, most commonly of the respiratory tract, ear, eyes and skin. These bacterial and viral infections far outweigh other causes of consultation.

Hospital

In all, 1 in 8 children is admitted between the ages of 0 and 4 years and 1 in 16 between 5 and 15 years. Many children are now admitted to hospital for relatively short periods. Over the last 50 years the total number of children admitted to hospital has increased whilst the total length of stay has gone down dramatically. Most of these children are acutely unwell and probably have an infection. A short period of admission to hospital, or day case observation, allows the child to be assessed and discharged home to recover once serious problems have been excluded. The major causes of admission to hospital, including during the neonatal period, are:

- Perinatal conditions 17%
- Disorders of the respiratory system 14%
- Disorders of the ear 11%
- Injuries and poisoning 10%
- Ill-defined symptoms, e.g. abdominal pain 9%
- Disorders of the digestive system 7%.

Outpatient attendance

In all, 1 in 5 children attends a hospital each year, either in accident and emergency or in the outpatient department. Major reasons for attendance are accidents, respiratory disorders, and neonatal, developmental and disability problems. In addition, 1 in 300 children will attend a child and adolescent mental health unit.

Influences on child health

Gender

At all ages boys have a higher death rate than girls. This is particularly true as boys get older, when the difference is largely due to increased danger from accidents.

Social factors

The socioeconomic status, usually measured by social class, is a powerful predictor of most aspects of child health and illness; for example, in the neonatal period there is a clear association between birth weight, neonatal outcome and social class. In the first year of life, sudden unexplained death in infancy (SUDI) is strongly influenced by social and environmental factors; the risk is of the order of 1 in 200 for high-risk families but 1 in 8500 for those of low risk. For the rest of childhood there is a clear association between social class and most causes of morbidity and mortality, including admission to hospital.

Maternal factors

Disease in the mother can directly affect the newborn baby. Examples of this are maternal diabetes (a baby may be born preterm with a disproportionately high birth weight) and thyroid disease (babies of thyrotoxic mothers may also have such symptoms in the newborn period). Drugs, e.g. antiepileptics, given to mothers during pregnancy can directly affect the fetus and newborn. Maternal influences are covered in Chapter 8.

Influence of fetal and infant life on adult life

Over the last few years increasing evidence has emerged of the effect of fetal and infant factors in adult disease. This was first described by Professor David Barker from Southampton and is known as the Barker Hypothesis. This states:

Under-nutrition in utero programmes foetal metabolism to produce a 'thrifty' phenotype. Thus babies who are small at birth are liable to become adults with increased susceptibility to hypertension, cardiovascular disease, central obesity, impaired glucose tolerance.

Barker has found a correlation between birth weight and other measures of fetal nutrition and the subsequent development of cardiovascular disease, hypertension and diabetes in later life. There seems little doubt that the Barker effect does exist but it remains to be shown what the total contribution is to adult disease. It is likely that adult lifestyle, e.g. tobacco smoking, lack of exercise and poor diet leading to obesity, is a greater and more easily remediable influence.

Skills needed for paediatric practice

All paediatricians need to have the basic medical skills as outlined in the General Medical Council's booklet on 'Good Medical Practice'. The principles apply to all doctors but have been amplified for paediatricians by the RCPCH in its publication, 'Good Medical Practice in Paediatrics and Child Health'. This again expands on the principles outlined in Box 1.1. The importance of working in teams and of recognizing the skills and contribution of other professionals must be acknowledged. All doctors must maintain professional etiquette and the particular needs of children and families need to be considered. A general principle in all medical practice is the need to communicate with patients and in paediatric practice this needs to involve both child and family. Children's level of understanding develops with age and also with stage of development, and the latter in particular must be assessed in order to ascertain an appropriate level of communication.

There are particular ethical and legal issues that need to be considered in the practice of paediatrics and these are covered in Chapter 11. Some of the most difficult areas are around issues of confidentiality and those relating to child protection have been summarized in the RCPCH document, 'Responsibility of Doctors in Child Protection Cases with Regard to Confidentiality' (see also Chs 21 and 37).

There have been significant changes in the way that medicine is practised compared to just 25 years ago. Medicine is now so complex that no doctor can expect to know everything in his or her particular field of expertise, let alone outside of it. Medical students are taught in a different way, so that they learn and understand the principles of medicine and how to find out about those areas where they are uncertain. The shorter time periods available for postgraduate training, along with this rapid expansion of knowledge, make the newly qualified paediatrician less experienced than in the past. It is important therefore not to work in isolation, to be part of a team, and not to be afraid to ask for a second opinion.

The environment in which we work has also changed and, partly because of greater public expectation, there is a greater tendency to complain when things have not gone the way that might have been expected. All doctors — and paediatricians are no exception — have to be prepared for complaints and must know how to handle them. Good communication is the key both to preventing complaints and to dealing with them well. Clear explanations of the aims and limitations of treatment and what is likely to be the outcome in a particular situation will do much to produce realistic expectations. If something does go wrong, then honesty and a clear explanation are important. The most important factor for patients and parents when adverse outcomes have occurred is to know what the reasons are and that every step has been taken to try to prevent the same outcome for future patients.

A career working with children is hugely rewarding and there can be no greater pleasure than to have an adult, whom you treated as a child, come into your consulting room and tell you about their life achievements and show you their own offspring.

2

Child development and developmental problems

Delyth Howard

LEARNING OUTCOMES

By the end of this chapter you should:
- Understand prenatal brain development
- Know the factors influencing a child's development
- Understand the process of normal development
- Know how to assess development in a child under 5 years of age
- Know the common patterns of developmental abnormality.

You should also take this opportunity to ensure that:
- You are able to perform a developmental assessment on a child under the age of 5 years
- You know how to perform basic assessment of hearing and vision
- You can recognize common patterns of developmental delay
- You know when to refer on for detailed developmental assessment.

MODULE ONE

Introduction

A knowledge of child development is integral to all of our work as paediatricians. It influences how we interact with our patients and how we manage their medical conditions. In addition, we need to be able to assess and diagnose developmental problems.

Basic science: the development of the nervous system

Prenatal development is an important factor in postnatal developmental issues. The developing brain is vulnerable to a range of influences.

BOX 2.1 Development of the nervous system

16 days	Neural plate forms from ectoderm
18 days	Neural groove
22 days	Neural tube
27 days	Neural tube closed, brain and spinal cord differentiation begins
4 weeks	Triencephalon: three-vesicle stage of brain development
6 weeks	Five-vesicle stage, with differentiation of cerebral hemispheres
From 4–9 months	Histogenesis, cell differentiation into neurons and supporting cells
	Cell proliferation and neuronal migration
Near term	Myelination

Table 2.1 **Malformations and timings**

Stage	Normal development	Failure
Stage 1 (weeks 3–4)	Formation and closure of spinal cord	Anencephaly Encephalocele Chiari malformation Spina bifida
Stage 2 (weeks 5–10)	Formation of brain segments	Holoprosencephaly Corpus callosum agenesis Dandy–Walker syndrome
Stage 3 (2–5 months)	Neuronal migration and cellular differentiation	Heterotopias Polymicrogyria Agyria-pachygyria Lissencephaly
Stage 4 (5–15 months)	Myelination	Developmental delay Dysmyelinating disease

Prenatal brain development (Box 2.1)

1st trimester

Differentiation of the nervous system starts with the development of the neural plate from the ectoderm, 16 days after conception. This plate, which stretches along the entire back of the embryo, lengthens and starts folding up, forming a groove at around 18 days. The neural groove then begins fusing shut into a tube at around 22 days post-conception. By 27 days, the neural tube is fully closed and has begun its transformation into the brain (cephalic portion) and spinal cord (caudal portion). Neural crests give rise to the peripheral nervous system. The brain undergoes further differentiation, but the spinal cord retains the tubular structure.

Defects in formation of the neural tube lead to major brain or spinal cord defects, often lethal. Incomplete closure (dysraphism), occurring in the first 3–4 weeks of gestation, may give rise to anencephaly, encephaloceles or spina bifida (Ch. 28). At 4 weeks the brain structures are differentiated into three vesicles: forebrain, midbrain and hindbrain. From 4 to 6 weeks further development of the forebrain takes place, with differentiation of the cerebral hemispheres. The next stage in brain development is histogenesis, with cells differentiating into neurons or glial cells. Neuronal proliferation begins at 2 months of gestation.

Neurological activity in the fetus is manifest by 6 weeks' gestation, with spontaneous arching of the body. Reflex limb movements follow at 8 weeks, with more complex coordinated movements by 10 weeks (hiccuping, yawning, thumb sucking).

2nd trimester

Neuronal proliferation continues. Neuronal migration spans a period between 4 and 9 months of gestation. Disorders in neuronal proliferation, migration and maturation result in a variety of brain malformations (Ch. 28). These include lissencephaly, schizencephaly and agenesis of the corpus callosum. These are generally associated with psychomotor delay and seizures. Microcephaly (p. 253) may be a manifestation of abnormal neuronal proliferation or migration.

The second trimester marks the onset of more neurological activity in the form of critical reflexes: continuous breathing movements and coordinated sucking and swallowing reflexes. These abilities are controlled by the brainstem. The brainstem is largely mature by the end of the second trimester, which is when babies first become able to survive outside the womb. The grasp reflex is evident by 17 weeks, with the Moro reflex seen from 25 weeks.

3rd trimester

By the 6th month, nearly all the neurons needed for life are present. Last to mature is the cerebral cortex. Myelination begins near term.

In the last trimester, fetuses are capable of simple forms of learning, like habituating (decreasing their startle response) to a repeated auditory stimulus, such as a loud clap just outside the mother's abdomen.

Brain malformations may result from exogenous and endogenous causes (Table 2.1). Exogenous causes may be nutritional, radiological, viral, chemical, medications or ischaemic. Endogenous causes are genetic.

Postnatal brain development

The nervous system continues to undergo further development and maturation for some time after birth. By birth, only the lower portions of the nervous system (the spinal cord and brainstem) are very well developed, whereas the higher regions (the limbic system and cerebral cortex) are still rather primitive. Although all of the neurons in the cortex are produced before birth, they are poorly connected. In contrast to the brainstem and spinal cord, the cerebral cortex produces most of its synaptic connections after birth. Synapses are formed at a very rapid rate during the early months of life, achieving maximum density between 6 and 12 months after birth. The infant's brain forms and retains synapses that are frequently used. Synapses decrease due to disuse or natural attrition (apoptosis). Early experiences are thus vital to the formation and retention of synapses. By 2 years of age, a child's cerebral cortex contains well over 100 trillion synapses.

Myelination continues throughout childhood and possibly onwards in adulthood. The timing of myelination depends on the area of the brain in question.

Factors influencing development

There are many influences on a child's development (Box 2.2). These influences interact to produce the picture we see in the child. Genes and environment interact at every step of brain development. Generally speaking, genes are responsible for:
- The basic wiring plan
- Forming neurons and connections between different brain regions.

BOX 2.2 Factors influencing development

Prenatal
- Toxins: infections, drugs, alcohol
- Ischaemia
- Nutrition
- Genetic: chromosomal disorders, single gene defects

Pre- or postnatal?
- Parental IQ: IQ may be partially genetically determined, but parental IQ may also influence parenting

Postnatal
- Social environment
- Personality
- Emotional factors: interaction with caregivers
- Cultural factors
- Nutrition
- Parenting
- Physical health

Experience is responsible for fine-tuning those connections. It is usually not possible to separate out the most significant influences on an individual's development: the 'nature versus nurture' debate.

Normal development

Normal development follows a recognized sequence in most children. Children have to acquire certain skills before being able to move on to the next skill (for example, the development of head control is a prerequisite for sitting). Previous mass observations of children have given us the typical sequence of acquiring developmental skills, as well as the range of expected ages for key developmental skills (known as 'milestones'). It is on these that we base our decisions about whether a child is developing normally. There are, of course, significant variations within the 'normal' range.

During your career, you will build up your own personal knowledge of normal development from interacting with hundreds of children. Nothing can replace this experience, but before you have built up this memory bank, you will need a foundation from which to start. Tables of developmental milestones can provide some guidance on expected developmental skills at certain ages. It is never possible to provide an exhaustive list of milestones. You must also be aware that suggested ages for certain skills may vary between authors. As you gain experience, you will get a feel for what is usual at each age. Nevertheless, it is helpful to learn some key milestones, as well as the normal sequence of skill development, which is perhaps more important.

Typically developing children may show slight variations in their skill levels in different areas of development. For example, they may be slightly more advanced in their gross motor skills and relatively less advanced in their speech and language skills, or vice versa.

Categories of development

Developmental skills can be grouped into the following four categories. These categories are not mutually exclusive, and some skills may span categories:
- *Fine motor and vision*: hand skills, including drawing, puzzles
- *Speech, language and hearing*: communication skills, including receptive and expressive language, and non-verbal communication
- *Gross motor*: large movements, including sitting, walking, running, going upstairs
- *Social behaviour and play*: including feeding, toileting, dressing and social relationships.

Fine motor and vision

A child's visual abilities are developing and changing along with other areas of development. Visual skills are closely linked to fine motor skills. During the first year of life, babies progress from only being able to focus on objects very close by, to rapidly developing distance vision. From a few months of age, visual abilities are being integrated with hand skills in reaching for objects. Subsequently infants develop the ability to focus on rapidly moving objects and to judge distances. Between 1 and 2, children will develop their visual interest in simple pictures, in addition to recognizing real objects. Refinement of hand skills continues, with development in grasp and control. Children often do not have a clear hand preference until around 3 years of age, with 90% demonstrating a clear preference by age 4.

Speech, language and hearing

Prelingual (1st year)

Babies in their first year are learning about communication, and have a variety of communication strategies before they develop language. From very early in life, babies will mimic the facial expressions of adults. Conversational exchanges occur, with babies learning about turn-taking in reciprocal vocalization. Vocalizations are shaped by the language babies hear. Humans have an inherent capacity to learn any language, but our speech sound system is shaped during the first year of life. Vocalizations start as open vowel sounds. Next comes double-syllable babble. Vocalizations become more expressive, varying in pitch and volume. Social communication is an important aspect. Babies use eye contact and facial expressions as part of their communication. Receptive language develops in advance of expressive language. Babies learn to recognize their own name. They develop situational awareness (e.g. when their coat is put on, they become excited about going out) before understanding single words in context. An understanding of an object's use (definition by use) develops prior to understanding object names.

Early lingual (1–2 years)

Receptive language or comprehension of single words begins in this phase. Initially a child can point to named familiar objects. This might include pointing to named body parts on themselves. The ability to recognize those same objects in photographs or pictures develops later.

Expressive language may start as sound labels (for example, 'mmm' at mealtimes, or animal noises). Single words come next. Single words may be used for a variety of purposes: to comment or label or to request. Next comes the ability to join two words together to create novel phrases (e.g. 'mummy car'). Common phrases do not count as joining words together (e.g. 'all fall down').

Non-verbal communication is an important part of this stage of development. Children will use gestures to communicate, particularly pointing to request or to show objects of interest.

Gross motor

Gross motor development proceeds in a cephalo-caudal direction. Typically developing children will all proceed along the same sequence of skill acquisition. Head, neck and trunk control is a vital prerequisite for sitting. Walking is usually achieved by moving through prone into four-point kneeling and then crawling. These actions develop prior to standing and walking. However, some children show a disordered pattern of motor development, which can be considered a normal variant. These are children who bottom-shuffle. They typically prefer the sitting to the prone position. They eventually get up and walk, but often have not crawled.

Social behaviour and play

Paediatricians are often very aware of the different stages of social behaviour in infants and children, from the skilful interactions required when trying to examine children of different ages.

The development of self-help skills, such as dressing and feeding, is likely to be influenced by experience and opportunity.

Developmental milestones

Centiles can be used to define the range of normal for each milestone, in a similar way to those used for growth or puberty. Often the median age or 50th centile is quoted (as here), which is the age by which 50% of children have achieved the skill in question. Sometimes it can be more useful to know the 95th centile (e.g. 18 months for walking), since if a skill has not been achieved by this age, it is very likely to be of concern. Below is a list of milestones, but this is by no means exhaustive and is intended as a guide only. You can find lists in many texts, often with slight variations in the age quoted.

Fine motor and vision

- Watches own hands in finger play   3 months
- Fixes and follows object through   3 months
  90 degrees laterally

• Grasps objects	4 months
• Passes toy from one hand to the other	6 months
• Inferior pincer grasp	9 months
• Looks for falling toys	9 months
• Bangs bricks together in imitation	12 months
• Refined pincer grasp	12 months
• Builds tower of two bricks	15 months
• Builds tower of three bricks	18 months
• To and fro scribble on paper	18 months
• Builds tower of six or seven bricks	2 years
• Circular scribble	2 years
• Copies vertical line and circle	3 years
• Builds tower of nine bricks	3 years
• Copies three-brick bridge	$3\frac{1}{2}$ years
• Copies cross	4 years
• Draws a person with head, body and legs	4 years
• Builds six-brick steps	4 years
• Copies square	$4\frac{1}{2}$ years

Speech, language and hearing

• Vocalizes when spoken to	3 months
• Babbles in repetitive strings of double-syllable babble	9 months
• Knows and turns to own name	12 months
• Uses 2–6 recognizable words	15 months
• Points to familiar objects when requested	15 months
• Joins two words together	2 years
• Understands commands with two key words	2 years
• Vocabulary of 200 words	$2\frac{1}{2}$ years
• Understands commands with three key words	3 years
• Talks in short sentences	3 years
• Asks 'what?' and 'who?' questions	3 years
• Able to tell long stories	4 years
• Asks 'why?', 'when?' and 'how?' questions	4 years
• Counts up to 20 by rote	4 years

Gross motor

• Lifts head and chest up, supporting self on forearms in prone	3 months
• Little or no head lag on pull-to-sit	3 months
• Rolls front to back (and usually back to front)	6 months
• Sits independently	8 months
• Crawls	10 months
• Walks independently	13 months
• Squats to pick up object	18 months

• Runs	2 years
• Walks upstairs holding on, two feet to a step	2 years
• Jumps with two feet together	$2\frac{1}{2}$ years
• Kicks a ball	$2\frac{1}{2}$ years
• Stands on one foot momentarily	3 years
• Walks upstairs adult fashion (one foot to a step)	3 years
• Pedals tricycle	3 years
• Hops	4 years

Social behaviour and play

• Smiles	6 weeks
• Responds with pleasure to friendly handling	3 months
• Stranger awareness	9 months
• Enjoys peek-a-boo	9 months
• Helps with dressing	12 months
• Waves bye-bye	12 months
• Takes off socks, hat	18 months
• Spoon-feeds self	18 months
• Plays alongside other children	2 years
• Eats with fork and spoon	3 years
• Helps adult around house	3 years
• Joins in make-believe play with peers	3 years
• Can dress and undress, except for laces	4 years

Developmental assessment

Developmental assessment is a vital skill for any paediatrician. When conducting a developmental assessment, you are aiming to answer several questions:

- Is the child's development normal for his or her age?
- If not, in which ways and to what degree is it abnormal?
- What is the diagnosis?
- What might be the cause(s)?
- What needs to be done?

Screening assessment

In many situations you might be seeking to answer only the first of these questions. This would be the case, for instance, if a developmental assessment were being conducted as part of child health surveillance. For this purpose, you would present the child with a number of tasks that you would expect him or her to be able to do at that age, and see whether he or she could achieve them. You would not be seeking to find out exactly what the child is able to do in each developmental area, but simply establishing whether he or she can perform a set range of age-appropriate tasks. If the child does not demonstrate the age-appropriate skills, you would refer him or her on for further evaluation. The Denver developmental screening test is an example of a structured assessment tool developed for the identification of children with developmental problems. It is not intended as a detailed diagnostic developmental assessment.

Detailed assessment

The aim of a detailed developmental assessment is to discover the child's precise skill level in each area of development.

Informal assessment

This type of assessment should be one of every paediatrician's skills as it is commonly used in clinical practice. A range of appropriate toys are used, although without a formal scoring system. Using your knowledge of normal development, it is possible to ascertain an approximate developmental age that the child has reached. It is important to realize that, even in typically developing children, there may be differences in age-equivalent scores in each area of development. It would be meaningless to give an overall developmental age when there is significant variation between different areas of development.

Formal assessment

There are a number of standardized assessments that can be used, such as the Griffiths Mental Development Scales (0–8 years; Box 2.3), the Bayley Scales of Infant Development (0–42 months) and the Schedule of Growing Skills (0–5 years). Some standardized assessments require attendance on a training course.

Box 2.3 Griffiths Mental Development Scales

- Developmental assessment tool for children aged 0–8 years
- Two separate modules: 0–2 years and 2–8 years
- Assesses development in six areas:
  Locomotor
  Personal/social
  Hearing and speech
  Fine motor
  Performance
  Practical reasoning
- Gives a score for each area of development (age equivalent)
- Overall developmental quotient is calculated from summary of individual scores

---

Why is it important to make a diagnosis?

Different developmental difficulties will have differing implications for the child's future. Therefore defining the developmental diagnosis is important. A diagnosis of specific language impairment has very different implications from a diagnosis of autism.

As in other aspects of medicine, diagnosis is important for several reasons:
- *Prognosis*. Diagnosis enables you to give more information about prognosis, based on other children with the same disorder.
- *Intervention*. Diagnosis will inform the most appropriate interventions.
- *Genetic*. Many conditions have a genetic basis, which will be particularly important for families with, or planning, other children.

A developmental diagnosis alone does not tell you what the cause is.

Principles of developmental assessment

General

- Explain to carer you do not expect child to be able to do all the tasks you set.
- Use a systematic/structured approach, completing one area of development before moving on to next.
- Use simple, clear language appropriate to child's age level.
- Unless you are assessing language and understanding, use visual/gestural clues to show child what you want him/her to do.
- Assess skills directly where possible, rather than asking carer about them.
- Do not assess 'irrelevant' areas, i.e. tasks that will not give you developmental information or tasks for which you do not know the age-equivalent.
- Keep pace going; do not leave long gaps between tasks or child may get bored and lose interest.
- Keep it fun; give lots of praise and encouragement.
- Observe children carefully throughout, even when you are not directly testing them; they may spontaneously demonstrate skills that will give you more information.
- Observe quality of how child performs a skill, not just whether he/she can do it; this includes looking at both hands for fine motor skills.

Structure

- Start with tasks you expect child to be able to do quite easily (i.e. below child's age level).

13

- If they cannot manage these, go down to simpler/younger tasks.
- Work up gradually, increasing age level of tasks in sequence until child can no longer do tasks.
- Save gross motor assessment till last (unless asked to do this specifically), as child is likely to get excited/not want to sit down afterwards.

Positioning and equipment

- Limit number of toys out at any one time.
- Use toys provided. Ask for specific items if you need them.
- Put yourself and child in optimal position to get best out of him/her (especially if this is fine motor or speech and language assessment):
  < 18 months: seated on carer's lap at table opposite you (*not* on floor)
  2–5 years: seated at small table opposite you.

Suggested assessment schema

This schema presents a bare minimum of tasks for estimating a child's developmental skills. Tasks should be presented in increasing order of difficulty. You will develop your own order of assessment, but this is suggested as a framework to get you started.

Infant

Equipment
- 1″ cubes
- Brightly coloured small toy
- Small object (e.g. raisin)
- Cup
- Cloth
- Paper and pencils
- Familiar objects (cup, sock, shoe, brush)
- Mat/blanket on floor

Fine motor and vision
- Ask if there are any concerns about infant's vision.
- Gain infant's visual attention with toy and move through visual fields, looking at fixation and following.
- Offer small toy, looking at reach and grasp, in-hand manipulation, transferring etc.
- Offer one cube to one hand then other hand.
- Offer second cube with child holding first.
- Demonstrate banging two cubes together to see if child imitates you.
- Demonstrate placing one cube on top of another to see if child imitates you.
- Offer third cube.

- Partially hide cube or toy under cloth to see if infant finds it.
- Totally hide cube or toy under cloth to see if infant finds it.
- Hide cube or toy under cup to see if infant finds it.
- Place raisin on table in front of infant (each hand). (N.B. Remove raisin quickly from infant's hand before it is eaten.)
- For older infants, offer pencil/crayon and paper.
- Visual assessment:
  Observed visual behaviour
  Detection of small objects
  Preferential looking acuity system (e.g. Keeler cards).

Speech, language and hearing
- Ask if there are any concerns about infant's hearing.
- Listen throughout assessment for any vocalizations.
- Observe non-verbal communication, including facial expressions, eye contact, gestures.
- Imitate vocalizations back to infant.
- Talk in double-syllable babble to see if infant copies.
- Call infant's name to look for response.
- Clap hands and encourage infant to imitate.
- Wave bye-bye and encourage infant to imitate.
- Offer familiar objects (sock, cup, brush) to look for definition by use.
- Assess understanding of simple instructions ('Give it to Mummy').
- Use limited number of familiar objects to look for single word recognition ('Where's the cup?').
- Hearing assessment:
  Otoacoustic emission and auditory brainstem responses (ABR) testing at birth
  Distraction testing from 7 months (see Ch. 32 for details).

Gross motor
- Lie infant supine on mat.
- Encourage infant to roll.
- Pull to sit.
- Place in sitting position.
- Pull to stand or to bear weight on feet.
- Observe and support stepping/walking.
- Downward parachute.
- Hold in ventral suspension or place in prone position.
- Forward parachute.

Social behaviour and play
- Observe throughout.
- Smile and interact with infant and watch responsiveness.
- Ask about self-feeding etc.

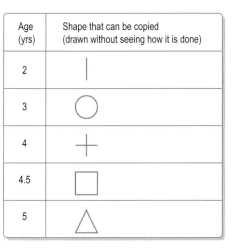

Age (yrs)	Shape that can be copied (drawn without seeing how it is done)
2	|
3	○
4	+
4.5	□
5	△

Age (yrs)	Tower of bricks (number of bricks in a tower)	Shape with bricks
1.5	3	
2	6	
2.5	8	Train
3	9	Bridge
4		Steps

A   B

Fig. 2.1 **(A) Shapes that can be drawn at different ages; (B) shapes that can be made with bricks at different ages**

Toddler

Equipment
- Small table and chairs
- 1″ cubes (at least 12)
- Paper and pencils
- Range of real objects (cup, spoon, brush etc.)
- Doll or teddy
- Picture book
- Miniature toys
- Beads or puzzle
- Ball
- Stairs

Fine motor and vision (Fig. 2.1)
- Offer 1″ cubes; encourage tower building.
- Build three-brick bridge for child to copy/imitate.
- Build train for child to copy/imitate.
- Build six-brick steps for child to copy/imitate.
- Offer paper and pencils; observe spontaneous drawing.
- Draw shapes for child to copy: horizontal and vertical line, circle, cross, square, triangle.
- Ask child to draw picture of a person (e.g. 'Draw Mummy').
- Look at manipulation/coordination using beads or puzzles.
- Visual assessment:
  Preferential looking acuity measure (e.g. Cardiff acuity test)
  Letter matching acuity systems (e.g. Sonksen–Silver, Sheridan–Gardiner).

Speech, language and hearing
- Lay out a number of objects/toys to test single word understanding.
- Increase complexity of questions gradually, to check two-word level of understanding, then three-word level, then prepositions, adjectives, verbs (e.g. 'Where's the duck?', then later 'Give me the spoon and the doll', 'Put the spoon in the cup and give me the car', 'Where's the big pencil?', 'Put the car under the table', 'Make teddy kick the ball' etc.).
- Listen for expressive language throughout.
- Observe non-verbal communication, including facial expressions, eye contact, gestures.
- Use picture book to gain sample of expressive language ('What can you see?').
- Hearing assessment:
  Performance/conditioning test — child is conditioned to 'perform' in some way when he or she hears a sound; this is done as a game, e.g. place brick in basket.
  Speech discrimination test (e.g. McCormick toy test) — child is asked to choose a named toy from a set of toys composed of pairs with similar names (e.g. 'tree' and 'key').

Gross motor
- Observe walking
- Place object on floor for child to pick up
- Running
- Jump with two feet together
- Stand on one leg
- Hop
- Kick a ball
- Up and down stairs

Social behaviour and play
- Observe throughout, looking particularly at social interaction.

- Ask about self-help skill.
- Ask about play with peers.

Developmental problems

Delay or disorder?

A child's development can be abnormal in many ways. Delayed development simply means that a child is acquiring skills at a later age than the norm. Development can be delayed in just one area (for example, speech and language delay), or in two or more areas — commonly called global developmental delay.

Children with global developmental delay may present initially with delay in one area of development, but on further assessment it becomes clear that they have more general delay. Disordered development means an unusual pattern or sequence of development. The term also suggests that the problem is due to an underlying developmental disorder, and the child is unlikely to 'catch up'.

Any child presenting with delayed (or disordered) development in one area needs careful evaluation of the rest of his or her development. Delay in one area can be the initial presenting feature of global developmental delay (Ch. 18).

Common patterns of developmental delay and their causes

Speech and language delay

Speech and language delay is the most common pre-school developmental problem, occurring in 5–10% of all children. It is more common in boys. This is discussed fully in Chapter 29.

You should understand the difference between speech delay (difficulties with speech sound production), expressive language delay (difficulties in choosing or using appropriate words to convey meaning) and receptive language delay (problems with understanding language). Children with developmental language delay or specific language impairment typically have difficulties in both receptive and expressive language. Usually understanding (receptive language) is in advance of expression.

Tongue tie is not an adequate reason for speech delay, and operative treatment is not indicated unless tongue movements are severely limited.

Delay in gross motor skills

Delay in gross motor skills may typically present with delayed sitting and poor head control, or with delay in walking. The upper limit of the normal age of walking is 18 months.

Possible causes of delayed sitting/poor head and trunk control include:
- Central neurological (brain) disorders, such as cerebral palsy, brain malformations
- Neuromuscular conditions, such as spinal muscular atrophy
- Severe global developmental delay (severe learning difficulties), which may sometimes present initially with delayed gross motor skills.

Possible causes of delayed walking include:
- Central neurological disorders, such as cerebral palsy, particularly of diplegic distribution
- Neuromuscular problems, such as Duchenne muscular dystrophy
- Spinal problems
- Orthopaedic problems, such as developmental dysplasia of the hip
- Global developmental delay.

Bottom-shuffling, a normal variant, is usually associated with a later average age of acquiring independent walking. Children who bottom-shuffle typically do not crawl, dislike the prone position, and are reluctant to take weight through their feet, adopting the 'sitting on air' position when held under their arms. Although it is a normal variant, bottom shuffling can also be associated with pathological underlying causes, such as cerebral palsy; therefore careful clinical examination is warranted.

Global developmental delay

Global developmental delay simply means delay in two or more areas of development. Many children presenting with global developmental delay are subsequently found to have significant learning difficulties (previously termed 'mental retardation'). Where the cause is environmental/social or secondary to ill health, children may 'catch up' with time and appropriate input/stimulation.

Possible causes of global developmental delay include:
- Environmental/psychosocial issues: lack of experience, deprivation, poor parenting, ill health
- Any condition causing learning difficulties, such as chromosomal disorders or syndromes.

www.guideline.gov/summary/summary.aspx?view_id=1&doc_id=4106

Guideline on investigations in children with global developmental delay

Further reading

Quality Standards Subcommittee of the American Academy of Neurology and the Committee of the Child Neurology Society 2003 Practice parameter: evaluation of the child with global developmental delay. Neurology 60(3):367–380

Sheridan M, Frost M, Sharma A 1997 From birth to five years: children's developmental progress. Routledge, London

Melanie Epstein

Psychological and emotional development

LEARNING OUTCOMES

By the end of this chapter you should:

- Know how early experiences affect brain development
- Be familiar with the stages of cognitive development
- Understand the links between the attachment system and attachment behaviours
- Know the differences between secure and insecure attachment styles
- Understand some of the long-term effects of trauma and neglect in the first few years.

Introduction

No variables have more far-reaching effects on personality development than a child's experiences within the family. As humans, with a long period of helplessness and vulnerability after birth, we rely on adult care longer than any other species. Our physical and psychological security is inextricably linked, and depends on our connections with other people. These connections are sought and maintained because our brains are particularly sensitive to social relationships and the need for psychological security. The key to this is the attachment bond.

Emotional development

The attachment to a newborn is built on prior relationships with an imaginary child, and with the developing fetus that has been part of the parents' world for 9 months. During pregnancy the developing neurobiological structure of the brain follows the genetic blueprint, barring adverse environmental circumstances such as intrauterine infection or teratogens, in particular maternal ingestion of alcohol or other drugs. After birth, brain development becomes experience-dependent. Newborn babies are genetically 'pre-programmed' to seek out and adapt to the relationship that they have with their parents. Interactions with the environment during sensitive periods are necessary for the brain to mature. The capacity of the developing brain to alter its neurobiological structure (neuroplasticity) in response to the environment is an adaptive mechanism that has evolved out of the process of natural selection. This allows the child to adjust to the infinite possibilities created within a family in interaction with the wider culture.

At birth, there are about 100 million neurons, which are not yet part of functional networks. Synaptogenesis occurs predominantly in the first 3 years, and by the age of 2 there is the same number of synapses as in an adult. Brain development is a refining process of strengthening certain synapses and eliminating redundant synapses in a selective way, depending on experience and interactions with caregivers. A popular neuroscientific soundbite is 'Neurons that fire together, wire together'.

Stages of cognitive development

Optimal cognitive development is best achieved when attachment needs are met. Jean Piaget (1896–1980) identified four stages in cognitive development, as shown in Table 3.1.

The attachment bond

The essential task of the first year of life is the creation of a secure attachment bond between the infant and caregiver. This depends on the mother or primary caregiver's pattern of response to the infant's physical and emotional needs. Winnicott saw healthy development as starting with the 'good-enough' mother, who through following her maternal instincts helps the baby learn to express needs and feelings without being overwhelmed by them. She synchronizes and responds to the emotional rhythms of the baby. She is adept at handling negative reactions, and her inevitable failures, in a constructive healing way. In the presence of good-enough parenting, we learn to regulate our emotional reactions and tolerate gradually increasing amounts of frustration. Winnicott distinguished this sort of parent from a 'perfect' mother who satisfies all the needs of the infant on the spot, thus preventing him or her from developing. The responses to cues from the infant are built into an internal model of what the infant expects from the carer. This forms a foundation for future relationships. By the end of the first year, the infant's behaviour is purposeful and based on specific expectations. This is because he has aggregated his past experiences with the caregiver, and

these are becoming 'hard-wired'. Attachment is not just a set of behaviours or a psychological construct; it forms the substrate of the developing brain. Neuroscientific research has demonstrated the synaptic circuitry and anatomical locations. If children grow up with dominant experiences of separation, distress, fear and rage, they will go down a pathogenic developmental pathway, not just psychologically but neurologically. Attachment experiences form the neurodevelopmental framework out of which we emerge, and are important in cortical, prefrontal system and limbic system development. They later form the basis for personality development.

The brain is at its most plastic for the first 2 years after birth. This is the reason for the current emphasis on early prevention and intervention in policy and practice. The older the child becomes, then the harder it can be to 'rewire' certain areas of the brain. Research on children adopted from Romanian orphanages suggests that the sensitive period for developing attachments ends at about 3. A child who has experienced abuse or neglect as an infant may unwittingly continue with patterns of responses that are engraved in the mind, even if circumstances change. Other relationships later in life can be crucial: for example, relationships with adoptive parents, a relationship with a supportive partner or a therapeutic relationship. The ability to attribute meaning to experience also helps to mitigate the effects of past experience. The best predictor of the pattern of attachment that will later emerge between a mother and her 12-month-old baby is the way the mother currently talks about her own mother and her experiences of being mothered as a girl. How she reflects on and interprets those experiences now is more important than the actual attachment circumstances at the time.

The biological function of the attachment system

The attachment system was first described by the British psychiatrist, John Bowlby. It operates as a homeostatic system with the goal of emotional regulation. It is activated by anxiety and distress, and deactivated by a subjective feeling of security. It operates analogously to other biological homeostatic mechanisms: for example, systems for thermoregulation. The biological function has been thought to be protection from predators. A feature of the attachment system is the *intensity* of the emotion that accompanies it. If all goes well, there is joy and security associated with being protected, comforted and understood. If threatened, there is jealousy, anxiety and anger. If broken, as occurs with loss, there is grief and depression.

Table 3.1 **Stages in cognitive development**

Stage	Description	Play	Example
Sensorimotor (infancy)	Intelligence is demonstrated through a baby's interactions with the environment and with the carer. These may be sensory (hearing, seeing, touch), motor (grasping, pulling) or expressions of feeling Knowledge of the world is limited (but developing) because it is based on physical interactions/experiences. Children acquire object permanence at about 7 months of age. Physical development (mobility) allows the child to begin developing new intellectual abilities. Some symbolic (language) abilities are developed at the end of this stage	'Practice play' to obtain mastery	A rattle *is* its colour when looked at, its texture when touched or sucked on, its sound when shaken; the baby demonstrates pleasure or another response, and may attempt to reach out to the rattle. Before object permanence develops, the rattle ceases to exist when out of sight
Preoperational (toddler and early childhood)	Intelligence is demonstrated through the use of symbols, language use matures, and memory and imagination are developed The child's world is concrete and absolute; things are as they seem. The child is influenced more by how things look than by principles of logic. This includes the belief that inanimate objects are alive Children tend to observe the world from their point of view (egocentrism)	Symbolic (make-believe play)	Chloe (age 3 years 9 months) speaking of a car in the garage: 'The car's gone to bye-byes. It doesn't go out because of the rain'
Concrete operational (primary school and early adolescence)	In this stage (characterized by seven types of conservation: number, length, liquid, mass, weight, area, volume), intelligence is demonstrated through logical and systematic manipulation of symbols related to concrete objects Egocentric thought diminishes, and the child is more able to conceptualize the world from another's viewpoint. This is linked to the child's emotional development	With rules. As thinking becomes more logical, rules are incorporated. These become more sophisticated as children go through their development	If an 8-year-old child is asked, 'If John is taller than Susan and Susan is taller than Charlie, who is taller, John or Charlie?,' he or she will need to use real objects, e.g. dolls, to solve the problem. He will not be able to solve this in his head before the age of about 11
Formal operational (adolescence and adulthood)	Intelligence is demonstrated through the logical use of symbols related to abstract concepts. Ideas can now be manipulated, rather than just objects Adolescents can think hypothetically about a situation that they have not experienced before, or even one that nobody has ever experienced before	With rules	Einstein developed the seeds of his theory of relativity when he was about 16. He imagined himself as a particle of light travelling away from a planet at the speed of light and then looking back, thinking how it would appear

Attachment behaviour

Attachment behaviour is any behaviour designed to bring children into a close protective relationship with their attachment figures when they experience anxiety (Fig. 3.1). This brings feelings of security associated with being protected, comforted and understood. Having this 'secure base' enables children to feel safe to explore. For most children, their primary attachment figure is usually their mother or main carer. Children may also have a small but limited number of attachment relationships with other family members, or other adults such as a teacher.

There are three broad types of attachment behaviour:
1. Signalling behaviours (smiling, vocalizing, laughter) that bring the mother to the child for social interaction
2. Behaviours that bring the mother to the child to give comfort (e.g. to stop the child crying)
3. Behaviours that take the child to the mother.

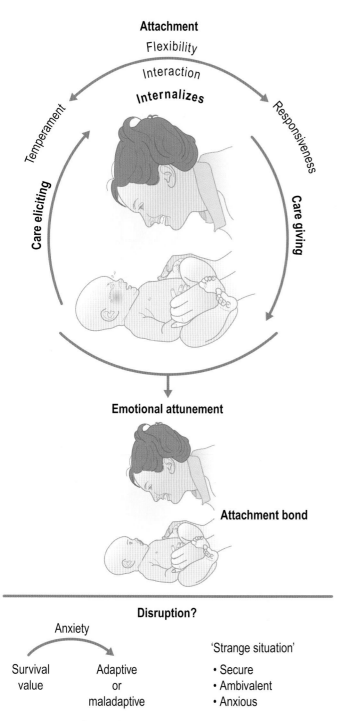

Fig. 3.1 **Attachment behaviour: the importance of early experiences**

Attachment

Flexibility

Interaction

Internalizes

Temperament

Responsiveness

Care eliciting

Care giving

Emotional attunement

Attachment bond

Disruption?

Anxiety

| Survival value | Adaptive or maladaptive | 'Strange situation' • Secure • Ambivalent • Anxious |

Separation from the mother in distance or time increases anxiety. This activates the attachment system. Attachment behaviours ideally help bring the mother back. When this occurs, the anxiety and behaviours diminish. The attachment system is also activated by:

- Pain
- Tiredness
- Frightening experiences
- Inaccessibility of the primary caretaker: this could be real or apparent, physical or psychological.

By the age of 3, there is less need for direct proximity to the attachment figure, and the child is starting to develop 'a secure base' inside.

When attachment behaviour is activated, a child is unable to engage in other important developmental experiences such as exploration, play and other social interactions. When persistent over time, this will have adverse consequences for social and cognitive development.

There are four styles of attachment behaviour (Table 3.2):

Table 3.2 **Styles of attachment behaviour**

Attachment style	Parenting	Child's behaviour
Secure	Consistently responsive	Approaches carers directly and positively Learns sense of trust; deals better with stress
Avoidant	Consistently unresponsive	Denies or stops communicating distress Leads to low self-esteem and later aggression
Ambivalent	Inconsistently responsive	Maximizes distress Lack of exploration
Disorganized	Cause of the distress*	No strategy can bring comfort or care

* This may occur when parents are abusive, are emotionally unreachable (major unresolved issues from the past, depressed, psychotic, heavy drug or alcohol users) or fail to protect the child. There is no coherent strategy that children can use to reduce anxiety. Children may then *freeze*, either physically or psychologically.

1. Secure attachment
2. Avoidant attachment
3. Ambivalent or inconsistent attachment
4. Incoherent or disorganized attachment.

Around 70% of children develop a secure attachment. Secure attachment with at least one adult is a necessary precondition for the development of resilience (p. 212).

If the normal routes to proximity and security are unsuccessful, children have to either develop psychological strategies that attempt to minimize anxiety (defences), or try to find alternative creative ways to secure the attachment figure psychologically. For example, if parents only respond to negative behaviour rather than to a child's expressions of sad feelings, a child might learn to hit out when he feels sad or insecure. He will then get some emotional security, but at the expense of 'burying' his real feelings.

Insecure attachment is a risk factor that will interact with other risks present in the emotional and physical environment of the growing child (Fig. 3.2).

Attachment behaviour is seen throughout the lifespan and is a key part of our psychological make-up. Parents experiencing a threat to their security associated with ill health in their child may respond with apparently undue anxiety or anger. In this context, it is helpful to consider the parents' emotional state as a normal expression of their attachment behaviour. In this case, the paediatrician is being asked to take the role of the good-enough parent in helping to regulate the parental distress.

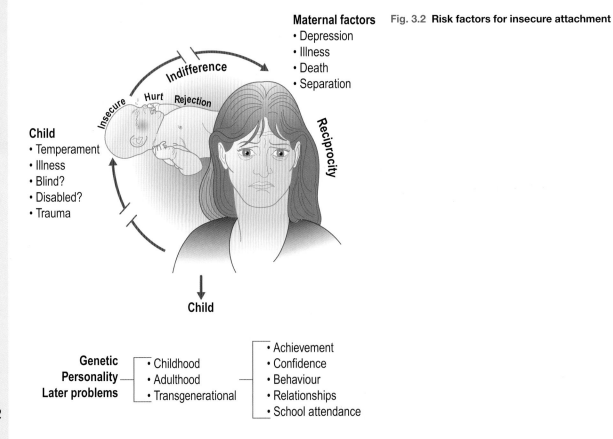

Fig. 3.2 **Risk factors for insecure attachment**

Maternal factors
• Depression
• Illness
• Death
• Separation

Indifference

Hurt   Rejection

Insecure

Reciprocity

Child
• Temperament
• Illness
• Blind?
• Disabled?
• Trauma

Child

Genetic
Personality — • Childhood
Later problems — • Adulthood
• Transgenerational

• Achievement
• Confidence
• Behaviour
• Relationships
• School attendance

The effect of trauma and neglect

Abuse and neglect in the first years of life have a particularly pervasive impact (see also Chs 21 and 37).

Disorganized attachment, frequently the result of maltreatment, becomes in itself a major risk factor that, in the 'wrong' circumstances, can disrupt many different areas of development. It is predictive of the development of behavioural problems at preschool and school age in both high-risk and normal samples.

Disorganized attachment in infancy has been linked to a number of severe mental health problems in adulthood. Other early attachment experiences are also linked with adult psychopathology. Loss predicts multiple disorders, including depression, anxiety and antisocial personality disorder.

The roots of violence

Delinquent, antisocial and violent behaviour, frequently associated with no sense of either empathy or remorse, has been traced back to being on the receiving end of abuse and neglect during the first 2 years of life. Violence 'is the manifestation of attachment behaviour gone wrong'.

The development of a secure attachment relationship protects against later aggression and violence in three ways:
1. Through learning empathy (the ability to be mindful of another's mind, and thus mind how you treat them)
2. Through learning self-control
3. Through learning to modulate feelings, particularly those that are destructive, and the ability to self-soothe.

The context of the attachment relationship

The parent–baby relationship is always located in a wider context, within which are found both risk and protective factors. These can harm the baby directly (e.g. pollution, unhealthy housing) but mostly they are titrated into the relationship via their effects on the parents' functioning, since they dictate the baby's immediate experiences. Box 3.1 summarizes the risk factors that affect parent–child relationships.

Conclusion

Successful parenting is a principal key to this and the next generation. As paediatricians we have the

---

BOX 3.1 Risk factors affecting the parent–child relationship

Child
- Prematurity or congenital abnormalities
- Difficult temperament
- Early problems making a baby difficult and less rewarding
- Language delay, coordination problems, physical or sensory disabilities
- Significant illness

Parents
- Lack of ability to attune to baby
- Lack of interaction or maltreatment
- Mental health problem or background of abuse, neglect or loss
- Addiction (this may be associated with the baby having cognitive/developmental/behavioural difficulties associated with addiction during pregnancy. Addiction is also an attachment-related disorder and may predispose to attachment difficulties in the baby)
- Family dysfunction
- Domestic violence
- Single teenage mother without support

Environment
- Poverty is a major risk factor. There is a high prevalence of depression, attachment difficulties and post-traumatic stress among mothers living in poverty. Associated poor nutrition has effects on the child in utero and during later development

---

privileged role of being offered a window to this part of people's lives. It is important to remember to support and help parents in this role at every opportunity, as well as to know when to intervene when a child is being harmed by inappropriate or dangerous parenting. Whilst our foremost duty is always to the child, the balance between protecting the parent–child attachment and protecting the child poses professional challenges at times for us all.

 www.aimh.org.uk

Association for Infant Mental Health UK; follow links to 'The Importance of the Early Years and Evidence-Based Practice'

www.zerotothree.org

Comprehensive interactive resource for parents and professionals on normal development 0–3 years

CHAPTER Charlotte M. Wright   Alison Kelly   Linda Wolfson

4

Nutrition, infant feeding and weaning

LEARNING OUTCOMES

By the end of this chapter you should:

- Understand the physiology and mechanics of breastfeeding and how this can best be supported
- Understand the characteristics of infant formula and its role as a breast-milk substitute
- Know how nutrient requirements change through early life to adulthood and how they relate to growth and maturation
- Know how dietary intake varies with the developmental stage of the child in order to fulfil those requirements
- Understand how nutritional status can be most effectively assessed in childhood.

MODULE ONE

Introduction

Nutrition is a balance between supply and demand. The intake of nutrients, including energy, fat, protein, carbohydrate and vitamins and minerals, must be sufficient to meet the body's needs. These requirements are determined not only by basic metabolism and activity levels but also, uniquely in childhood, by the demands of growth. This chapter will consider how this balance of supply and demand is achieved at different stages and how it may be upset. It will consider how nutrient requirements change through childhood, reflecting the varying pace of growth and changing activity levels, from the immobile but rapidly growing infant to the more active but slower-growing child. In parallel we will consider how dietary intake varies with the developmental stage of the child in order to fulfil those requirements. Finally we will consider how the nutritional status of children can be most effectively assessed, from the simple measure of weight and estimates of dietary intake through to more complex measures of body composition and energy expenditure.

Pregnancy and fetal nutrition

The growth of an individual begins in utero, and maternal health and nutrition can impact on the nutritional status of the fetus in a number of ways. During pregnancy, nutritional requirements are increased as a result of the physiological changes in the mother as well as the energy costs of the growing fetus and placenta. Average weight gain in pregnancy is around 12.5 kg and the total energy cost of a normal pregnancy has been estimated as around 50 000 kcal. This necessitates intake of an additional 200 kcal per day above normal requirements in the third trimester. Requirements for vitamins and minerals increase during pregnancy and can normally be ingested through the diet, although iron deficiency is common and iron is generally supplemented. Folic acid is an essential co-factor for DNA synthesis and is recommended as a supplement preconceptually to reduce the risk of neural tube defects.

Low maternal weight gain in pregnancy correlates with lower infant birth weight and increased perinatal mortality, but maternal under-nutrition as a *cause* of low weight gain is only seen in conditions of extreme starvation, because of the fetus's preferential access to maternal nutrients. The placenta is a highly active organ metabolically, producing hormones essential for maintenance of pregnancy and growth factors. Additionally active transport mechanisms deliver nutrients from the maternal circulation to the fetus.

Fetal life is the period of most rapid growth and change in body proportion and composition. During early life, the fetal water content is high, and there is a predominance of extracellular ions such as sodium and chloride. With organogenesis and increasing cell mass the content of intracellular ions, such as potassium, increases. During the third trimester the fetus triples in weight and doubles in length, and this period is associated with accretion of minerals such as calcium and iron. Protein stores increase and fat deposition occurs prior to birth. If an infant is born prematurely, before this phase of growth is completed, nutrient stores are low and it is difficult then to achieve tissue and mineral accretion at in utero rates.

Intrauterine growth restriction

This is a failure to achieve growth potential, and can be defined as birth weight below the 2nd centile for gestational age. Ultrasound estimation of fetal weight has shown two patterns of growth restriction. Symmetrical growth restriction, commencing early and resulting in low weight, length and head circumference, is more usually related to intrinsic characteristics or pathologies in the fetus. Asymmetric retardation, with late flattening of the growth curve and low weight but relative sparing of length and head circumference, is more likely to result from placental insufficiency. This may be caused by maternal hypertension, pre-eclampsia or, commonly, smoking. Rapid catch-up growth usually occurs in early infancy.

Infancy

At birth the average weight is 3.5 kg and length 50 cm. The normally grown newborn needs sufficient stores of energy and nutrients to deal with the transition from the uterine environment with its constant nutrient supply, to intermittent oral feeds which must be ingested, digested and absorbed. During the first year of life growth is rapid, particularly the brain, and the infant lays down

considerable fat stores. The normal infant requires around three times more energy per kilogram than an adult reflecting both higher metabolic requirements and energy requirements for growth. Later in the first year requirements for growth diminish, but are matched by the cost of rising activity levels.

The benefits of breastfeeding and hazards of breast-milk substitutes

Breast milk is the sole and essential food for newborn infants. Fresh human milk is a live and complex substance that provides far more than just basic nutrition (Box 4.1). No breast-milk substitutes can completely replicate its physiological role, as a source both of nutrition and of immune protection. For this reason, the use of breast-milk substitutes remains one of the most important worldwide causes of preventable mortality in infancy. Recent studies have demonstrated the association of bottle feeding with increased morbidity in the UK and excess infant mortality in the USA. In low-birth weight and sick infants, breastfeeding is associated with reduced mortality from necrotizing enterocolitis and advantages

BOX 4.2 Key factors in establishing breastfeeding on maternity units

- Skin-to-skin contact
- Rooming in
- Feeding on demand, not to the clock, for as long as the baby wants
- Good positioning and correct attachment at the breast
- Skilled support when needed

in cognitive function. The protective effect of breast milk is greatest in the early weeks of life, but continues throughout the first year.

Unfortunately only a minority of children in the UK currently receive breast milk for more than the first few weeks. Breastfeeding rates fell to their lowest point in the 1970s, due to over-confidence in the safety of formula milk. Although increased promotion of breastfeeding has resulted in a substantial improvement, over 30% of infants still never receive any breast milk, with only 42% still breastfeeding at 6 weeks and only 21% beyond the age of 6 months. There are also marked social class gradients, which means that children already facing multiple adversities predominantly start life without the protective benefits of breast milk.

In 1981, to overcome a lack of professional support and the effects of marketing of formula, the World Health Organization (WHO) launched the International Code of Marketing of Breast-milk Substitutes to protect and promote breastfeeding and to ensure the proper use of breast-milk substitutes. In 1989 the WHO and the United Nations Children's Fund (UNICEF) published the 'Ten Steps to Successful Breastfeeding' to establish effective breastfeeding practices amongst professionals. Mothers who deliver in hospitals and communities who have implemented the ten steps are more likely to breastfeed successfully (Box 4.2).

Establishing breastfeeding

For breastfeeding to be established successfully, the mother needs to produce enough milk, but the baby must also remove it frequently and effectively (Box 4.3). Many breastfeeding problems have their roots in the newborn period, when breastfeeding is being established. Ideally this should start with skin-to-skin contact at birth, leading to the first feed when the baby is ready. For lactation to be successful, mothers must learn to recognize signs of hunger, respond to the baby's needs and feed on demand. After birth, mothers should be encouraged to feed for as long and as often as the baby wants. The expected pattern of feeding changes at different stages and varies between babies, but frequent

BOX 4.3 The physiology of lactation

The endocrine control of lactation

The anterior pituitary gland secretes prolactin, directing the acini cells to produce milk and priming the prolactin receptor sites for future milk production. Prolactin levels stay high after a feed and stimulate the breast to produce milk for the next feed. Levels are higher at night and therefore night feeding is good for milk production. Inadequate stimulation may lead to sites shutting down and reduced milk capacity.

The hormone oxytocin assists milk ejection. The posterior pituitary secretes oxytocin, causing the myoepithelial cells around the alveoli to contract and leading to the 'let-down' or 'milk ejection' reflex. Milk collected in the alveoli flows along the ducts to the lactiferous sinuses. Oxytocin opens the ducts and helps the milk to flow easily.

The autocrine control of lactation

After the early weeks, milk production is controlled more locally within the breast. The feedback inhibitor (FIL) is a protein within the milk, which enables the breasts to work independently. FIL protects the breast from the harmful effects of being too full; conversely, frequent suckling or expression causes the inhibitor in milk to fall, so that the breast makes more milk. If the baby prefers one breast, this breast will make more milk.

feeds may be needed, particularly in the early days. However, babies may sometimes need to be wakened for a feed when the mother's breasts are overfull, or the baby demands so infrequently that the breasts are under-stimulated. Most mothers need to offer both breasts at every feed, but this is variable. On the maternity unit babies should normally stay with their mother ('roomed-in') at all times, except when the mother's or baby's condition prevents this. Of all of the 'ten steps', there is the strongest link between rooming-in and successful breastfeeding.

Positioning and attachment at the breast

For a breast to continue to produce milk, it must be emptied frequently and effectively; therefore establishing correct attachment is essential (Fig. 4.1). Babies remove milk by compressing the lactiferous sinuses in the breast, creating a vacuum between the mouth and breast. The breast response of ejection or 'let down' will only occur when the baby can correctly attach and coordinate suckling. Correct positioning also plays a crucial role in the prevention of sore nipples. Each mother will have individual preferences, abilities and needs, but the principles are as follows:

Correct

Incorrect

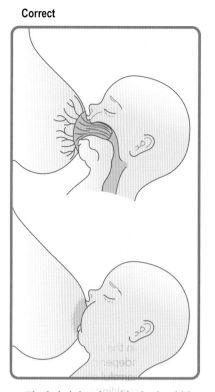

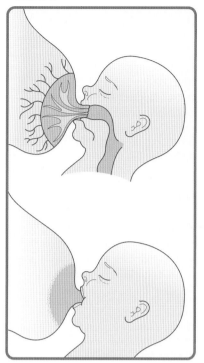

Fig. 4.1 Signs that a baby is correctly attached at the breast.

The baby has a wide gaping mouth. Generally, more of the upper areola should be seen above the baby's mouth than below. The baby's lower lip will be flared out against the breast and the chin will be directly in contact with the breast. The baby's neck will be slightly extended. The jaw muscles work rhythmically and this movement can be seen extending to the ears. If the cheeks are being sucked in, the baby is not correctly attached. The baby sucks deeply with pauses, rather than continually.

- *The baby's head and body should be in a straight line (without restricting the baby's head from slightly extending backwards).* Babies cannot suckle or swallow easily if their head is twisted or bent, and will not open their mouth or put their tongue forward widely if their head is unable to tilt back.
- *The baby's mouth should face the breast, with the top lip opposite the nipple.* The maternal nipple points to the baby's nostrils, and the head is slightly extended backwards, allowing the baby's chin to come to the breast in advance of his nose.
- *The mother should hold the baby's body close to hers.* The angle at which she holds the baby, directly facing her chest or angled under her breasts, depends on the size and shape of her breasts and the direction her nipples point.
- *The position should be sustainable.* If the baby is newborn, the mother should support his or her whole body, and not just the head and shoulders.

The role of the doctor in maintaining breastfeeding

For most women, normal lactation is possible, even if temporarily affected by the labour and delivery process; true milk insufficiency occurs in only 0.2% of mammals. Despite this, many mothers still fail to establish effective feeding, and breastfeeding cessation most often occurs in the first few days. While this may partly reflect the lack of a breastfeeding culture, particularly in poorer areas, mothers are easily undermined by poor or conflicting information and a lack of support. Effective support for breastfeeding requires a basic understanding of lactational physiology, effective newborn feeding behaviour and confidence in normal neonatal adaptation (Box 4.4), as well as a practical understanding of the mechanics of feeding.

Women most commonly give up breastfeeding very early due to a perception that they are 'failing' at it. They may have sore nipples and breasts or difficulties getting the baby to attach effectively or at all; if so, the baby may be fretful and apparently unsatisfied by feeds. Nursing and medical staff can also inadvertently induce a sense of failure by excessive concern about weight gain or blood sugar levels, or by separation of mother and baby for medical procedures. Confidence in breastfeeding is severely undermined if supplementary formula milk feeds are recommended, particularly in the first days. This has been recognized to be such a problem that most maternity units operate a non-supplementation policy. Doctors should support this policy wherever possible, and neonatal procedures and policies should be designed to ensure minimal interruptions to feeding. Doctors should familiarize themselves with common problems that may arise and what practical interventions can be tried (Boxes 4.3 and 4.4). Supplementation may appear to solve a short-term problem, by removing the immediate perceived risk of underfeeding. However, this may lead to permanent cessation of breastfeeding and its protective benefits, exposing the child to more substantial long-term risks; it may also deter breastfeeding of subsequent children.

Metabolic adaptation

At birth, the baby must adapt to the abrupt cessation of placental nutrition and to the introduction of milk feeds. In the healthy full-term infant, changes after birth in hormones and enzymes allow energy-providing fuels such as glucose and fat to be released from body stores. Fat is broken down in the liver, forming ketone bodies that are important alternative fuels to glucose, particularly in the first 2–3 postnatal days until feeding is established. Healthy term babies can sustain themselves for several days until demand feeding is established. Some groups of infants (e.g. low-birth weight infants, infants of diabetic mothers) are at risk of failure of metabolic adaptation, resulting in low levels of glucose and fatty fuels in the blood.

Osmoregulation

Most newborn babies lose weight as they excrete surplus interstitial fluid. Colostrum is the ideal way to provide nutrients in concentrated form, allowing the baby to make this adjustment easily. The amount of breast milk available at a feed gradually increases, provided feeding is frequent. Using biochemical means to assess fluid balance can be misleading, as during this period of adaptation later norms may not apply and small rises in sodium and urea may be without significance or consequence. During early infancy fluid requirements are high, due to higher obligatory losses from the skin and respiratory and renal tracts, and this makes the infant susceptible to dehydration, but breastfeeding provides sufficient fluids and does not need to be supplemented in the healthy infant.

Common feeding problems in the neonatal period

Taking a full breastfeeding history and assessing breast-feeds are important, and the assistance of an infant feeding advisor or lay breastfeeding counsellor is helpful. Weighing babies can be a simple way of assessing crude fluid balance but is only accurate if measurements are correctly recorded on accurate scales. It is also important to assess stool and urine output and other signs in a baby, which determine establishment of lactation and effective feeding.

Delay in establishing feeding

Some babies may initially be too sleepy to attach and suck at the breast. This is not uncommon and over-medicalized management can lead to unnecessary breast-feeding cessation, since it rarely reflects underlying illness or metabolic disturbance. The mother may have had sedatives in labour or have been separated from her baby and missed feeding cues. Breast milk may need to be expressed by hand (at least eight times in 24 hours) to stimulate lactation and keep the mother motivated. Babies who are still unwilling to feed after 48 hours should be examined carefully and investigated if indicated. If alternative feeding is needed, this should consist of expressed breast milk, given by cup, unless the baby is unwell. Tubes are rarely necessary and bottle teats may interfere with the normal imprinting of correct attachment.

Hypoglycaemia

Hypoglycaemia should be identified and treated in sick, symptomatic or high-risk infants. Concerns may arise in the slow-to-feed or sleepy breastfed baby, but generally speaking, healthy term babies are unlikely to have problems and usually supportive breastfeeding measures and supervision are all that is required. Hypoglycaemia in the high-risk or sick neonate is discussed in Chapter 48.

Excessive early weight loss

Most infants lose weight after birth, generally 4–7% of birth weight with the nadir around 48–72 hours. Birth weight is normally regained by 2 weeks. Greater weight loss will be seen in relatively large infants, while growth-retarded infants commonly show none. Standard growth charts do not allow for neonatal loss and thus cannot be used in the first month. Where weight loss is greater than 10% at any stage, the baby should be fully examined and feeding assessed, but there is rarely a need for supplementation with formula or intravenous fluids, unless the baby is unwell or has severe hypernatraemia. With most babies, the feeding technique can be improved and expressed breast milk can be given. This is preferred to formula, as breast milk has the lowest renal solute load and is more easily digested; therefore larger volumes can be given safely. It also encourages continued breast stimulation and effective milk removal.

Jaundice (see also Ch. 48)

Physiological jaundice of the newborn can be more pronounced if feeding is delayed or restricted.

Formula feeding

Types of formula milks and their preparation

If a mother needs or chooses to use a formula milk, it should be one that meets with the UK formula and follow-on milk regulations. All formulae recommended for general use are made from modified cow's milk. Whey-based infant formulae ('first' milks) are all that is required for the first year of life. Manufacturers are

Table 4.1 Complementary feeding stages and associated problems

Age range	Skills to be acquired	Food types used	Common problems	Solutions
3–6 months	Form a bolus of food and pass it to the back of the mouth so that it can be swallowed without choking	First-stage foods: smooth bland cereal purées, gradually thickened over time	Chokes when fed	May be too young: if under 6 months, suggest waiting Adjust consistency of purée and start with very small amounts
4–6 months	Become accustomed to new flavours and smells	Addition of puréed fruit or vegetables to feeds	Refuses new flavours and foods	Most infants require repeated exposures to new tastes before accepting them
6–9 months	Chew lumpy foods	Second-stage foods: coarse purées and sloppy foods with lumps	Gags on lumps	Avoid foods with discrete lumps: offer progressively thickened purées of even consistency
6–12 months	Bite and chew solid foods Finger feeding	Solid foods that can be easily softened in the mouth, e.g. potato, pasta	Refuses to be fed from spoon Won't chew solids	Offer dry finger foods suitable for self-feeding: bread, fruit, biscuits, processed meat Avoid very resistant foods Keep offering solids and avoid excessive milk intake

keen to promote casein-dominant formulas ('second' milks), which are nearer to cow's milk and thus require less modification, but they are less physiologically similar to breast milk. Mothers should thus be advised to continue whey-based formulae until the child switches to doorstep cow's milk after the age of 1 year. Formulae milk can be purchased in a 'ready to feed' form or dried for reconstitution with boiled, cooled water. Each feed should be made fresh and not stored, to reduce the risk of contamination. Formula-fed premature and sick babies should be fed initially on sterilized 'ready to feed' milks. All equipment used in the preparation and feeding should be washed thoroughly and sterilized.

Other breast milk substitutes

Soya milk formulae have been available since the 1980s, but they have many potential problems, particularly in relation to their phytoestrogen content and the use of glucose syrup in place of lactose, which has the potential to damage teeth. These formulae should thus not be recommended without sound medical reasons. Vegan parents would usually breastfeed and should be strongly advised to continue as long as possible. Hypoallergenic formulae are available for proven allergy, but again should not be recommended without detailed medical and dietetic assessment. A goat's milk formula is commercially available but this does not yet meet the requirements of the formula and follow-on milk regulations, and parents should be advised that it is unsuitable and potentially unsafe.

Complementary feeding

Complementary feeding ('weaning') is the process by which solid foods are progressively added to the sole milk diet, at the time when breast milk alone can no longer supply all nutrient needs. The optimal timing for first solids is much debated. If started too early, solid foods may stress the immature gut, kidneys and immune system and reduce breast milk intake, lessening its immune protective effects. Starting too late may result in under-nutrition and food refusal. Until recently the officially recommended age in the UK was not before 4 months, but this has recently been revised to 6 months in line with WHO recommendations. In practice, at present, most UK infants are weaned around the age of 4 months.

Solid foods require a range of new skills that need to be learnt by infants with the help and encouragement of their carers. The skills needed and the types of foods that allow their acquisition are shown in Table 4.1, along with the sorts of problem that may present at different stages. Breast milk remains the main nutrient source until the age of 6–9 months and is an important component of the diet until the age of 2 years. Bottle-fed infants should continue to take formula milk until the age of 1 year, to ensure adequate iron intake, as cow's milk is a poor source of iron and may cause gastrointestinal blood loss. Breast milk has relatively low absolute levels of iron, but this is in a highly bioavailable form.

The toddler diet

Problem-orientated topic:

feeding problems in a toddler

Chelsea, a 2-year-old girl, has been found to be iron-deficient and mum describes her as always being a bad feeder, particularly since solids were introduced. Now she eats 'nothing', though she will drink large amounts of milk.

Continued overleaf

Table 4.2 Nutrient contents per 50 g of typical infant and toddler food

Type of food	Energy (kJ)	Fat (g)	Carbohydrate (g)	Protein (g)	Vitamin C (mg)	Iron (mg)
Breast milk	145	2.1	3.6	0.65	2	0.04
Puréed carrot	46	0.20	2.2	0.3	1	0.2
Small banana, mashed	202	0.15	11.6	0.6	5.5	0.15
Mashed potato with margarine	219	2.2	7.8	0.9	2.5	0.2
Mince beef, stewed	870	13.5	0	21.8	0	2.2
Chicken, boiled	384	3.7	0	14.6	0	0.6
Sugared cereal + milk, 1/2 bowl	271	4.6	11.3	1.8	0.4	0.7
Toast and butter, 2 slices	439	6.0	11.4	1.9	0	0.4
Fromage frais, 2/3 small pot	276	2.9	2.7	2.7	0	0.04
Apple slices	76	0.05	4.5	10.2	7	0.05
Digestive biscuits, 3	890	9.4	30.9	2.8	0	1.4

Q1. What should a child be eating at this age and what is the usual main source of iron?

Q2. How will you assess her nutritional status?

Q1. What should a child be eating at this age and what is the usual main source of iron?

During the second year of life the rate of growth slows, but children become increasingly mobile and activity levels rise. Overall nutrient needs are slightly reduced per kilogram body weight compared to the first year of life, but are still around double adult requirements for body weight. From the age of 1 year, children should progress to family foods, including all the main food groups. Energy requirements remain high, so that starchy, high-fat foods are often preferred, while fruit and vegetables, which are low-energy, are rejected (Table 4.2). It is important to continue to offer small amounts of these and other new foods to establish familiarity, but unrealistic to expect most toddlers to eat large amounts. Red meat is an important source of haem iron, which is easily absorbed; solid meat can be challenging for toddlers, but minced and processed meats are popular. Milk remains an important part of the diet, supplying both energy and calcium, and toddlers should have 500 ml of full fat milk per day. Follow-on formula milks are available and provide additional vitamins and minerals, but should not be necessary if a varied solid diet is taken. Occasionally, when toddlers consume very large volumes of milk and refuse solid food, the volume or frequency of milk feeds may need to be restricted to stimulate appetite. Drinks should be given from a cup from 1 year.

Vitamins and minerals

Vitamin and mineral deficiencies are rare in healthy infants but may occur in higher-risk groups, such as premature babies. Being fortified, breakfast cereals, bread and margarine are important sources of various vitamins and micronutrients, as are citrus fruit juices. If the diet range is poor, vitamin supplements should be given and supplemental vitamin A and D drops are recommended from 6 months of age onwards. Vitamin D stores are usually sufficient at birth and levels are increased with sunshine exposure, but deficiency can occur in high-risk groups where there has been maternal deficiency or late introduction of complementary feeding. Infants of South Asian origin are still at high risk of rickets, because of their pigmentation and relative low intake of routinely fortified foods. Vitamin D drops are essential for these infants. Vitamin K is routinely given at birth to prevent haemorrhagic disease of the newborn.

With increasing age, the pace of growth continues to slow. By the age of 5, children should ideally be eating the same range of family foods as their elder siblings and parents, and usual healthy eating guidelines should apply. Food consumed should be less energy-dense than in the early years and consumption of lower-fat, higher-fibre foods should be encouraged (Box 4.5). As eating habits develop, a healthy eating pattern should be adopted, with plenty of fruit and vegetables and sparing amounts of high-fat and high-sugar foods.

Q2. How will you assess her nutritional status?

Although it seems logical to assess nutritional status by measuring what is eaten, this in fact supplies very limited useful information. There are two reasons: firstly, each individual's nutrient requirements vary, depending on many factors, few of which can be accurately estimated;

In recognition of the contribution of diet to cardiovascular diseases, cancer and the rising problem of obesity, policies have been developed to improve the health of the nation through encouraging healthier eating. In England, 'Choosing Health' (Department of Health white paper 2004) plans to review the following areas:

- Educational campaigns, e.g. '5 a day', salt reduction and obesity awareness
- Simplification of food labelling to allow consumers to make healthier choices
- Review of the advertising and promotion of unhealthy food and drink products to children
- Continuation of work with industry to improve the nutritional content of processed foods (e.g. salt and sugar reduction in breakfast cereals)
- Healthy Start programme, which provides disadvantaged pregnant women and mothers with vouchers for fresh fruit, vegetables and milk
- Healthy schools initiative, e.g. provision of free fruit to 4–6-year-olds

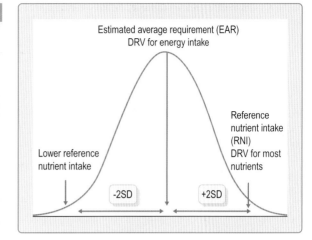

Dietary reference values (DRV)
- These are the reference ideal nutrient requirements set for adults and for different ages of children
- Calculated from amount of nutrients eaten by healthy normally growing individuals
- Values are designed to avoid inadequacy in the diet

Estimated average requirement (EAR)
- The mean value of the requirement for a group of individuals (this is assumed to follow a normal distribution curve)
- Intakes of this amount should be sufficient for 50% of the population

Reference nutrient intake (RNI)
- Intakes two standard deviations (SDs) above the EAR
- Should be sufficient for almost all the population

Lower reference nutrient intake (LRNI)
- Intakes two SDs below the EAR
- Intakes below this level are inadequate for most of the population

Recommended requirements
- Defined as the RNI for most nutrients, where consumption of excess is not harmful
- EAR used for energy, since excess energy intake above average requirements leads to obesity
- DRVs can be used in food labelling or to assess intake and guide dietary prescription

Fig. 4.2 How nutrient requirements are calculated

secondly, dietary assessment is intrinsically inaccurate. Thus dietary assessment cannot be safely used to diagnose nutritional insufficiency, although food diaries can provide helpful information about the range and type of foods eaten and the meal pattern, and may act as a guide to dietary advice once a problem has been identified (Fig. 4.2). In contrast, measurements of weight and height provide essential, objective information about nutrient balance, particularly if used in combination (Table 4.3).

Serial measurements of weight and height can be highly informative as long as the degree of natural variation is understood. In infancy moderate deviations in weight are common and 1 in 20 infants will fall (or rise) through two intercentile spaces (1.3 SD), but only 1% will drop though three (2 SD). Different criteria apply to very large and small infants, for whom specialist charts are available. Obtaining accurate height (and length) measurements in the preschool years is intrinsically difficult, so that apparent decelerations are most commonly due to measurement error. After the age of 5 (and before puberty) variations in height of more than one centile space occur in less than 5% of children. A full assessment should always involve calculating body mass index (BMI = weight/height^2) and plotting this on a centile chart, since BMI values vary greatly through childhood. Anthropometry cannot distinguish between different body compartments; thus a muscular athletic child with a low fat mass could have a high BMI, while a child with cerebral palsy with a very low muscle mass could have a low BMI but a high fat mass. However, the current gold standard measure of body composition, using stable isotopes, is expensive and not generally available. Less direct measures, which may prove useful in future, are not yet adequately standardized for routine use in childhood. In practice, in the assessment of obesity, a high BMI (> 98th centile) equates closely with high adiposity.

Energy expenditure can also be measured accurately in a research setting using stable isotopes, but there are currently no standard methods for field or clinical use, although accelerometers are providing interesting research data.

Assessment of micronutrient status presents different challenges. Serum levels usually only partly reflect whole

Table 4.3 Strengths and limitations of different nutritional assessment methods

	Method	Strengths	Limitations
Dietary assessment	24-hour recall, 3–7-day diary or weighed record	Allows targeted dietary advice	Individual requirements vary greatly Portion size uncertain in unweighed records Diet during recording period may not be representative, particularly weighed records Exact nutrient content of foods vary
Anthropometry			
Weight	Naked weight on electronic scale	Summary of overall growth, particularly in infancy Serial measures can identify changes in nutritional status Easy to measure accurately	Cannot distinguish between bone, fat and muscle mass
Height	Standing or lying, without shoes on rigid measure or stadiometer	Indicator of stunting if used serially, or related to parental height Easy to measure	Most variation in height not nutritionally determined Inaccurate in preschool children
Weight for height (BMI)	Weight (kg)/height (m²)	Indicator of both wasting and overweight Allows variations in weight to be interpreted in growing child	Cannot distinguish between fat and muscle mass Gives no measure of growth over time Large intrinsic measurement error
Body composition			
Stable isotopes	Deuterium-labelled water given by mouth and concentration in urine measured by mass spectrometry	Gold standard method, highly accurate	Expensive and labour-intensive
Dual-energy X-ray absorptiometry (DXA)	Absorption of low-dose X-ray estimates bone and muscle mass	Provides fairly robust, accurate estimates	Costly equipment, not portable Normal range for children not well delineated
Bioelectrical impedance	Conduction of current though limbs and body used to estimate non-fat mass	Portable, cheap, reliable	Current childhood formulae not robust Normal range for children not well delineated

body content, particularly where the nutrient is stored, as with iron, or in a deficiency state where the nutrient may be cleared from plasma very quickly. Signs of frank deficiency may be distinctive but are rare and, ideally, insufficiency should be identified before they occur. The markers and diagnostic criteria for the most common childhood deficiency states, iron deficiency and rickets, are described above in the relevant sections.

Religious and cultural dietary restrictions

Families may have special dietary practices or exclusions that reflect a religious or other affiliation. These will vary between apparently similar ethnic groups (e.g. Sikh as opposed to Muslim Punjabis), and within a religious group depending on their degree of adherence (e.g. ultra-orthodox as opposed to reform Jews). Most Muslim and Jewish families will avoid all pork and any non-halal or non-kosher meat respectively, leading sometimes to the false impression that they are vegetarian.

Families who do describe themselves as vegetarian may range from avoidance only of meat (but not fish) to those who avoid all meat, fish, eggs and dairy products. Other families may exclude particular foods due to personal beliefs about the risks associated with them.

Thus it is essential to ask all families about their usual diet and any possible exclusions, and not to make assumptions. In practice dietary variations that lead to nutrient deficiency are usually extreme and rarely religiously determined, with diets that exclude dairy products (an important source of energy) most likely to lead to problems.

www.doh.gov.uk/PolicyAndGuidance/fs/en
www.healthyliving.gov.uk/healthyeating
www.scotland.gov.uk/Topics/health
www.wales.gov.uk

Further reading

Morgan Jane B, Dickerson JWT (eds) 2003 Nutrition in early life. Wiley, Chichester

Committee on Medical Aspects of Food 1994 Annex IV to Weaning and the weaning diet, Report 45. HMSO, London

Department of Health 2005 Dietary reference values for food energy and nutrients for the United Kingdom: Report on Health and Social Subjects. HMSO, London Report 41

Hamlyn B, Brooker S, Oleinikova K, Wands S 2002 Infant feeding 2000. TSO, London

Wright CM 2002 The use and interpretation of growth charts. Current Paediatrics 12:279–282

MODULE ONE

Edited by Jonathan Darling

Toolkit for child health and disease

MODULE TWO

Mark Bradbury   Alan Cade

History-taking and physical examination

MODULE TWO

LEARNING OUTCOMES

By the end of this chapter you should:

- Be able to take a paediatric history
- Be able to conduct an age-specific general examination of children
- Be able to examine each organ system in detail
- Be able to recognize common and important paediatric conditions and syndromes
- Be able to recognize the pathognomonic features of the more common conditions in childhood
- Know the normal range of physiological parameters in children.

Introduction

The skills of history-taking and physical examination in children are an essential part of your paediatric toolkit. You need to develop and hone these skills through constant practice, and your competence in them will be tested when you sit postgraduate clinical examinations in paediatrics and child health.

Rather than blindly asking the same questions and performing the same examination sequence by rote in every consultation, you need to develop a logical and strategic approach focused around the child's problem.

At the outset of any consultation, you establish the nature of the child's presenting problem(s) and construct a hypothesis of what might be the most likely cause, along with other possible causes. This initial broad differential diagnosis is then modified as you proceed through the history and examination. Throughout the process, you are seeking evidence for and against your various differentials, and this mental list may continually be reordered as you acquire new information. You thus adapt your clinical approach to what you find as you go along, as well as to the individual circumstances of the child and family. Professional examinations look for this thoughtful and logical approach.

At the end of the process, you need to make sense of what you have discovered, construct a problem list and management plan, and communicate with the child and family about these. These aspects are covered later in this module (pp. 59 and 63).

Remember that the process of history-taking and examination can be powerfully therapeutic in its own right through the way you interact with the child and family. Attention to detail, careful listening, treating people with empathy, sensitivity and respect, clear explanations and finding time for questions can all make a difference.

History-taking

In order to formulate a diagnosis and an effective management plan for a child who is ill, it is important to have an appreciation of the problems which the child is presenting with and the context in which they are arising. The foundation for this formulation is a thorough history. An effective history-taking interview utilizes communication skills (active listening, good questioning and observing non-verbal communication) in a structured information-gathering process. The greater the history-taker's skill, the more accurate the differential diagnoses and the greater benefit to the patient.

The objectives of a history-taking interview include:
- Developing an appreciation of the presenting difficulties, their severity and the impact on the child and family
- Reaching a diagnosis or differential diagnosis, including an understanding of what factors may have triggered, exacerbated or maintained the presenting problem
- Consideration of the strengths of the family and child and whether they are able and motivated to work at resolving the presenting complaint, and what opportunities the healthcare team have to support the child and family
- Understanding what expectations, ideas and concerns the child and family have about the illness and its treatment.

Communication skills and the interview process

The initial communication during a history-taking interview offers the opportunity of establishing a good rapport at the same time as demonstrating professional competence and a respect for confidentiality. Good communication skills and practice at the interview process enable treatment to begin as soon as the family has entered the room.

With older children and teenagers it is good practice to take the story in their words first, then to repeat the questions to the parent(s). Unfortunately some parents interrupt, trying to be helpful, and at times it is necessary to conduct the interview with parent and child separately. With younger children, always have age-appropriate play materials on hand to entertain and relax the child and siblings. Gaining the child's interest and confidence can have a positive effect when it comes to the physical examination. It will also help parents to answer questions if they do not have to distract or comfort their child.

A simple ABCD approach can be used to plan the interview process:
- *Accepting*
- *Broadening*
- *Clarifying*
- *Deepening.*

Accepting

Accepting describes the strategy used at the opening of the interview. The factors to consider are:
- Greeting the child and each parent. It is worth asking at this stage how each of the adults and other children present are related to the child. This avoids the very embarrassing situation of mistaking an older parent for a grandparent or younger parent for a sibling later in the interview.
- Establishing a warm friendly atmosphere.
- Trying to maintain privacy and reduce distractions, switching off mobile phones and adjusting emergency bleeps to the vibrate setting.
- Sustaining eye contact and avoiding getting buried in a set of notes.
- Asking a simple question to prompt the presenting complaint and listening carefully to the reply.
- Observing the child–parent interaction during this early stage.

Often we cannot change the physical environment in which the interview takes place, but try to avoid the barrier of a desk, arranging the chairs in a less formal but practical configuration.

Broadening

At this point in the interview, open questions are useful:

- How?
- What?
- Why?
- When?
- Where?
- Who?

These allow the parent or child to do the majority of talking, again in their own words, about the presenting problems. Avoid jargon or more complicated medical words, and define terms that may be misunderstood. After this stage of the history, a broader understanding of the problem exists but specific details are often required, leading to the next stage.

Clarifying

With a long or complicated history, it is often helpful to summarize it and tell it back to the history-giver to check for errors. Important details regarding the presenting complaint may not have been mentioned spontaneously, and can be asked about using more direct, closed-style questions and often saving time. The additional information needed in the other sections of the history may be obtained using the same style of questions.

Deepening

This describes the questions that probe deeper into areas of concern, ideas and expectations, trying to uncover:

- Any hidden agendas
- Self-blame felt by the parents in relation to things they may have done or not done
- The extent of any frightening experiences of the illness for the parents and child
- Any unarticulated fears of death or bad outcomes.

This phase also presents an opportunity to ask about the impact of the illness on family life.

Using rather vague general questions and statements — for example, 'Other parents I have spoken to have said how worrying it was that…', — and then pausing for a response is a method of deepening the interview.

How long should it take to elicit a history?

If you are presented with a child who is acutely ill with severe asthma or major trauma, take a short focused history, enquiring about the current problems, past medical history, and drug and allergy history only. This can be completed in minutes, not delaying the start of treatment. When the situation is under control, a more complete history can then be taken. This contrasts with a complex history in the outpatient department that may require 30 minutes or longer to complete.

Taking notes during the interview

It is often helpful to limit yourself to writing down a few important details during the history. This will help avoid long pauses for writing, improves eye contact and allows you to observe non-verbal communication. When writing in the medical notes, ensure your entry is timed and dated, and that you clearly identify yourself. If for any reason you wish to keep notes of the history for your own files, then it would be good practice to anonymize the history and keep it in a secure folder to protect confidentiality.

Organizing the content of the interview

A systematic method of organizing the content of a history-taking interview into separate sections is outlined below:

1. General information
2. Presenting complaint and history of the presenting complaint
3. Past medical history
4. Pregnancy and birth history
5. Feeding and dietary history
6. Growth
7. Developmental history
8. Medications and allergies
9. Immunizations
10. Family history
11. Social history
12. Review of systems.

This structure is familiar from adult history-taking but adds extra sections specifically relevant to children.

1. General information

Note the date, time and location of the interview. Ask or check identifying data, including name, age and birth date, gender, race and referral source. Record the name of the adult giving the history, and his or her relationship to the child. Note who else is present, and record when an interpreter is being used.

2. Presenting complaint and history of the presenting complaint

Record the main complaint in the informant's or the patient's own words, and the history of the presenting complaints in chronological order. Questions should include:

- Description?
- Recent examples, focusing on main factors, context and exacerbating and relieving factors?
- When did it start?
- Frequency?
- Severity?
- Change of symptoms over time?
- What effects do these symptoms have?
- What help was sought previously and how helpful was this?
- What ideas and concerns about the causation of the symptoms do the child and the family have?
- Are there any other associated symptoms?

3. Past medical history

This is a detailed list of the child's previous illnesses, visits to casualty departments, times in hospital and operations. It is worth noting whether these problems are ongoing/active or resolved/inactive.

4. Pregnancy and birth history

Factors important in this section include:

- Health and age of mother in pregnancy
- Antenatal scans and tests
- Length of gestation
- Type of delivery
- Birth weight
- Condition of the baby at delivery
- Any immediate health problems after birth
- Any health problems in the first few weeks of life.

If there were problems prior to, during or after delivery, then more detailed questioning in these areas will be required.

5. Feeding and dietary history (Ch. 4)

Ask whether the baby was breast- or bottle-fed, and how well the baby took to feeding after birth. If the infant has been bottle-fed, enquire about the type of formula milk used and the amount taken during a 24-hour period. Any vomiting, regurgitation, colic, diarrhoea or other gastrointestinal problems should be noted. Ask at what age the child was started on solid food and if supplementation with vitamins was given. For an older child, ask about the range of foods

- When presenting or analysing measurements of a continuous variable (such as height), it is sometimes helpful to group subjects into several equal groups.
- Growth charts often display the cutoff values that split the data such that there is 1% of the observations in each group. These cutoff points are called *centiles*, and there are 99 of them (the middle one also being called the median and the 25th and 75th centiles also representing quartiles).
- If the physiological variable is normally distributed (e.g. height), the centiles can be related to the standard deviation (SD). The growth charts in common use display the centiles that correspond to the intervals two-thirds of a standard deviation from the mean:

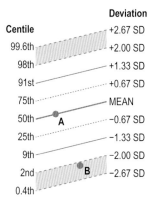

- A child whose height falls on the 50th centile (A) is average for his/her age.
- A child whose height falls just below the 2nd centile (B) is well below average for his/her age, such that he/she is in the bottom 2% of the population. To help parents' understanding, it may be useful to say, 'If a class of 100 pupils were asked to line up, such that the tallest was at one end and the shortest at the other, your son/daughter would be standing next to the shortest pupil.'

Fig. 5.1 Normal distribution: principles of centile charts

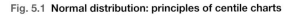

eaten and some examples of meals and snacks from the last few weeks.

6. Growth (Ch. 22)

Parents may have brought along the parent-held child record to the interview. This contains details and plots of previous weights and lengths/heights (Fig. 5.1) that will allow assessment of the child's physical growth. For older children and teenagers, it is important to ask about the onset of puberty.

Be familiar with the parent-held record. You may find it useful to refer to when you are taking a history, particularly with regard to growth and immunization.

7. Developmental history (Ch. 2)

The developmental history needs to be appropriate to the child's age. For younger children, questions about milestones in gross motor skills and locomotion, fine motor skills and vision, hearing and speech, and social development are appropriate. In older children, details about school performance are more appropriate.

8. Medication and allergies

List the child's current medications accurately, including dosage and frequency, and (if possible) when they were commenced. Highlight any specific drug allergies or sensitivities. These also need to be recorded in a specific location in the medical records.

9. Immunizations (Ch. 16)

Ask about and make a list of the child's immunizations. If any have been omitted, enquire about the reasons. If parents are unsure, then the parent-held child record may contain helpful information. Many areas of the UK have a computerized immunization record that can be checked at a later date, if required.

10. Family history

Record family structure and draw a genetic family tree, including parents, siblings and grandparents with their ages, health or cause of death (p. 88). A question such as 'Are you and your partner related?' is a helpful way to detail consanguinity. A positive family history may link to shared genes, infections or environment.

11. Social history

Ask about who makes up the household. Details about the size and type of accommodation may be helpful. Occupation of the parents and whether they smoke are covered in this section. Major or psychiatric illness affecting parents can be clarified at this stage. It is worth asking whether there are any financial problems and what benefits the family are currently receiving. It may be relevant to know if the family has any pets. Further details about the child's school, school work and school friends, as well as any problems at school such as bullying or teasing, can also be checked out at this stage.

This can be a difficult and sensitive area. It can be helpful to practise some clear questions that you can ask in an unembarrassed way.

12. Review of systems

This section serves as a checklist for any information that may have been omitted up to this point in the history. The questions that are relevant to the presenting complaint are best asked earlier in the history when clarifying the further details relating to the presenting compliant.

Enquiries concerning each system can be introduced with a question such as 'Are there any symptoms relating to your/his/her…?':

- Head (e.g. injuries, headache)
- Eyes (e.g. loss of vision, squint, discharge, redness, puffiness, injuries, glasses)
- Ears (e.g. difficulty with hearing, pain, discharge, ear infections, surgery/grommets)
- Nose (e.g. discharge, difficulty in breathing through the nose, nose bleeds)
- Throat (e.g. sore throat or tongue, difficulty in swallowing)
- Neck (e.g. swollen glands, masses, stiffness, symmetry)
- Breasts (e.g. lumps, pain, early puberty)
- Chest (e.g. shortness of breath, exercise tolerance, cough, wheezing, haemoptysis, pain in chest, noisy breathing/stridor)
- Heart (e.g. collapse, murmurs, sweating, poor feeding in infants)
- Gastrointestinal system (e.g. reduced appetite, nausea, vomiting with relation to feeding, amount, colour, blood- or bile-stained, projectile, bowel movements with number and character, abdominal pain or distension, jaundice)
- Genitourinary system (e.g. dysuria, haematuria, frequency, oliguria, urinary stream, wetting day or night, urethral or vaginal discharge)
- Extremities (e.g. weakness, deformities, difficulty in moving limbs or in walking, joint pains and swelling, muscle pains or cramps)
- Neurological system (e.g. headaches, fainting, dizziness, clumsiness, seizures, numbness, tremors)
- Skin (e.g. rashes, hives, itching, colour change, hair and nail growth, easy bruising or bleeding)
- Mood and behaviour (e.g. usual mood, nervousness, tension, possible substance abuse).

When you have completed the history, it should be possible to develop a problem list. This will include physical, genetic, developmental, emotional, cognitive, educational, family and social components. With this information a detailed physical examination can be performed and a differential diagnosis developed (Ch. 6).

Principles of the physical examination

Examination of children of different ages presents unique challenges. Without sensitivity to the child's perspective, the examination will be difficult and incomplete. You need to adapt the set routines used in adults to the age,

- Always wash your hands
- Introduce yourself to the patient and carer
- Do not take the child away from the environment that he or she is comfortable with
- Involve the parent/carer
- Allow time for children to get used to you before placing a hand/stethoscope on them
- Use visual clues to build up a picture of the child's problems, e.g. crutches, helmet, ankle foot orthoses, inhalers, medications
- Do not hurt the child; ask the child/carer if there is any pain or discomfort prior to commencing your examination

mood, level of understanding and state of health of the child (Box 5.1).

Be both structured and opportunistic, checking on completion that you have not missed any important signs. If faced with an uncooperative child you may have to return later, although this is obviously not possible in clinical examinations.

Preparation and approach

You will learn much about a child and his or her state of health simply by observation. The child's interaction with environment, carer, siblings (if present) and yourself will give you important clues about developmental progress, physical and mental abilities, and desire to be examined. There may be clear visual clues to an underlying problem:

- The presence of spectacles/hearing aids
- The school-age child wearing nappies: physical and developmental problems
- The presence of central cyanosis/dyspnoea at rest: cardiovascular, respiratory and neurological causes
- Nasogastric tubes in situ: eating disorders, swallowing difficulties, gastrointestinal disease
- The nutritional and pubertal state of the child
- Dysmorphic features
- The presence of a rash: psoriasis, dermatomyositis, eczema, erythema nodosum
- The physical characteristics of a parent: achondroplasia, myotonic dystrophy, neurofibromatosis.

At the outset you may well have a clear idea of what you might find and what in particular you need to look for. However, a general physical examination is always advisable, except for when you are directed otherwise in clinical examinations. Do not forget that a child may have co-morbidities.

The general examination

Be confident and take control. Do not ask young children whether you can examine them, because if they say 'no' you must then go against their wishes. Adequate exposure whilst retaining modesty will ensure nothing is missed. Both the environment and your hands should be warm. Get down to the child's level and talk in an age-appropriate manner. Avoid technical terms and unrealistic requests (e.g. 'Take deep breaths' to a 2-year-old). Continue to talk to children whilst examining them, encourage and praise them, and thank them afterwards.

A full and thorough examination of a child, including ears, throat and perineum (if appropriate), should take no more than 3 minutes. This will not include a detailed system or developmental examination but these should be carried out if concerns are raised through either the history or the general examination. The general examination includes assessment of puberty and nutrition.

Growth and nutrition (see Ch. 22)

Accurate measurement of length in a non-walking infant requires two people and a horizontal rigid stadiometer. Height is measured without shoes on and weight in only light clothing, e.g. underwear. Head circumference is the maximum achievable distance around the head in the occipito-frontal plane and should be measured using a non-stretch tape measure! For more detailed assessment of nutritional status, measure mid-arm circumference and skinfold thickness, but this is not routinely necessary. Isolated growth parameters mean little and should be interpreted in the context of previous recordings and position on centile charts.

Child protection concerns (see Ch. 21)

Occasionally such concerns arise during the examination. Observe the following:

- State of dress, hygiene and dentition
- Behaviour: 'frozen watchfulness', fear of strangers, unwillingness to undress
- Relationship with carer: fear, obedience, lack of respect
- Nutritional state: failure to thrive
- Thorough examination, including frenulum, fundi and all of the skin
- Perineal examination — this may be best left to a more experienced colleague to avoid repeated examinations.

Your documentation should be accurate and complete, and should include relevant verbatim statements from carers and child, and any discussions with carers. Confronting the carer with your concerns may again be best left to a colleague with greater experience of child protection matters, when your suspicions have been verified.

Cardiovascular examination

This system examination is included in every Membership of the Royal College of Paediatrics and Child Health (MRCPCH) part II clinical examination. You have 9 minutes to demonstrate an ability to examine a child's cardiovascular system and interpret the clinical signs.

General inspection and visual clues

Look for visual clues first: supplemental oxygen, wheelchair, medication, TED stockings, a parent's appearance (Marfan's or Holt–Oram syndrome). Children with cardiac disease may have developmental delay because of their underlying syndrome or because of the heart disease itself. If delay is present, you should comment on this at the outset, and although in an examination you may not have time to do a detailed developmental assessment, you should offer to do this. Similarly, mention the state of a child's dentition (risk of endocarditis).

Look for dysmorphic or other features consistent with an underlying specific cardiac lesion:
- *Down's syndrome*: atrioventricular septal defect, Fallot's tetralogy, atrial septal defect, ventricular septal defect
- *Alagille's syndrome*: jaundice, pulmonary stenosis
- *Turner's syndrome*: short stature, coarctation, aortic stenosis, bicuspid aortic valve
- *Williams' syndrome*: peripheral pulmonary artery stenosis, pulmonary or aortic stenosis.

Does the child have any cardiorespiratory distress at rest (or feeding)? Is there peripheral or central cyanosis? Demonstrate whether the child has finger clubbing (cyanotic heart disease — right-to-left shunt), splinter haemorrhages (infective endocarditis or just trauma!), and comment on the colour and temperature of the hands.

Peripheries

Feel the brachial pulse in all ages for rhythm, character and volume, and measure the heart rate over at least 15 seconds. Heart rate will increase during inspiration as venous return increases. Normal values for age-specific heart rates are found in Table 5.1. (Beware if the child is on β-blockers.) Palpation of the femoral pulses is mandatory but can be left until examination of the abdomen

Table 5.1 Age-appropriate heart rate

Age (years)	Heart rate (beats per minute)
< 1	110–160
1–2	100–150
2–5	95–140
5–12	80–120
> 12	60–100

(hepatomegaly — heart failure, splenomegaly — infective endocarditis), provided it is not forgotten.

Specific inspection

Expose the chest wherever possible. Look for evidence of asymmetry and surgical scars:
- *Left lateral thoracotomy*: coarctation repair, left Blalock–Taussig shunt, patent ductus arteriosus (PDA) ligation, pulmonary artery (PA) banding
- *Right lateral thoracotomy*: right Blalock–Taussig shunt, tracheo-oesophageal repair
- *Central sternotomy*: reconstructive surgery, valvular surgery
- *Submammary*: atrial septal defect repair in girls
- *Infraclavicular*: pacemaker insertion.

Palpation

Localize the apex beat (normally mid-clavicular line, 4–5th intercostal space). Displacement of the apex is seen in left ventricular hypertrophy and dilated cardiomyopathy. Feel for thrills and heaves. If you can feel a thrill you will be able to hear a murmur very easily.

Auscultation

Auscultate the precordium (do this opportunistically earlier in the examination if the child is likely to become uncooperative). Listen in the four areas (Fig. 5.2) and be clear by the end of auscultation what the characteristics of the heart sounds are, and whether any additional heart sounds are systolic, diastolic or pansystolic; early or late in the cardiac cycle; radiating to anywhere; and pathological or not.

Radiation may be detected in:
- *Aortic stenosis*: neck (thrill may be palpable in the suprasternal notch)
- *PDA and coarctation*: interscapular region of the back.

Splitting of the second heart sound is normal and may be exaggerated during inspiration. Fixed splitting is heard in atrioventricular septal defects.

43

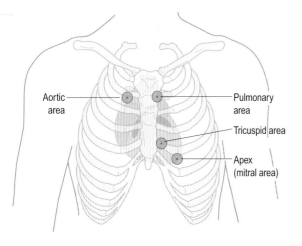

Fig. 5.2 Surface anatomy of auscultation points for the four heart valves

Aortic area

Pulmonary area

Tricuspid area

Apex (mitral area)

Table 5.2 Age-appropriate systolic blood pressure

Age (years)	Systolic blood pressure (mmHg)
< 1	70–90
1–2	80–95
2–5	80–100
5–12	90–110
> 12	100–120

Extras

To complete the examination of the cardiovascular system, listen to the lung bases (pulmonary oedema in left heart failure), look for peripheral oedema (right heart failure), and measure the blood pressure. This must be done using an appropriately sized sphygmomanometer cuff (to cover two-thirds of the upper arm) on the right arm (unless a four-limb recording is indicated: for example, in coarctation or interrupted arch). Normal values are difficult to remember but as a general rule the systolic blood pressure should be less than 115 mmHg in the under-10s (Table 5.2). A simple formula to use for calculating normal values for systolic blood pressure is:

Systolic blood pressure = 80 + (age in years × 2)

Centile charts exist for age-appropriate means and normal ranges for systolic blood pressure.

Presentation of findings during examination of the cardiac system must concentrate on positive signs rather than compiling a long list of negative or normal ones. Nine minutes will give more than ample opportunity to undertake a full cardiac examination and discuss the findings and/or implications. If your findings are incorrect or misinterpreted, you may be asked to examine the child again.

Respiratory examination

This is commonly required in paediatric postgraduate clinical examinations. As for cardiac examinations, opportunism should be employed to auscultate the chest of a potentially uncooperative child, provided no other part of the examination is compromised or missed.

General inspection and visual clues

13–14

Clues to aid diagnosis include sputum pots (productive cough suggestive of bronchiectasis), inhalers, spacer device and peak flow meter (asthma), suction catheters and machine (ineffective cough due to underlying neuromuscular disease) and non-invasive ventilation equipment (neuromuscular disease). Graduates of neonatal units who have bronchopulmonary dysplasia requiring supplemental oxygen often help with exams. Pointers to prematurity include scaphocephaly, glasses, evidence of previous line insertions and PDA surgery.

Be vigilant throughout to pick up further clues. A child's weak voice may indicate a vocal cord palsy (?any surgical evidence of previous cardiac surgery and damage to a recurrent laryngeal nerve), or an inability to generate enough airflow through the vocal cords secondary to underlying lung or neuromuscular disease.

The nature of a chronic cough can be helpful:
* *Moist*: lower respiratory tract infection (LRTI) or bronchiectasis
* *Barking*: laryngotracheobronchitis or psychogenic
* *Paroxysmal*: whooping cough.

Stridor is indicative of upper and large airway narrowing, and the level is suggested by whether it is expiratory (below the thoracic inlet) or inspiratory (above the thoracic inlet). Duration and variability (persistent/intermittent) give clues to causation.

Peripheries and specific inspection

After looking for finger clubbing and noting whether the child has peripheral or central cyanosis, expose the chest fully where possible and comment on chest shape if abnormal. Note any hyper-expansion, asymmetry, pectus excavatum and carinatum, Harrison's sulci, kyphosis or scoliosis. Look for evidence of previous surgery (chest drains, lobectomy, tracheostomy). The presence of axillary and cervical lymphadenopathy may be relevant.

15

Children with respiratory distress may feature in the video section of the clinical exam. Note the nature, pattern and rate of respiration. Normal respiratory rates are given in Table 5.3. Assess the work of breathing by checking for suprasternal, intercostal and

Table 5.3 Age-appropriate respiratory rates

Age (years)	Respiratory rate (breaths per minute)
< 1	30–40
1–2	25–35
2–5	25–30
5–12	20–25
> 12	15–20

Table 5.4 Interpretation of percussion notes

Percussion note	Interpretation
Resonant	Normal
Hyper-resonant	Pneumothorax
Dull	Consolidation
Stony dull	Pleural fluid

Table 5.5 Interpretation of breath sounds

Breath sounds	Interpretation
Vesicular	Normal
Absent breath sounds	Pleural effusion
Decreased breath sounds	Collapse
Bronchial breathing	Consolidation

subcostal recession (and abdominal breathing in the under-1s). Nasal flaring and use of accessory muscles may be present. Prolongation of either component of the breathing cycle should be noted.

Palpation and percussion (Table 5.4)

16 Check the position of the apex beat and the trachea (for mediastinal shift).

Percussion of the chest can be frightening to the younger child so explanation is necessary. Do not forget to percuss (and auscultate) in the axillae.

Auscultation (Table 5.5)

Assess air entry and breath sounds. Additional noises include fine and coarse crepitations, inspiratory and expiratory wheezes, transmitted upper airway noises and pleural rub.

Chest wall expansion and tactile vocal fremitus are difficult in the younger child, but worth trying in a cooperative school-age child.

Extras

17 Palpate and percuss for the liver to assess hyper-expansion further. Normally the edge of the liver may just be palpable, and dullness to percussion may extend up to the nipple line. In hyper-expansion, this area of dullness will be shifted down and the liver more easily palpated.

Table 5.6 Signs of disease in abdominal examination

Condition	Signs to look for
Cystic fibrosis	Portal hypertension
Alagille's syndrome	Liver disease
Inflammatory bowel disease	Colectomy, enterostomies, malnutrition, perianal fissuring
Wilson's disease	Liver disease
Nephrotic syndrome	Scrotal oedema, ascites
Prematurity	Umbilical and inguinal herniae
Hereditary spherocytosis	Splenomegaly and jaundice
Thalassaemia	Splenomegaly ± hepatomegaly
Sickle cell disease	Splenomegaly up to school age → autosplenectomy

Finally, in school-age children, measure peak expiratory flow rate (PEFR). This should be undertaken on three occasions whilst the child is standing, taking the best recording. There has been a recent change in the peak flow meters used in the UK, which now give slightly different values to the commonly used mini-Wright meters (Ch. 42).

www.peakflow.com

A useful way of calculating expected peak flow based on height of the child is:

Predicted PEFR (litres/min) = (height (cm) $\times$ 5) – 450

Abdominal examination

This is often done badly in clinical examinations. Signs are misinterpreted and children who have nothing wrong with them are 'diagnosed' as having a non-existent pathology. Examination can be difficult because young children do not like to be laid down, and older children find it difficult to relax their anterior abdominal wall musculature. Older children tend to have less subcutaneous fat than the average adult and so it is easier to feel a normal liver edge or slightly loaded descending colon.

General inspection and visual clues

Although an enormous variety of conditions will have intra-abdominal manifestations in childhood, there are a number that lend themselves very well to paediatric examinations (Table 5.6).

Many of these have extra-intestinal stigmata that may direct you towards a diagnosis before examining the abdomen. Some haematological conditions that result in abdominal organomegaly occur in certain races. For example:

- *Caucasian*: hereditary spherocytosis
- *Mediterranean*: thalassaemia
- *Afro-Caribbean*: sickle cell disease.

Assess basic nutritional status, and plot height and weight (offer to do this as a matter of course in clinical examinations). Look at the face for skin colour, evidence of dysmorphism, and features of chronic liver disease including jaundice, bruising, spider naevi and xanthelasma. Jaundice is clinically detectable when the serum bilirubin rises above 35 μmol/l. It can be subtle, even at much higher levels and particularly in artificial lighting, and is most easily seen in the sclera.

Peripheries

Look at the hands for evidence of liver disease, including palmar erythema, koilonychia and leuconychia. Clubbing is found in inflammatory bowel disease. Examine the mouth for dentition, ulceration (Crohn's and Behçet's disease), lip swelling (Crohn's disease) and lip pigmentation (Peutz–Jeghers disease).

Specific inspection

If modesty allows, expose the child's abdomen fully and lay the child flat on the bed or parent's lap. Look for spider naevi in the distribution of the superior vena cava. Note any abdominal distension and look for scars, especially in the groin and flank where they can be difficult to see. Diabetes may lead to a number of physical features, including lipoatrophy and multiple injection sites.

Palpation

18 Prior to palpating the abdomen, ensure that the child does not have any pain or tenderness. This can be checked by asking the child to draw the abdomen in and then out — 'make yourself as thin and as fat as possible.' This will not only demonstrate the level of likely discomfort the child is in, but may also reveal larger abdominal masses if the child does not have a lot of subcutaneous fat.

Perform light then deep palpation of all four quadrants of the abdomen, without unnecessary prodding and without causing discomfort (if possible). At completion, you should be able to describe the size, texture and consistency of the liver, spleen and kidneys, if palpable, and any other masses, e.g. bladder, colon, transplanted kidneys. A palpable spleen is abnormal except in the young infant. Differentiate between a normal-sized liver pushed down by over-inflated lungs and hepatomegaly (see above).

Percussion and auscultation

19 Percussion for evidence of ascites should normally be rapid; it does not require the demonstration of shifting dullness or a fluid thrill if there is no abdominal distension or oedema when the child is in the supine position, and no other reason to suspect ascites. Auscultation over the liver, spleen and renal arteries may rarely detect bruits. Listen for bowel sounds if obstruction is suspected.

Extras

20
21 Get the child to sit up and look at the back for evidence of spina bifida, Henoch–Schönlein purpura and striae. In the clinical situation it may be appropriate and necessary to examine the perineum fully. In young boys, early diagnosis of undescended testes can prevent future infertility. Testes may retract due to cold hands. In a chubby baby it can be very difficult to palpate the testes but with perseverance and a relaxed infant it should be possible to clarify the situation. For infants an assessment of the hips to exclude developmental dysplasia of the hips is necessary (p. 78).

In the MRCPCH/Diploma of Child Health exam situation you should always offer to examine the perineum as part of the abdominal system examination. You may or may not then be invited to do so by the examiner. Rectal examination is not a standard part of the clinical examination and should never be performed in the exam situation.

To complete the examination, urinalysis should be requested. A variety of 'multistix' exist, the best of which include measurement of nitrites and leucocytes. A urine sample that contains both leucocytes and nitrites gives a sensitivity and specificity of 95% and 60–70% respectively for a urinary tract infection.

Neurological examination

22 ### Limbs and gait (Tables 5.7 and 5.8)

This is an examination that can be enjoyable for the child, and hopefully for you as well. The child should have as little clothing on as possible besides underwear. Look for:
- Asymmetry (unless both arms or legs are abnormal)
- Contractures
- Posture
- Muscle mass
- Involuntary movements
- Fasciculations
- Scars
- Skin abnormalities.

Table 5.7 Joint movement innervations

Joint	Movement	Root value
Shoulder	Abduction	C5
	Adduction	C5–C8
Elbow	Flexion	C5, C6
	Extension	C7, C8
Hand	Flexion	C8, T1
	Extension	C6–C8
Hip	Flexion	L1–L3
	Extension	L5, S1
Knee	Flexion	S1
	Extension	L3, L4
Ankle	Dorsiflexion	L4, L5
	Plantar flexion	S1, S2

Table 5.8 Muscle power grading

Grade	Power
0	No movement
1	Flicker of contraction
2	Movement if gravity removed
3	Movement against gravity but not resistance
4	Movement against resistance
5	Normal power

Table 5.9 Reflex nerve innervations

Reflexes	Root value
Ankle	S1, S2
Knee	L3, L4
Biceps/supinator	C5, C6
Triceps	C7, C8

Then check tone, power, coordination, sensation, reflexes (Table 5.9) and for clonus. Much of this can be tested by getting the child to walk normally, walk on their toes, walk on their heels, walk heel to toe (over 3 years), hop, jump, run, squat and rise, and climb steps for the lower limb examination. If a child can do all of these with no apparent difficulty, it is unlikely that you will find any abnormality on further testing.

Tone is assessed by moving the limb around the joint in an unpredictable manner. Coordination has already been assessed by walking heel to toe and climbing steps etc., but can be more formally assessed by the finger-to-nose and heel-along-the-shin manoeuvres. Sensation is assessed by means of a piece of cotton wool touched lightly on to the skin, working in a systematic order through the dermatomes (Fig. 5.3).

It would be unusual in the exam to have to proceed to assessing abnormalities of pain (spinothalamic tracts), vibration and proprioception (posterior columns). However, you should be proficient in these skills for your clinical practice.

A number of eponymous tests should also be carried out:

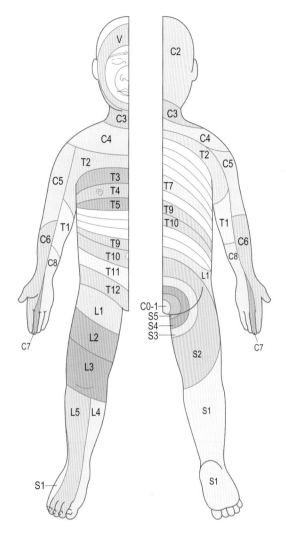

Fig. 5.3 Dermatome distribution

- *Gower's sign.* Lay the child supine and ask him or her to stand. A child with proximal muscle weakness will first turn prone and then 'walk up' the legs with the hands.
- *Trendelenburg's test.* Ask the child to stand on one leg. The pelvis should rise on the side of the elevated leg. If not, this indicates a problem between the femur and pelvis on the weight-bearing side.
- *Fogg's test.* Ask the child to walk on the outsides and then the insides of the feet and observe the associated arm and hand movements; a subtle hemiplegic arm may adopt the typical posture (flexion at the elbow and wrist).

Tremors and abnormal movement disorders

Abnormal limb movements can be confusing, but if described and interpreted correctly, can lead to precise localization of brain pathology.

Tremors

- *Essential tremor*: present only on initiation of movement and maintenance of posture. This is a common condition of adulthood that is inherited in an autosomal dominant fashion and can present in childhood. Other causes include thyrotoxicosis, phaeochromocytoma and Wilson's disease.
- *Intention tremor*: seen at the end of movements, due to cerebellar disease including Wilson's disease.
- *Static tremor*: seen at rest and disappears on movement. Occurs in Wilson's, Parkinson's and Huntington's disease.

Movement disorders

- *Myoclonus*: brief, sudden muscle contractions. Seen in seizure disorders, metabolic disorders, brain infections, brain injury and degenerative conditions.
- *Chorea*: random rapid movements, seen most commonly in cerebral palsy, Sydenham's chorea, Wilson's and Huntington's disease. Due to damage to the corpus striatum.
- *Athetosis*: slow writhing movements, seen in cerebral palsy and Wilson's disease. Due to damage to the putamen.
- *Dystonia*: sustained disturbed muscle contraction causing abnormal posturing. Seen with certain drugs (anticonvulsants), trauma, infections, and vascular, metabolic and degenerative pathologies.
- *Hemiballismus*: random gross proximal limb flailing due to contralateral subthalamic brain damage.
- *Tic*: spasmodic stereotypic involuntary repetitive movements, typically of the facial muscles. Gilles de la Tourette is an inherited form with associated vocal tics, obsessive–compulsive behaviour and attention deficit hyperactivity disorder (ADHD).

Cranial nerves (Table 5.10)

Although often feared as a station in the Membership exam, cranial nerve examination is straightforward in compliant, cooperative children. It is important to be clear about what you want of them. If necessary, demonstrate on yourself. For the younger child, improvisation is required, but with imaginative use of toys most cranial nerves can be assessed.

Visual acuity

With older children who can read or recognize pictures, ask them to hold a reading/picture book and to read

Table 5.10 Cranial nerve functions

Cranial nerve	Function
I Olfactory nerve	Smell
II Optic nerve	Visual acuity Visual fields Fundoscopy
III Oculomotor nerve	Efferent fibres to superior, inferior and medial recti, inferior oblique and levator palpebrae superioris muscles Parasympathetic supply to pupil
IV Trochlear nerve	Efferent fibres to superior oblique muscle
V Trigeminal nerve	Motor: muscles of mastication Sensory: to the face. Ophthalmic, maxillary and mandibular divisions. Corneal sensation
VI Abducens nerve	Efferent fibres to lateral rectus muscle
VII Facial nerve	Motor: muscles of facial expression Sensory: taste to anterior $2/3$ of tongue
VIII Vestibulocochlear nerve	Hearing, balance and posture
IX Glossopharyngeal nerve	Motor: stylopharyngeus muscle Sensory: tonsillar fossa and pharynx, taste to posterior $1/3$ of tongue
X Vagus nerve	Motor: pharynx and larynx Sensory: larynx
XI Accessory nerve	Trapezius and sternomastoid muscles
XII Hypoglossal nerve	Movements of the tongue

or point out small objects on the page. The distance they hold the book from their face will give you an indication as to whether they are hypermetropic or myopic. Whilst they are reading, cover one of their eyes and then the other to check for binocular vision. With the infant and toddler, get the child to fix and follow a light or small object and to pick a small object from your open palm. Formalized testing of visual acuity (e.g. using a Snellen chart or Stycar matching letters) should be done at 6 metres if requested.

Visual fields

In the older child, test as for adults by confrontation, moving a wiggling finger in from the peripheries and comparing against your own visual field. With younger children, try bringing objects like a brightly coloured ball on a string into view from behind, or ask when a toy starts to move. Test with both the child's eyes open and then individually if possible.

Pupillary reaction

Shine a torch at one eye twice and then the other twice, looking initially for a direct light reflex and then a consensual reflex.

Fundoscopy

This is probably best left to the end of the examination, certainly in the younger child. There are likely to be only limited conditions or abnormalities on fundoscopic examination, and familiarization with these by means of picture atlases or attendance at paediatric ophthalmology clinics is worth while. These conditions include coloboma, aniridia, false eye, cataract, optic atrophy, papilloedema and retinitis pigmentosa.

Eye movements (III, IV and VI)

It is important to ask children whether they have diplopia at any point during testing. Ask the child to follow an object or your finger through the letter 'H' manoeuvre, finishing off by bringing your finger or the object close towards the child's face to test accommodation. Look for nystagmus throughout testing. A third nerve palsy will give a unilateral ptosis, fixed dilated pupil and an eye that looks down and out. Fourth nerve palsies cause diplopia when looking down and in, causing particular difficulty with walking downstairs.

Fifth nerve

Ask the child to open and close the mouth without and then against resistance, move the jaw sideways against resistance, and clench the teeth to assess the muscles of mastication (masseters, pterygoids and temporalis). Complete the motor component of the nerve by trying to elicit a jaw jerk. Assess sensation using cotton wool on the face, testing all three branches of the nerve. The corneal reflex should not be tested in the exam setting, but mention it.

Seventh nerve

Test the muscles of facial expression by asking children to raise their eyebrows, screw their eyes up tight, blow their cheeks out and show you their teeth (or smile). Preservation of normal muscle movement in the upper face and forehead with a facial palsy is indicative of an upper motor neuron defect due to bilateral innervation. Taste testing is not undertaken routinely.

Eighth nerve

Ask about hearing difficulties in any child, and in the older infant (7–9 months) be prepared to perform a hearing distraction test. The Rinne and Weber tests are done to try to elucidate the nature of a hearing loss, i.e. conductive or sensorineural. For the Weber test, place the vibrating tuning fork on the child's forehead and ask in which ear it is heard loudest. For conductive hearing loss it is loudest in the affected ear, and for a sensorineural defect it is loudest in the normal ear. For the Rinne test, place a vibrating tuning fork close to the child's ear and then on the ipsilateral mastoid process. For conductive hearing loss, bone conduction is better than air conduction, but the opposite is true if hearing is normal.

Ninth to twelfth nerves

The ninth and tenth cranial nerves can be assessed together. Observe the child swallowing and talking, look inside the mouth, and ask the child to say 'aah' if old enough for you to look at palatal movement. The gag reflex has a sensory component (IX) and a motor component (X), but is not normally tested. The eleventh nerve is easily tested by asking the child to turn the head sideways and to shrug the shoulders against resistance. Finally, inspect the tongue both inside the mouth and on protrusion. The tongue will protrude to the side of weakness.

Eye and squint examination

This has largely been covered in the assessment of the cranial nerves. However, the eye examination is not complete without looking for the presence of a squint (strabismus).

There are five questions that need answering:

- Is there a squint or not?
- Is it convergent or divergent?
- Is it latent or manifest?
- Is it intermittent or permanent?
- Is it paralytic or not?

Start by direct observation of any obvious abnormality of the eye, size, shape, the cornea, sclera, iris or pupil. Hold a light source approximately 30 cm from the face and look for symmetry of the light source reflected from the pupils. Asymmetry would suggest a manifest squint that you will clarify by means of the cover/uncover test. Sit with your eyes at the same level as the child. Ensure that the child is looking at your face and cover one of his or her eyes with a hand or piece of card. If there is a manifest squint of the uncovered eye, there will be movement of that eye as it takes up fixation on your face (because the good eye is covered). When you uncover the good eye, it should take up fixation again unless the squint is alternating (i.e. involving both eyes). If there is no manifest squint, then cover one eye and look for movement of the eye as you uncover it. If there is movement, then there is a latent squint of this eye, induced by it losing fixation on your face when it is covered. Repeat the test on the other eye.

www.mrcophth.com/eyeclipartchua/clipart.html
Demonstration in animated format of the ocular nerve palsies and squints

Cerebellar function

27 Signs of cerebellar disease include truncal ataxia, dysarthric speech, horizontal nystagmus, intention tremor, dysdiadokinesia and dysmetria (inability to coordinate accurate movements, resulting in overshooting the mark). Introduce yourself to the child and encourage him or her to speak. Cerebellar disease may produce stuttering dysarthria. Have the child walk in a straight line, heel to toe if old enough. A child with a unilateral cerebellar lesion may stumble towards the side of the lesion. Undertake the finger–nose test. You will detect an intention tremor and past-pointing with disease. Test for dysdiadokinesia but bear in mind that young children without pathology find this manoeuvre difficult. Finally, ask the child to perform the heel-to-shin manoeuvre.

Examination of the joints

28 Expose the joints proximal and distal to any affected joint(s), together with the corresponding contralateral joint for comparison. Inspect the joints for symmetry, swelling, deformity, scarring, erythema and wasting of adjacent musculature.

Ask about joint pain before palpating the affected joint for alteration in skin temperature, tenderness, swelling or synovial thickening. Movement in the first instance should be active, putting the joint through the full range of anticipated movement. Only if there is limitation should you go on to passive movement, but do not hurt the child unnecessarily. Measure limb circumference at the same place on both limbs for objective assessment of muscle mass. Finally, assess function by asking the child to undertake everyday actions. For example, if assessing hand function, ask the child to shake hands with you, hold a knife and fork, write his or her name, and touch the thumb to each finger pad of the same hand.

Examination of the skin

Examine the skin every time you review a child. This should be straightforward because it is simply a description of what you see. However, the plethora of terms and descriptions can be confusing. The more common ones are listed in Table 5.11 (see also Ch. 36).

Where modesty and environment allow, examine all the skin, and the hair, nails and mucous membranes

Table 5.11 Terms used to describe skin lesions

Term	Description
Macule	Area of discoloration or textural change, any size, not raised, e.g. vitiligo, freckle
Papule	Small (< 5 mm), solid, raised lesion, e.g. lichen planus, xanthoma
Nodule	Large (> 5 mm), raised lesion, e.g. dermatofibroma
Petechiae	Haemorrhage in the skin (< 2 mm), non-blanching
Purpura	Haemorrhage in the skin (2–10 mm), non-blanching
Ecchymosis	Large bruise, non-blanching
Vesicle	Small blister (< 5 mm), elevated, fluid-filled
Bulla	Large blister (> 5 mm), elevated, fluid-filled
Wheal	Transient, compressible papule or plaque due to dermal oedema
Pustule	Elevated blister, pus-filled
Lichenification	Thickened skin, accentuated skin creases

in good natural light. Describe the site, distribution, appearance, size and texture of the rash or lesions identified.

Site and distribution

- Localized or widespread
- Symmetrical or asymmetrical
- Centripetal or centrifugal distribution
- Area of the body: limbs, trunk, scalp, palms and soles
- Pattern: flexures, extensor surfaces, sun-exposed areas, nappy area.

Appearance

- Pattern of lesions: linear, grouped, annular or demonstrating the Koebner phenomenon
- Monomorphic (all lesions of similar appearance) or pleomorphic, e.g. chickenpox
- Colour
- Size
- Shape: regular or irregular, discoid, linear
- Characteristics: macular, papular, vesicular etc.
- Borders: clear or ill-defined, any surrounding changes.

Texture

29
30
- Macular or raised lesion
- Blanching or not
- ?Nikolsky sign: separation of layers of the epidermis on slight shear pressure.

Hair

Again, description is all that is necessary and a number of terms can be used:

- Hypertrichosis: excessive hair growth in a non-androgenic pattern
- Hirsute: excessive male-pattern hair growth
- Alopecia: absence of hair:
  - Alopecia areata/totalis/universalis
  - Telogen effluvium (diffuse hair loss: for example, after illness)
  - Trichotillomania (due to the child pulling at the hair)
  - Infection, e.g. ringworm.

Describe the site, distribution (localized or diffuse) and appearance of hair changes, and comment on the scalp.

Nails

Check fingernails and toenails for:

- Pitting: psoriasis, eczema, lichen planus
- Leuconychia: hypoalbuminaemia
- Koilonychia: iron deficiency
- Thickened, discolored nails: fungal infection
- Clubbing
- Beau's lines: transverse lines/grooves due to temporary arrest in growth associated with severe systemic illness.

Mucous membranes

Describe any changes you see, which may include ulceration, inflammation and pigmentation.

On completion of a full skin examination, it may be necessary to go on to the examination of other organ systems, depending upon clinical symptoms and signs.

N.B. Areas of skin depigmentation may only be visualized under ultraviolet light using the Woods lamp.

Examination of the neck

31 Thyroid disease is uncommon in children but the examination of a child's neck is commonly requested in paediatric exams. Typically there may be nothing to find, apart from some shotty cervical lymphadenopathy of little consequence (Fig. 5.4).

Goitre

32 With hyper- or hypothyroidism there will typically be evidence of disease beyond the examination of the neck. Shake the child by the hand, looking for

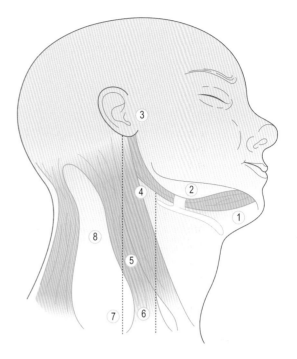

Fig. 5.4 Anatomy of the cervical lymph nodes.
(1) Submental; (2) submandibular; (3) parotid; (4) upper cervical, above the level of the hyoid bone and along the internal jugular chain; (5) middle cervical, between the level of the hyoid bone and cricoid cartilage, and along the internal jugular chain; (6) lower cervical, below the level of the cricoid cartilage and along the internal jugular chain; (7) supraclavicular fossa; (8) posterior triangle (also known as the accessory chain).

evidence of a tremor and feeling for skin temperature (hypothyroidism — cool, hyperthyroidism — warm). Ask the child's name to assess voice quality (deep, hoarse voice — hypothyroidism) and address to assess mental sluggishness. Inspect from the front, looking for eye disease, facial coarsening, hair thinning/thickening, previous surgery and goitre. Describe any swelling in terms of symmetry, size, shape, and whether there are overlying skin changes. Ask the child to take a drink to ensure that the thyroid gland moves with swallowing. Move around to the back of the sitting child to palpate the thyroid gland, making a point of looking down on the child from above to assess whether exophthalmos exists. Palpate the thyroid gland gently, as it can be tender if inflamed. Come back around the front to feel for tracheal deviation and percuss over the manubrium for dullness, both of which signify retrosternal extension of the goitre. Auscultate over the thyroid gland for the presence of a bruit.

Pubertal assessment (Figs 5.5 and 5.6)

This is part of the normal examination, but be sensitive and respect modesty. It is important to recognize pre-

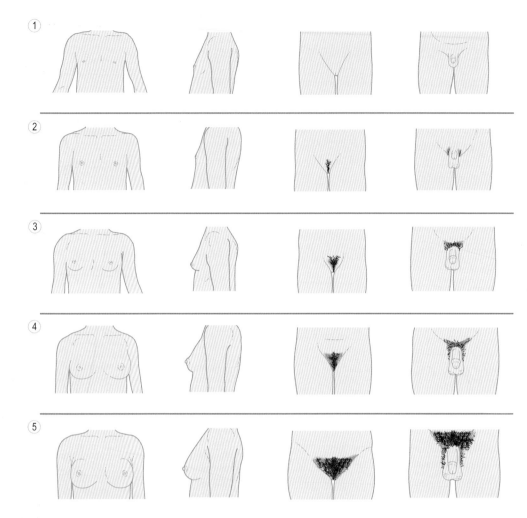

Fig. 5.5 Tanner stages of puberty

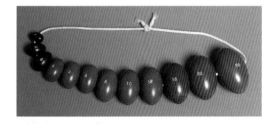

Fig. 5.6 Orchidometer

cocious puberty, which is the onset of pubertal changes before 8 years in girls and 9 years in boys.

Testicular size is measured with an orchidometer, and varies from 2 ml (prepubertal) to an average adult testicular volume of 15 ml.

Examination of the ear, nose and throat

Examination of the ears and throat, and to a lesser extent the nose, is a standard part of the assessment of every child. In the older child, it is straightforward. For the infant and toddler, leave it until last because, to ensure adequate and safe assessment, the child needs to be held tightly on a parent's lap, and he or she may object to this. Correct positioning is key (Fig. 5.7). Gently pull the pinna backwards and upwards to straighten the external auditory canal and visualize the tympanic membrane. Brace with fingers against the cheek. For the mouth, turn the child to face you and gently depress the tongue, with a tongue depressor if required, to visualize the pharynx, taking note of the dentition, gums and buccal mucosa.

Do not examine the throat of a child with signs of significant respiratory obstruction, as this may precipitate complete obstruction.

Dysmorphology (Fig. 5.8)

It is difficult to learn this from a textbook. Avoid the pitfall of stating that a child is dysmorphic when in fact the child simply looks like other family members

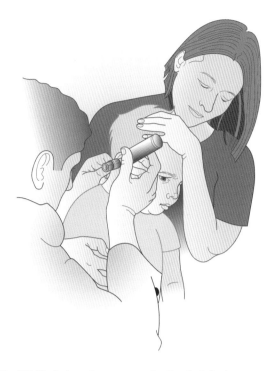

Fig. 5.7 Technique for ear examination in infants

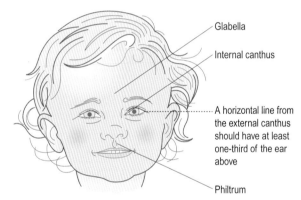

Glabella

Internal canthus

A horizontal line from the external canthus should have at least one-third of the ear above

Philtrum

Fig. 5.8 A normal face

who are all normal! Examine the whole child, and avoid 'spot' diagnoses based only on the face.

Whilst asking some questions, such as name, address and school (to assess developmental progress), look at stature and body proportions. Measure height and lower segment length (pubic symphysis to the floor) to calculate the upper segment to lower segment ratio. Measure weight, head circumference and arm span. The latter should approximately equal height (± 4 cm). Look for limb asymmetry, limb shortening, and hand and digit abnormalities. Ask the child to make a fist to see if there is a short fourth metacarpal (pseudohypoparathyroidism) or if the thumb can extend beyond the ulnar border

of the hand (Marfan's syndrome). Look at the trunk for evidence of skin abnormalities (ash leaf macules, neurofibromas, café au lait spots) and kyphoscoliosis. Briefly assess pubertal status. Now it is useful to move on to the head and face, by which time the possibilities for diagnosis will have been honed considerably.

Measure head circumference and assess the shape of head and face (triangular in Russell–Silver syndrome, frontal bossing in achondroplasia, mid-facial crowding in Down's syndrome). Describe the features of the hair, eyes, nose, mouth, palate, ears, teeth and chin. A number of terms are used in dysmorphology and ease the description of abnormality:

- Hypertelorism: distance between the internal canthi > length of the eye
- Slant of the palpebral fissures:
  - Normal: horizontal or upward-slanting with an angle < 10°
  - Upward-slanting: angle > 10°
  - Downward-slanting: external canthus lower than the internal canthus
- Synophyrs: meeting of the eyebrows in the midline.

It may not be possible by the end of the examination to give a certain diagnosis. However, provided the dysmorphic features have been described correctly, they can be entered into an electronic database to obtain a differential diagnosis.

Summary

The breadth and depth of the physical examination of children is entirely dependent upon the clinical situation and the willingness of the child. For the general practitioner or senior house officer/foundation doctor in paediatrics who is seeing a hot, fractious child with a likely upper respiratory tract infection, a brief but thorough 'top-to-toe' examination, including in particular the lungs, skin, ears, nose and throat, together with a measure of the body temperature and hydration status, may be all that is required. Provided you are dealing with a compliant child, this may take no more than 3–5 minutes. Clearly, any untoward finding or sign that does not fit with the likely diagnosis warrants further, more detailed examination. Because the examination can never be entirely thorough in an uncooperative child, the full examination may have to be undertaken at a different time, should the situation allow this. However, as long as the limited extent of the examination is made clear in the notes, this is acceptable. The chance of a failed or incomplete examination will be minimized by following the principles set out in this chapter.

Ragbir Thethy

Diagnosis and management

LEARNING OUTCOMES

By the end of this chapter you should:
- Understand an approach to differential diagnosis
- Know how to select and interpret diagnostic tests
- Be able to draw up a management plan
- Understand the importance of family involvement
- Understand psychosocial factors.

Introduction

Reaching a diagnosis is what, as doctors, we all aim for, so that the appropriate treatment can be instituted. The process is not as easy as it first seems, especially for those starting out in paediatrics. This chapter aims to show you the different steps that are required to achieve a differential diagnosis, then a definitive diagnosis, and then an approach to management.

A child does not come into clinic or accident and emergency department with a label or letter saying, 'I have …. Please give me the following treatment….' Rather, by using a number of processes, the differential diagnosis is arrived at, followed by the final diagnosis.

The process involves the use of:
- A good history and examination
- Reaching a diagnosis or differential diagnosis
- Investigations
- Management planning.

All of these are interlinked (Fig. 6.1).

History and examination

The ability to take a good history and conduct a thorough examination is the cornerstone of being a good doctor. These aspects have been discussed earlier (Ch. 5). Once the history has been obtained, 90% of the diagnosis should have been reached, so findings on examination should not come as a surprise. The ability to take a good history is dependent on the doctor being able to communicate with the parent/carer and the child. Use an interpreter if necessary. Your examination findings are crucial to confirming your thoughts as to what may be wrong with your patient.

Reaching a diagnosis or differential diagnosis

Putting your findings from the history and examination together into a differential diagnosis depends on your

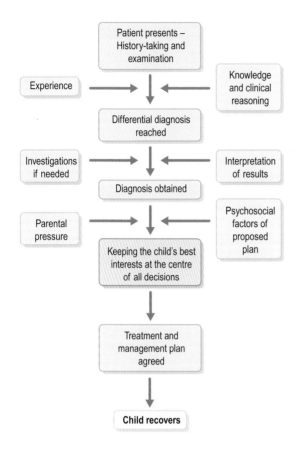

Fig. 6.1 Diagnosis and management

Flow chart contents:

Patient presents – History-taking and examination

Experience → Differential diagnosis reached ← Knowledge and clinical reasoning

Investigations if needed → Diagnosis obtained ← Interpretation of results

Parental pressure → Keeping the child's best interests at the centre of all decisions ← Psychosocial factors of proposed plan

Treatment and management plan agreed

Child recovers

---

knowledge base, clinical reasoning skills and use of other sources of help. These enable you to make sense of the clinical information and to formulate a diagnosis or differential diagnosis that then guides further investigation and management.

Knowledge and pattern recognition

Knowledge will stem from the training you received at medical school, tutorials, reading and experience. In fact, the majority of your knowledge will be from the patients you have seen; it is, in essence, pattern recognition. Obviously, at the beginning of your career, the number patients you have seen will be small, and therefore your 'data bank' will not be extensive and your knowledge will mainly be that obtained from bookwork and teaching sessions. However, as you progress and see more patients, then your 'personal knowledge bank' will increase, and there will be more and more pattern recognition. This is how your consultant may impress you by arriving at a diagnosis on just hearing the history. It is because he or she has seen patients with a similar condition before. The experienced clinician may be more concerned to rule out rarer causes of common presentations based on

small variations from the usual pattern. For example, a senior house officer might see a child with a stiff neck and might diagnose the child as having a muscle strain causing torticollis. However, the consultant might want further investigations for other causes such as a malignant tumour. To increase your knowledge, follow up each patient you see with reading to reinforce what you have learnt.

Tutorials, ward rounds, teaching sessions and bedside teaching all aim to increase your knowledge base. Then, when you meet a patient with the same or a similar constellation of symptoms, you will be able to recognize the pattern and make a reasonable stab at a diagnosis. Pattern recognition through experience is essential to becoming a good doctor.

Clinical reasoning

To complement your knowledge base, you need sound clinical reasoning skills. When the clinical information does not fit a pattern you recognize, or contains puzzling elements, you need to go back to first principles and consider what clinical and pathological processes might be involved. This is why an understanding of the basic science behind symptoms, signs and disease processes is emphasized in professional exams, and also in this course. A helpful starting point is to list all the major categories of pathological processes (sometimes called the 'surgical sieve'), and for each in turn consider whether there is any way it could explain some or all of the symptoms and signs. Look for the best clinical 'handles' — features that will best enable you to get to grips with what is going on. Symptoms and signs that are *generally unusual* in the patients that you see are most likely to help you.

Once you have your list of differential diagnoses, you need to add your best estimates of the prevalence of the various conditions you think of. 'Common things are common', and so odd presentations are more likely to be unusual manifestations of a common disease than a rare one. Finally, bear in mind the 'rule of parsimony', by which you seek the fewest number of diagnoses (a single one, if possible) to explain all the clinical features. If you have to invoke multiple unrelated pathologies all occurring coincidentally to explain the patient's illness, beware! You are probably missing something. Look hard for a unifying diagnosis. Once you have been through this process, write down your list of differential diagnoses in order of likelihood, briefly citing the key features that support each one. This discipline helps to clarify your thoughts, and if noted in the clinical record, allows others to follow your reasoning easily with regard to further investigation and management.

Other sources of help in diagnosis

Books and journals

Do not be too embarrassed to look things up — you are not expected to know everything! Ideally, the clinical areas that you work in should provide access to a reasonable range of up-to-date texts and journals, along with Internet access to Medline or an equivalent and to electronic journals. Pubmed is a free service provided by the US National Library of Medicine, which provides access to Medline and links to full-text articles. Read the clinical descriptions of conditions on your differential list with which you are less familiar.

www.ncbi.nlm.nih.gov/
Pubmed

Colleagues

Discussion of interesting and puzzling cases with colleagues is an excellent way to broaden your knowledge, improve your diagnostic skills and help you make difficult diagnoses. Do this informally on the wards and in clinics, as well as more formally at clinical meetings. Discussion groups and forums on the Internet are another way of doing this, but take care to follow General Medical Council guidance on confidentiality, avoid using information that is identifiable to a patient, and only participate in groups run by trustworthy professional organizations. Paediatric forums are available at www.doctors.net.uk, and the RCPCH has its own discussion list.

www.doctors.net.uk

Computer-based diagnostic aids

A number of computer-based systems have been developed to assist in diagnosis. These are likely to become more widely available and more sophisticated, and you should check whether there are any in your local area. Some hospital trusts subscribe to 'Isabel', which suggests a checklist of likely diagnoses based on clinical features and age. There are some excellent, though costly, dysmorphology databases (e.g. the London Medical Databases) that can assist in the diagnosis of syndromes.

www.isabelhealthcare.com
Isabel

ww.lmdatabases.com
London Medical Databases

| BOX 6.1 | Test characteristics |

- *Sensitivity* is the proportion of patients with confirmed disease who have a positive test result
- *Specificity* is the proportion of patients without the disease who have a negative test result
- *Accuracy* is the percentage of tests that correctly identify the presence or absence of disease
- *Positive predictive value* is the probability that a patient with a positive test result actually has the disease
- *Negative predictive value* is the probability that a patient with a negative test result does not have the disease.
- *Likelihood ratio* is a good measure of a test's usefulness, and in effect combines sensitivity and specificity. The *pre-test probability* is the chance that the person has the disease before the test is done, and this will partly depend on prevalence of the disease in your population, and partly on your clinical findings. The likelihood ratio tells you how likely the test is to alter this probability significantly: for example, by making the diagnosis nearly certain or extremely unlikely. When a test's likelihood ratio is 1, this means it will not alter the pre-test probability at all, and therefore means the test is not clinically useful. High likelihood ratios (e.g. above 10) and low likelihood ratios (e.g. below 0.1) usually indicate clinically useful tests. To calculate the likelihood ratio, the true positive rate (i.e. the proportion of patients with the disease who have a positive test) is divided by the false positive rate (i.e. the proportion of patients without the disease who have a positive test)

Investigation

Deciding whether to use a test

Use an evidence-based approach wherever possible (Box 6.1 and see also Ch. 13). Consider the questions below before ordering any test.

Is the test any good?

For the particular question you are asking (e.g. does the patient have disease X?), what are the characteristics of the test (Box 6.1)? It helps to have an idea of the prevalence of the condition you are considering in the population you see, since this influences how well a test performs. In general, the rarer the condition, the worse a test will perform.

Will the test help to make (or rule out) a diagnosis?

Consider how sure you are of the diagnosis, based on the information you already have from the history, examination and other investigations. This is the pre-test probability. If you are already very sure, there may be little point doing the test, particularly if its likelihood ratio is near 1. If you do not know the likelihood ratio, think in these terms: 'If I get a very strongly positive result, how much surer will I be that this patient has the disease or not?' Similarly, what will be the effect of a negative result, or one that is somewhere in the middle? If a test is quite likely to make a difference to how sure you are, then it is likely to be worth doing, provided it is not too costly (see below).

Will the result of this test change the patient's treatment or management?

If you really think that the test result is unlikely to change the patient's treatment or management, you should think twice about doing the test. The patients and parents may benefit from simply knowing what the diagnosis is, and of course this can be a significant benefit in its own right, but appropriate explanation of the possibilities may be all that is needed.

Is there any contraindication to doing the test?

Some tests are contraindicated in certain situations. For example, lumbar puncture should not be performed when a child has suspected raised intracranial pressure or fluctuating consciousness level.

How costly is the test?

This includes cost to the patient and parents, in terms of distress, inconvenience and transport; cost to the medical team, in terms of time taken to arrange and perform the test; and cost of materials and processing. If it is costly in any of these ways, then think twice before doing it and carefully consider any alternatives.

 www.cebm.net/likelihood_ratios.asp
Oxford Centre for Evidence Based Medicine site, giving more information and examples

'Might-as-well' testing

When you have success with a technically difficult venepuncture, there is a temptation to send off extra tests because you feel you 'might as well' while you are in the vein. You reason that you will spare the child further distress, because you are less likely to have to come back and do further blood tests. *This is not good practice.* For many tests, you are more likely to get false negative results if you do them without clinical indication, since the prevalence of the condition being tested for will be lower and so the test performs less well. If the upper and lower boundaries of normal are placed at +2 and −2 standard deviations from the mean, as is common practice, then for a normal distribution this will encompass only 95% of tests. Thus, if you do 100 tests in healthy individuals, on average you can expect 5 to be abnormal. You have not helped the child if you have to repeat a test that was not indicated in the first place.

Key investigations

Some common investigations are reviewed here. See later in this module (Ch. 12) for further information on practical procedures and investigations.

X-rays

The main risk is increased exposure to radiation. The radiation dose from a chest X-ray is about the same as the average person receives from background radiation in 10 days. An abdominal X-ray is equivalent in radiation dose to 75 chest X-rays. If you request an X-ray, then you also need to be able to read and interpret its significance, at least acutely. Take advantage of every opportunity to review X-rays with radiologists, in review meetings or informally, in order to improve your skills. A chest X-ray may show up an infection that is otherwise undetectable apart from an increase in respiratory rate, particularly in young children.

Blood tests

Some of the basic tests are listed here.

Blood culture

This is the gold standard for diagnosing a bacteraemia and should be taken prior to any antibiotic therapy. The result of this investigation will influence your choice of antibiotic.

Full blood count (FBC)

In acute paediatrics, an increased white cell count usually indicates infection. An increase in lymphocytes suggests viral infection, while a neutrophilia points towards a bacterial cause. The white cell count is also raised in times of stress, e.g. after a convulsion.

Low haemoglobin indicates anaemia. The red cell size (mean cell volume, MCV) and the mean haemoglobin concentration (MCH) will give an indication as to the cause of the anaemia. If these are low (i.e. microcytosis and hypochromia, respectively), this suggests iron deficiency (or more rarely, β-thalassaemia trait). A macrocytosis is seen in vitamin B_{12} and folate deficiency.

If the haemoglobin, white cell count and platelet counts are low, this indicates a pancytopenia and implies bone marrow failure, e.g. due to leukaemia.

Urea and electrolytes (U&Es) and creatinine

These are useful in cases of dehydration, the urea and creatinine rising with increasing levels. The creatinine also gives an indication of renal function. Derangements of sodium and potassium may give diagnostic clues, and if significant, may need urgent action.

C-reactive protein (CRP)

This is a non-specific indicator of inflammation. The higher the value, the more likely that the patient is suffering from a significant illness. Remember that there is a lag of about 12 hours before the CRP starts to rise, so do not be reassured by a normal CRP if the duration of illness is less than this. In acutely febrile children, a CRP of above 80 mg/l is reasonably specific and sensitive for bacterial sepsis.

Blood glucose

A blood glucose level under 2.6 mmol/l indicates hypoglycaemia and needs immediate treatment and further investigation to establish the cause. If determined by 'BM stix', then ensure that a true laboratory glucose measurement is taken to confirm this; consider saving and freezing plasma for later metabolic testing if the hypoglycaemia is confirmed. It can be much harder to make a diagnosis if this opportunity is lost. The causes of hypoglycaemia are discussed in Chapter 35.

Lumbar puncture (LP)

This is required in all children under 3 months old who attend with pyrexia of over 38°C; it should also be considered in any infant in whom there is a fever with no focus (Ch. 44). Know the contraindications to lumbar puncture (p. 118). Cerebrospinal fluid (CSF) is sent for:

- *Microscopy and culture*. The white cell count will give an indication of meningitis/encephalitis (normal polymorph count $< 1 \times mm^3$).
- *Gram staining*. If anything is seen on Gram staining, then the child definitely has a bacterial infection and will need intravenous medication. It will also give an idea as to what the organism is.
- *Biochemistry and protein*. An elevated protein content (> 1000 mg/l) indicates a bacterial

infection. A protein content between 400 and 1000 mg/l is usually associated with viral meningitis, as long as the CSF glucose is normal.
- *Glucose testing*. The level is normally the same as the serum glucose, or at least two-thirds of it. A level much lower than this is associated with a bacterial infection. Do not forget to send a blood sample at the same time as the LP to check this.

Urine

A urine sample is often helpful.

Urinary tract infection (UTI)

This can present in a child who is non-specifically unwell, or with symptoms such as diarrhoea and vomiting, or just a temperature. A clean-catch urine is ideal. A normal dipstick test for protein, blood, leucocytes and nitrites will effectively rule out infection, but if any of these is positive or there is high index of suspicion, urine should be sent for microscopy, culture and sensitivity. An increased number of white cells might be an indication that the child has a urinary tract infection. Culture will confirm this and is the gold standard. Antibiotics can then be rationalized, according to reported sensitivities. A urinary tract infection is diagnosed if there is a pure growth of $> 10^5$ organisms/ml in the presence of pyuria (> 50 white cells per high-power field). Mixed growth, lack of pyuria, or lower numbers of organisms may all indicate a contaminated sample, and a repeat should be arranged.

Metabolic defect

Obtaining the first-passed urine in children with a low blood sugar is mandatory. The urine sample is used to rule out or diagnose metabolic defects (see also Ch. 34). If, as is often the case, the child is admitted or only passes this first urine out of hours, then the urine can be frozen until the next working day. Urine testing for metabolic screening should be considered in any acutely ill child.

Other tests

These will depend on the previous results obtained and the underlying problem.

Management

Once you have reached a diagnosis or differential diagnosis, you need to devise a plan of action. This plan may well be discharge but, even then, you have to take into account whether it is safe for the child to go home. Is the child safe from the illness, and indeed from the carer if there are child protection concerns?

Problem lists

Use of a problem list is a helpful way of ensuring that you address all the issues, particularly in more complex cases, and indeed in clinical examinations! Succinctly list all of the child's problems and then, for each, outline how you plan to deal with it, either through further investigation, initiation of treatment, reassurance or explanation, or referral to other services. Do not forget to find out how each is impacting on the child and family, and ascertain which they see as most important. If your view of what is most important is different, you will need to take time to discuss why, but it is important that you address the family's main concerns.

Management plan

Whatever the decision as to where the child is to be looked after, consider the following:

- Are any investigations required? If so, which ones and why?
- Does the child need any medications? If so, which ones?
- How will the medication be given? Oral, intravenous, per rectum?

For illnesses that follow a predictable course, a management plan can be applied that is specific for that disease. For example, for bronchiolitis, the following criteria could be assessed:

- O_2 saturations > 92%?
- Feeding OK?
- Little respiratory distress?
- Old enough to cope?
- No other coexisting morbidity?

If the answer to these questions is 'yes', then the child can probably be discharged home with the carer. However, there may be other factors specific to the patient that mean it is not appropriate for him or her to go home, e.g. anxious parents, prematurity etc. Therefore, each management plan needs to be adapted to the individual patient. 'One size does not fit all.'

To be able to implement a treatment package, parents must be on board and should be kept informed of their child's condition from the beginning. To obtain this level of parental cooperation, you need excellent communication skills (Ch. 7). In the majority of cases, parents care about their child and are extremely worried. They want to know what is wrong. You need to allay unnecessary fears and understand the parents' expectations. Then you should explain the investigation and management steps clearly and empathetically, including the reasons they are being taken and what they will involve. Conversely, when no test or treatment is required, explaining this to parents can be hard if they have come along with an expectation that their child needs some form of treatment. For example, a child may have a pyrexia and the carer seeks medical attention. The child is found to have an inflamed tympanic membrane. The carer is informed of this diagnosis. As the child has an infection, the carer expects antibiotics to be prescribed. However, the recognized treatment for otitis media is pain relief and temperature control with paracetamol and ibuprofen. The doctor has to explain that the infection is usually caused by a virus, how best to treat it, and the fact that antibiotics are not required since any benefits are outweighed by risk of side-effects. This conversation must be conducted with diplomacy and tact but also, most importantly, with empathy.

Such conversations with parents and children need to be conducted in a language that they are fluent in, via an interpreter if necessary. Lord Lamming's review into the death of Victoria Climbié recommended that a sick child must not act as a translator between parents and doctor. An interpreter should be an independent person skilled in translating medical terms, who the carer trusts, and who appreciates the need for confidentiality. If an interpreter is not available within the hospital setting, then one can be obtained via telephone translator services. These services are available 24 hours a day and are usually able to put you through within minutes to someone, somewhere, who speaks the same language as the carers. This is particularly useful in areas where a large number of languages is spoken, e.g. in parts of London where there are reported to be over 100 different languages and dialects. Check local arrangements each time you start a new job.

Psychosocial factors

Being ill is an unpleasant experience for anyone but for a child it is particularly distressing. Children are unable to articulate their feelings and worries. There are strangers talking to their carers, who may themselves seem anxious, upset and disempowered. The child has to undergo a range of experiences that vary from the strange to the embarrassing and the downright unpleasant. Children have little say in what does or does not happen to them. The process of history-taking, examination and investigation can be a frightening experience for the child, if performed without sensitivity to the child's needs and feelings. Each investigation or procedure involves further psychological stress. Consider carefully whether each one is necessary.

Admitting a child on to a hospital ward is a decision that must not be taken lightly. It must be a last resort, in view of the inherent risks and problems with admission, which include hospital-acquired infections. The majority of patients on general paediatric wards have infectious

BOX 6.2 Summary of diagnosis and management: an example

In a clinical examination, you have 13 minutes to take a history. You are given the GP letter to read, which is brief:

> *Please could you see William, who is 6 years old and wets the bed most nights? Past drug history: lactulose. Thank you for seeing him, Yours etc....*

You are to take a history from William's mother. You know you will be given a warning at 9 minutes that you have 4 minutes to go, and you plan to use at least 2 minutes at the end to prepare your problem list and management plan.

Phase 1: Take the history

Follow the ABCD approach outlined in Chapter 5, taking time for introductions. Find out what the problems are, using open and then closed questions to clarify. Make sure that you know which are most important to William and his family and why, as well as their impact on him and the family. Find out about any treatment already tried, the child's response to it, and what he and his parents thought of it. Complete the rest of the history in a logical focused manner. Be empathetic and avoid rushing. You have nearly completed this stage when you are given your 4-minute warning.

Phase 2: Checking and closing

If you have not already done so, summarize the key points back to William's mother to make sure that you have understood correctly. Explain that you are going to spend a short time thinking things through, but you may want to ask a few more questions.

Phase 3: Diagnosis or differential diagnosis, problem list and management plan

Spend the next few minutes writing a brief summary and then listing the problems in approximate order of priority, including key points relating to each, and your main diagnoses (and differentials where relevant). At this stage, you may wish to ask William's mother a few more questions that come to mind as you 'process' the history in this way.

Summary

William is a 6-year-old boy whose main problem is daytime wetting; this occurs randomly through the day, including when he is at school but especially when he is engrossed in activities. The wetting is accompanied by mild urgency and frequency. He also has primary nocturnal enuresis, and there is a background of mild but longstanding constipation.

Problem list

Problem	Comment
1. Daytime wetting with mild detrusor instability Differential: emotional upset, UTI	Although not mentioned in the GP's letter, this is the biggest problem for both William and his parents. There is very mild urgency and frequency. Wetting tends to happen when he is engrossed in activity. He has not had any UTIs or any treatment. There are no particular triggers such as bullying; he is happy at school
2. Functional primary nocturnal enuresis	There is a strong family history. The parents are taking a low-key approach and the problem does not trouble William much at the moment. He wears pull-ups at night. He has occasional dry nights (approximately once per week). He has had no treatment. He has never been reliably dry
3. Mild constipation	Although mild at present, it has been more significant in the past. It started 2 years ago. His mother gives him some lactulose once a week or so. His diet lacks fibre and fluid

Management plan

Problem	Investigation and management
1. Daytime wetting with mild detrusor instability	Dipstick urine to rule out infection and glycosuria
	Daytime reminder alarm set to go off every 90 minutes at first with a star chart. See William again soon (2–3 weeks)
	General behavioural advice about avoiding punishment and rewarding desired behaviour
	Consider a trial of oxybutinin later, but this is unlikely to be necessary

BOX 6.2 Summary of diagnosis and management: an example (*cont'd*)

Management plan

Problem	Investigation and management
2. Functional primary nocturnal enuresis	Dipstick urine (as above)
	General advice and reassurance
	No other action for now since it is better to focus on either the daytime or the night-time wetting, and it is the daytime that is the priority for the family
	Return to this later once the daytime wetting has resolved; consider starting a chart or possibly an enuresis alarm once he is 7 years old
3. Mild constipation	General advice to improve dietary fibre and increase fluid intake
	Start a small regular dose of lactulose 2.5–5 ml b.d., since it is important to avoid constipation while working on the daytime wetting

This approach helps you generate a clear and useful summary of the problems and a logical management plan. Note that a pitfall in this case would be to focus on the nocturnal enuresis while ignoring (or relegating to low priority) the daytime wetting, since this is not mentioned by the GP. There are, of course, a number of ways in which William's problems could be addressed. The examiners are looking for a sensible and logical approach that takes all the key problems into account. Candidates who do not allow themselves any time to organize their thoughts prior to presenting to examiners are unlikely to do well.

illnesses, e.g. viral gastroenteritis, viral upper respiratory tract infections and impetigo. Most hospitals have had to close wards to admissions to control infectious outbreaks such as norovirus (Norwalk) gastroenteritis. Infection control is hard enough on adult wards but can be even more challenging on paediatric wards, where children are more likely to ignore restrictions. Those in isolation soon become bored and lonely, wishing to leave the cubicle and mix with other children on the ward. Then there are also psychosocial factors for the child and the family. Being admitted to hospital can be a traumatic time for child, parents and siblings.

For the child

The hospital stay can be an episode of separation for the child and for the parent who cannot stay with him or her. It was only as recently as the 1950s and 1960s that attitudes to the admission of children changed and the importance of parental presence and involvement was appreciated. Seminal films by the Robertsons played an important role, documenting the adverse impact of separation from parents on children. These remain highly recommended viewing for anyone embarking on a paediatric career (for example, *Laura goes to Hospital*). Children are seen to go through phases of protest, despair and denial during hospitalization and, on their return home, they exhibit greater behavioural problems.

For the family

Not only is it traumatic for the child when he or she is admitted to hospital, but it can also be a traumatic and stressful time for the family. Parents often feel anxiety, fear and self-blame. A parent is expected to stay with the child during his or her stay in the hospital. This can add to the burden on parents. They have to arrange care for any other children they may have, which can be particularly difficult for single-parent families. They often have to sleep in suboptimal conditions (at best, they can expect a Z-bed next to their child; at worst, a chair next to the bed). Facilities for washing may be limited, and parent rooms are not always provided. Even when these are available, many parents choose not to stay overnight with their child or are unable to do so. In 1959, the Platt report advocated greater parental participation within hospital. In 1991, the Department of Health adopted this as official policy. Parental involvement in a child's hospital care carries a cost. This is partly financial — travelling, subsistence and loss of earnings — but it is also social, in arranging care for siblings. It leads to a loss of privacy and autonomy in family relationships. There is also the personal distress parents suffer from witnessing their child or other children in pain.

Summary

Box 6.2 summarizes the process of diagnosis and management.

Making a diagnosis, then deciding what investigations to conduct and what treatment to institute, are not as clear-cut as they may first seem. After obtaining a good history and conducting an appropriate examination, you need to combine the results of these with the knowledge you have obtained from books, tutorials and experience and with your clinical reasoning skills, in order to arrive at a differential diagnosis. After the patient has been subjected to the appropriate investigations (if needed), these are analysed and a diagnosis is obtained. From these results a treatment and management plan, tailored to the needs of the patient and carer, is established. To arrive at this final point, a good rapport must be developed between doctor, parents and child. Parents and child must be kept fully informed in a language they can understand, which may well require the use of an interpreter. Throughout this whole process, both carer and child must be 'on board' with the treatment and management plan instituted.

Richard Hain   John Hain

Communication skills

7

LEARNING OBJECTIVES

By the end of this chapter you should:

● Understand how to communicate with families, particularly with respect to breaking bad news

● Be able to review best practice in communicating with colleagues, including the writing of GP letters.

Communication with patients and families

The medical care of children is perhaps unique in the extent to which it relies on collaboration with the family. When considering a treatment plan for children, paediatricians take it for granted that the child's parents will always be available to the child, that they will usually have the child's best interests at heart, and that they will be able to work alongside medical and nursing staff. In effect, parents are expected to be colleagues with the paediatric team.

If this collegiate relationship is going to work safely and effectively, it is essential that families feel both confident and competent. It is the aim of communication with patients and their families to facilitate this, both by imparting information and by encouraging confidence. In many conditions, particularly those that persist for many years, families will come to see themselves as experts not only in their individual child, but also their child's condition. At the time of diagnosis, however, it is important to be able to impart not only facts, but also an understanding of them, in an effective manner.

Factors that can make this more difficult include prior understandings (and misunderstandings), emotional coping mechanisms such as denial, and simple differences in the way information is given and received, such as

vocabulary. It can be complicated by difficulty in remembering information. Devices for helping memory, such as audio recordings, diagrams or hand-written notes, are all important.

In this chapter we consider ways of reducing misunderstanding, and of optimizing the transfer of information and understanding, not only from doctor to family but also from family to doctor.

The most common communication scenario is one where the doctor is expected to impart news or information (Box 7.1). It is often the situation in which doctors feel most comfortable. There are always communication needs beyond simple information transfer, however, many of which the doctor will be unaware of but which will inevitably complicate the discussion if they are not acknowledged.

In general, in any communication, the doctor has two responsibilities to the family and patient. The first, and the simplest, is the passing on of the information that the doctor holds and the family needs. This needs to be done clearly and honestly.

The second, more nebulous but often more important, is to ensure that the family feels 'valued' by the professional. There is a power imbalance inherent in the relationship between doctor and patient since the doctor has the knowledge and is in his or her own environment. One of the goals of good communication exchange is to redress this imbalance.

MODULE TWO

An 8-year-old boy, Huw, attends children's accident and emergency with a week's history of tiredness, pallor and easy bruising. Today he had a prolonged epistaxis.

On examination, in addition to bruises over his legs and pallor, there is hepatomegaly, splenomegaly and widespread lymphadenopathy. A full blood count reveals haemoglobin of 6.8 g/dl, white cell count of 1.2×10^9/l and platelets at 9×10^9/l. The diagnosis of leukaemia is strongly suspected.

Before reading on, take a moment to consider your response to the following questions:

- What information do you need to give Huw's mother?
- How will you find out how much she understands?
- Why is it important that she should understand?
- What fears do you think she might already have?
- What do you think will make it difficult for her to understand?
- What techniques can you use to explain things more clearly?

This is more than good manners; families or patients who feel that their concerns have not been understood or taken seriously are less likely to work well in the team. Empathy — not only a capacity to understand something of what they are going through, but also an ability to communicate back to the family that you have understood — is a highly effective way to ensure this sense of being valued.

With this in mind, the process of giving news or information can be considered in five stages.

1. Set the scene

Communications should take place in an environment that is conducive to the exchange of information. This needs planning. Of course, this is not always possible and communication may at times have to be impromptu, but this should usually be avoided — if necessary, by arranging a discussion at a specified later time.

Families may find discussions with doctors quite intimidating and will need positive encouragement to volunteer information. The aim of setting the scene is to provide a physical and temporal space in which communication is facilitated.

Physical space

- *Privacy*. This helps families feel comfortable enough to discuss important issues.
- *Quiet room*. One should be reserved for the purpose (and the door shut).
- *Comfortable furnishings*. Sofas/armchairs are preferable to institutional chairs, allowing professionals and family to be on the same physical level.

Temporal space

- *Unhurried atmosphere*. It is important for families to feel that the doctor has put some time aside specifically for them. Creating this 'space in time' is, paradoxically, time-saving, allowing more efficient information exchange so discussions can be shorter without sacrificing effectiveness.
- *Minimize interruption*. Switch off mobile phones and bleeps or hand them to someone outside the room. This sends the message to the family that, for this period of time, its concerns are the most important.
- *Avoid consulting a watch* during the discussion. This gives an impression of hurry.

Remove barriers

Make a positive effort to remove barriers to avoid unintentionally discouraging contributions from family members:

- *No desk* should separate you from the family.
- *Eye contact* on same level emphasizes equality rather than a power differential.
- *Do not stand* while the family sits, or sit in a higher chair.
- *Maintain eye contact*. This is difficult when breaking bad news, but important. Loss of eye contact gives a sense that information is being withheld, or that you are not being entirely truthful. It can be hard to dispel this misconception once it has taken root.

Have the facts straight

- *Recognize the importance* attached by families to discussions with doctors.
- *Communicate results accurately*. Have the relevant printed reports in front of you, and if uncertain, admit this, rather than discuss a half-remembered result.

Who else should be there?

- *Both parents*. For discussions of any significance, this is ideal but not always possible. Their presence enables mutual support and minimizes the risk of misunderstanding. Alternatively, arrange a second

interview to cover the same ground, or make an audio recording for the spouse.
- *A member of the nursing staff*, especially one from the ward to which the child has been (or will be) admitted. This also helps the family identify another person to whom they can turn for information, once they have had time to digest the conversation. The underlying message that you are part of a team can be reassuring for families when everything else seems disturbing and new.
- *Child*, often ideal but not always possible or appropriate.

2. Alignment

It is tempting to start the discussion with what we want to say, but this would be like aiming a gunshot without first looking at the target. Instead, establish what the family already knows or understands by inviting them to talk first. Alignment essentially means understanding what things look like from the family's perspective. Aim to understand the following:

- *What they have already been told.* Many families will have considered leukaemia, perhaps because it has been mentioned as a possibility by the referring GP or other doctor. Others will have no idea that this is a possibility, while some will be afraid to mention their fear of it.
- *Any prior experience and its impact.* Leukaemia in childhood is cured in around 75% of cases. Most families who have considered it as a possibility will extrapolate from their own knowledge of cancers, which are usually in adults and carry a much worse prognosis. What started as a discussion to 'break bad news' can become an opportunity to reassure. People look for explanations for illness, and in their absence will often assume that inheritance, upbringing and/or contagion might be a factor.
- *What they understand.* Even those with no prior experience usually have preconceptions that may be unhelpful, particularly regarding the implications of the diagnosis and prognosis. Many families assume a diagnosis of leukaemia is universally fatal, or at least always causes long-term damage, or that a bone marrow transplant (often thought to involve surgery like a solid-organ transplant) will be necessary.
- *What vocabulary they use.* Note how the family uses language. Which words are used and which are avoided? The term 'tumour' (which can be benign or malignant) is usually synonymous with 'cancer' to lay people. Some families studiously avoid using the term 'cancer' or 'leukaemia', preferring instead 'tumour of the blood'. If this is the phrase

that the family already understands and which accommodates their coping mechanism, forcing them to use a more precise term may jeopardize both their understanding and their coping. Unnecessary corrections are discourteous and emphasize the power imbalance between doctor and patient.

Tools that assist alignment

Open questions
These encourage a person to define the agenda of the discussion by allowing them free rein to decide how to interpret the question. There are different ways of doing this; a good one is to start by saying, 'We haven't met before, so it would help me if you could summarize for me what has happened up until now'. The family can interpret the question in whatever way it chooses. Such an approach can often be dramatically revealing, such as the response, 'Well, it all started when we moved near some power cables after my husband left us four years ago.'

Closed questions
These are often considered less helpful, as their object is to narrow down the discussion and focus on specific issues. Carelessly used, their effect can be to restrict discussions to what the doctor wants to talk about, rather than what the family needs to hear. Nevertheless, closed questions can be crucial. Consider, for example, the importance of an answer to the question, 'Has anyone in your family suffered from leukaemia?' Discussions with no closed questions can be poorly focused and unsatisfactory.

Summarizing and checking
Since the purpose of the alignment phase is to gain an understanding of the perspective of patient and family, it is important to confirm that your understanding is accurate. This can be done, for example, by using the formula, 'From what you have said, it seems that you already suspect/understand/are worried about etc....' Families can then correct you or confirm your summary. The family then knows that you have listened, and you gain a better sense of their information needs.

3. Imparting information

Although it is important that families feel listened to, this is rarely enough. The family has to trust you and to understand the information you give accurately, since competent collaboration is necessary in patient care. Both level and pace need to be appropriate.

Appropriate level

What information does the family need to deal with the immediate situation, and to allay its major fears and anxieties? At the time of diagnosis of leukaemia, for example, it is important that the family should understand the nature of the disease, the immediate tests that are required and the significance of their results. Families will commonly ask about increasingly remote possibilities, and there is a balance between providing answers and avoiding an unhelpful discussion of things that are very unlikely to happen. Too much information makes it harder to take in what is really important. It can be helpful to make a further appointment at a specific date and time, once further results are available. This avoids a sense of premature closure.

Often, questions raised at the initial interview will reveal more general concerns that need to be addressed. For example, detailed questions about the side-effects of chemotherapy before leukaemia has been confirmed, let alone classified, may indicate a concern that, even if the child is cured, he or she will be left with long-term damage. Whilst addressing the specific detail of different chemotherapy protocols may not be appropriate, reassurance that most cancer survivors are healthy usually is.

There is often surprisingly little difference in the understanding of practical care between families with a high level of education and those without. What is often needed, however, is for the same concepts to be explained in different ways. The danger here is of sounding either patronizing or incomprehensibly technical. One way of minimizing the risk of either extreme is to avoid using jargon words, preferring instead the terms chosen by the family themselves. Most families will need more or less the same amount of information, irrespective of their educational level.

Appropriate pace

The rate at which people can assimilate information depends on many uncertain factors. These include prior understanding and what has already been explained. A useful way of ensuring that information is being given at the appropriate rate is to use summaries. These serve to reiterate what has been said, to punctuate the discussion and provide a pause, and also provide a chance to invite questions. A typical summary would be something like this:

So, we've talked about the two different sorts of leukaemia, lymphoid and myeloid, and the fact that they are treated quite differently and that lymphoid is, on the whole, easier to treat than myeloid. We've also spoken about the fact that before we can know which it is, we will need to do a bone marrow examination, and we talked a little bit about what that will

involve and in particular the fact that he will be asleep when it is done. Is there anything you would like to ask about those things before we go on?

Written materials

These can be valuable adjuncts to communication. Drawings can help to clarify what is being said; if complex, practise them beforehand. Good-quality written materials to take away can provide ongoing information that can be accessed at an appropriate pace and without pressure. However, written material should not usually be given without an opportunity for discussion with a knowledgeable person. It is difficult for any process of alignment to take place before printed materials are read, so that families may find themselves presented with a series of words that are unfamiliar but carry a message of dire news they are not yet prepared to hear. Poor written information may be positively harmful, but there are many printed resources of great quality.

Written materials also give an opportunity for families to access their own reference resources outside the meeting in order to clarify or expand on what has been written. The Internet is a mixed blessing in facilitating the development of expertise among families. Much of what is published on the Net is strongly held opinion rather than fact. Nevertheless, there are some extremely valuable resources. It is best to acknowledge that families may want to search for the topic on the Internet, provide three or four reputable websites, and invite them to bring anything else they discover back for further discussion.

4. Checking

Once all the information has been imparted, ask the family if they have had enough information, if their concerns have been addressed, and if they have any further questions. Summarizing is again useful at this point.

Reassure families that they will not be thought stupid if they do ask a question: 'No one expects you to remember everything first time and we are perfectly happy for you to ask again. If I am not here, my nursing colleagues will be around and will usually be able to answer your questions.' This also empowers and supports your nursing colleagues as sources of expert information in their own right. Avoid inviting questions in a way that actively discourages them: 'You don't have any questions, do you?' Generally, families need positive encouragement to ask.

If checking reveals that some issues have not been understood as well as you had thought, go back over the information again. This may need to be done many times. Rarely, it may be necessary to guillotine the discussion: for example, if it becomes clear that the family is simply unable to take in the information at that time.

5. Future plans

Do not let the family feel they are being abandoned at the end of the interview. Most families will feel reassured and more secure, simply knowing that there are plans for further conversations. Introduce other members of the team and refer to them during the conversations, so that families recognize yours is not the only expert voice. Assurances such as 'The nurses who work on this ward are very familiar with children with leukaemia and are always available to answer questions while you are here' can be both encouraging for families and supportive for colleagues. It may be helpful to add that if your colleagues are not sure of the answer, they will know whom else to ask; this allows staff to involve senior members of the team without feeling they have lost face in doing so.

For children who are to be discharged home, the contact may be the primary care team or a nursing outreach team. Provide a contact phone number if at all possible.

Families will appreciate knowing that there will be a second opportunity to discuss things with the person who has initially given them the information. This could be either on the ward (set a time and day) or as an outpatient. Remember that these appointments will be of enormous significance to families, so should not be undertaken lightly. For example, if it is not possible to be sure of the exact time when the next meeting should take place, it is better to say 'I will be there some time on Tuesday afternoon but can't say exactly when', rather than giving a spurious appointment time and then not being able to attend. Families understand that doctors' lives are busy and often unpredictable, and that they may not be able to give an exact time.

Finally, ensure that the plans for meeting again are acceptable to the family. This is particularly important if the child is being discharged since, if the plans are impractical for the family, the child will simply default and be lost to follow-up. So, once again, the conversation should finish by summarizing what has been said and inviting questions.

Summary (Box 7.2)

The discussion of bad news begins with a process of finding out how the situation is seen by the patient and

> **BOX 7.2 Goals of communication with the family**
>
> To enable the family of a child or young person to become competent colleagues in his/her medical care through:
> - Imparting factual information and understanding:
>   - To an appropriate level
>   - At an appropriate pace
>   - Using appropriate language
> - Imparting a sense of participation in the team through:
>   - Seeking their perspective
>   - Empathic acknowledgement (implied and overt) of their concerns
>   - Soliciting their views in decision-making

the family (alignment). This is followed by a period when the doctor gives information at a pace, level and amount that the family can assimilate accurately and easily. Check for understanding during the discussion and on completion, and repeat the information if necessary. Finally, make future plans, including arrangements for a follow-up meeting. This should allow the twin purposes of communication with families — the passage of information and establishment of a sense of being 'valued' — to be achieved.

Communication with colleagues

Colleagues, too, need to be treated with courtesy and respect. This is more than simple etiquette; it is essential to good communication and therefore impacts directly on patient care. Brusqueness or rudeness irritates, closing the door to further discussion. Courtesy helps avoid positions becoming entrenched, and instead encourages exchange of professional views.

For situations in which important patient data is to be passed on to colleagues, a combination of verbal and written communication is ideal. Verbal communication is the most effective means of exploring, explaining or clarifying a difficult clinical situation. A verbal handover, for example, allows information about patients to be passed on but, compared with a written handover, can more easily communicate less concrete aspects: relative urgency, non-specific worries, a condition that is improving or worsening, or other diagnostic possibilities that have been considered.

Written information is best when data needs to be stored for easy and repeated access by different professionals. Writing in the notes is usually done by a junior member of the team, and is often seen as a chore. As the only permanent record of most of the clinical decisions, it is

- Date and sign all entries (name legible)
- Include role (e.g. 'Paeds SHO') and contact bleep/extension number
- Structure with brief summaries of the following:
  - Problem list (existing and new)
  - Important medications (e.g. 'Ribavirin day 4')
  - History and examination findings
  - Status that day (e.g. 'Generally better, but some respiratory problems remain, cause unclear, nasopharyngeal aspirate awaited')
  - Plans (bullet-point list).
- This is sometimes known as the 'SOAP' system: subjective (i.e. what others and the patient tell you), objective (i.e. what you find on examination), analysis (i.e. how you interpret the situation) and finally plan.

imperative that entries in medical notes are well written, accurate and legible (Box 7.3).

In outpatients, the main record of an appointment is the letter to the GP. This is usually more easily legible than hospital notes, as it is typed, and provides a valuable cumulative narrative over months, years or even decades. GP letters are typically written by diverse doctors, of all levels of seniority, many of whom will have moved on from the team at the time their letter is read. Letters need to be clearly and systematically written, and the SOAP system works well. Keep letters to less than one side of paper where possible. The two most important elements are a problem list or introductory paragraph summarizing the issues, and a closing paragraph detailing the plan. This should include further possibilities (e.g. 'If tramadol is ineffective or poorly tolerated, we should consider introducing a small dose of morphine').

It is perhaps ironic that, for paediatricians, the main role of a GP letter is often seen as that of providing a record for other members of the paediatric team rather than for the GP. Such a letter may not be enough if you are asking the GP to become actively involved in the child's follow-up care in the community. GPs receive a huge number of letters each day, more than they can read in detail, and it is difficult to identify in this deluge those that are for action, rather than simply for information. Even when you are not asking the GP to undertake a specific task, it is the primary care team who will usually renew the prescriptions you have started. They are in the position of needing to write up the medications you have prescribed, on patients they may not have seen for some time. If a child is to be managed safely by collaboration between hospital and primary care teams, the GP needs to have information

presented in a way that is clear, accurate and quickly assimilated. You can readily derive a set of 'do's and don'ts' of writing to GPs, simply by imagining yourself in the position of the GP who has to read the letter.

Do's and don'ts of writing to GPs

1. Do ask the patient which GP should receive the letter

Until recently, every patient was registered with a single GP, but nowadays patients are registered with a practice, and soon may be able to register with two or more practices. Most hospital computer systems, however, automatically insert the name of the registered GP and this is unlikely to change in the near future. Despite changes in GP cover, most patients will continue to have a preferred or 'usual' doctor, so ask the patient or parent who this is, or reply to the referring GP. A GP tends to read a letter bearing his or her name more thoroughly. The same applies to addressing the letter to the current registering practice.

2. Do begin the letter with a statement of the diagnosis

Where available, a diagnosis (or diagnoses) should be stated at the beginning of the letter. GP notes are usually computer-based and use a diagnostic code for diseases, such as the Read code. Where there is a locally agreed disease coding system, including the relevant code in the GP/clinic letter is helpful, particularly for new diagnoses.

3. Do keep it short and well organized

A short letter is more likely to be read thoroughly. There is potential conflict between the two roles of the clinic letter: a record for hospital notes on the one hand, and communication with the GP on the other. A particular bugbear for GPs is having the contents of their own referral letter regurgitated in a clinic letter. These details do need to be recorded among the outpatient letters, but this is really only necessary on the first visit. Reiteration on subsequent occasions is unnecessary and results in a letter that is turgid and difficult to read, for primary care and hospital teams alike. To enable GPs easily to skip what they already know, one solution is to preface this paragraph with 'to summarize the background' and/or to use subheadings (e.g. 'GP action') to draw attention to the relevant sections.

4. Do not use specialty-specific jargon

Avoid terminology or abbreviations seldom used outside paediatrics. GPs should not need a dictionary of paediatrics to translate your letter! Courtesy, as well as the interests of effective communication, demands that you use a professional vocabulary you have in common. Even among paediatricians, some abbreviations are ambiguous; for example, a patient who needs a 'PEG' may end up with a gastrostomy, laxatives or a form of asparaginase chemotherapy.

5. Do write a management plan

This facilitates effective and efficient collaboration between professionals, both between primary and hospital teams and within them. A management plan along the lines of 'If X fails, I would recommend Y or Z' allows others to see what your long-term strategy is. It also allows the primary care team to continue your management plan without the child needing to wait until the next visit. Include a clear plan for follow-up, whether for primary or secondary care.

6. Do give clear, consistent and constructive messages to the family

Where a specific 'GP action' is recommended, spell out what has been said to the patient. If a GP reads that he or she should be altering medication, this will be translated into a change on the patient's prescription list. The GP needs to know whether the patient/parent has been told the prescription will be ready, whether they are expecting the GP to call first to let them know it is ready, or whether the prescription is contingent on follow-up investigations/examinations etc. Care of the child is through collaboration with the primary care team, and it is important that their working relationship with the family is not jeopardized by unclear or undermining messages from the hospital.

It is rarely appropriate to collude with families who castigate their GP. Apart from anything else, families with this habit will probably be representing the hospital team in a similarly critical light in parallel discussions with the GP. It often appears that some agreement is required with the observation, 'I kept telling them that there was something wrong but they wouldn't listen.' The need for families is usually for their anger to be acknowledged and understood, rather than encouraged and fuelled. Most feel more anxious and uncertain if professionals indulge in uninformed criticism of one another. It is better to acknowledge the importance of the issue with an empathic 'That must have been frustrating' or even 'I can see that made you angry.' Such an acknowledgement is true, helpful and supportive irrespective of the actual circumstances, but does not imply that you agree that the GP (to whose care they will soon return) is incompetent. Once their anger is expressed and understood, families will often not feel the need to mention it again, and the collaborative relationship between family and professionals in primary care and hospital teams is unscathed.

8. Do draw attention to changes in prescription

Any change in medication should be typed in bold, listed before the body of the letter, or highlighted at the time the letter is signed. An exhaustive and up-to-date medication list is useful, but can be misleading unless strictly accurate. Patients may be under several different consultants, so your knowledge of their medication list may be incomplete. Remember that after the first month of a hospital prescription, what the patient will actually be prescribed, and will therefore be able to take, depends upon what is entered on to the GP's computer.

9. Don't always wait for the letter to go through the mail

Even if you dictate a clinic letter the moment you have seen the patient (as is ideal), there will usually be a delay of around a week while it is typed, signed, posted, and finally received and read. If the GP may need to know the outcome of the clinic appointment sooner, fax your letter, or better still, contact the GP by telephone. Most receptionists will quickly recognize the need to put another doctor through. A useful phrase is 'I need to speak directly to Dr X about a patient of ours'. State at the outset whether the urgency is such that the GP should be interrupted during a consultation. If urgent and the GP is out on visits, ask for a mobile telephone number. Messages are less satisfactory; you will have no way of knowing whether or not they have got to their recipient. If you have the address, email is the obvious solution, but is still beset by fears about confidentiality.

Summary

Like patients, professional colleagues are part of a collegiate relationship which, in order to function smoothly, demands communication that is sensitive and affirming. Underlying the practical suggestions above is the principle that people should feel they are valued as part of a team supporting and caring for the child. Information exchange should be not just accurate, but also accessible and easily assimilated. Whilst this can be challenging, particularly when communicating with colleagues outside the hospital, it is an essential part of clinical care. It is not simply an issue of politeness, or professional courtesy and etiquette; children's safety depends on it.

An example of a good and a bad letter to a GP is shown on the website.

Colin Morgan

CHAPTER

8

Evaluation of the newborn

LEARNING OUTCOMES

By the end of this chapter you should:
- Be able to assess the newborn infant competently by history and examination
- Be able to manage/refer minor congenital abnormalities appropriately
- Be able to offer appropriate advice regarding feeding the newborn infant
- Be able to describe the screening programmes in place for newborn infants.

You should be able to recognize:
- Major congenital abnormalities and their clinical significance
- The features of innocent cardiac murmurs
- The features of serious congenital heart disease presenting on the postnatal ward; you should also understand the immediate management pathway.

MODULE TWO

Introduction

The principles outlined in Chapter 5 also apply to the newborn, but this chapter deals with special considerations.

Evaluation of the acutely unwell newborn infant is covered in the neonatology chapters (Volume 2, Module 8). All newborn infants are assessed and evaluated by midwifery and/or medical professionals in the first few days. This includes a formal assessment within the first 24 hours, as well as providing routine postnatal care. This contact with healthcare professionals mostly provides reassurance to parents that their infant is healthy and that minor abnormalities (which can create much parental anxiety) are not of clinical importance. However, in a minority of cases, this assessment identifies a problem or an infant at risk. For example, a thorough history may identify healthy infants at risk of medical problems, prompting screening for infection, hypoglycaemia or jaundice, or parental social problems requiring multidisciplinary support or intervention before discharge. A careful routine examination may reveal previously unsuspected but clinically important abnormalities, such as congenital heart disease.

History

A thorough history should include all available detail in the following areas.

Maternal history (Table 8.1)

- Age
- Social background/occupation

Table 8.1 **Maternal disease that affects the neonate**

Maternal disease	Neonatal effects
Diabetes	Increased risk congenital abnormalities Macrosomia Hypoglycaemia Increased risk of surfactant-deficient lung disease

Maternal antibodies
  Graves' disease
  Systemic lupus erythematosus (SLE)
  Myasthenia gravis
	Neonatal thyrotoxicosis
	Complete heart block, haemolysis, thrombocytopenia
	Congenital myasthenia gravis

Chronic maternal disease, e.g. Crohn's disease, chronic renal failure	Intrauterine growth retardation

- Medical problems and chronic maternal disease
- Medical treatment and drugs
- Recreational drugs/alcohol/smoking.

Family history

- Father's age/occupation
- Family history of genetic conditions and congenital abnormalities
- Previous pregnancies: dates and outcomes
- Health of siblings.

This pregnancy

- Medical conditions that have complicated the pregnancy, e.g. diabetes, depression, steroid therapy
- Pregnancy-related complications, e.g. pre-eclampsia, hyperemesis, cholestatic jaundice
- Maternal/medical expected delivery date (EDD) and any discrepancy
- Routine screening tests, e.g. ultrasound scan, haematology and infection status at booking
- Non-routine tests (why performed), e.g. additional/specialist ultrasound scans
- Special diagnostic procedures, e.g. amniocentesis.

Labour and delivery

- Maternal health during labour (including length of labour)
- Evidence of fetal distress:
  - Reduced fetal movements
  - Cardiotochograph (CTG) abnormalities
  - Low arterial and venous cord pH (especially < 7.0)
  - Fresh meconium-stained liquor
- Infection risk (most neonatal services have a protocol to assess risk factors for neonatal sepsis with thresholds for performing a septic screen and treating with intravenous antibiotics):
  - Prolonged and/or preterm rupture of the membranes
  - Maternal pyrexia, chorioamnionitis
  - Maternal group B streptococcal colonization (or previous infected infant)
  - Intrapartum antibiotics given < 4 hours before delivery
- Drugs/anaesthesia given
- Mode of delivery.

Infant history

- Condition at birth with details of any resuscitation
- Age, sex and gestational age
- Progress since birth, including feeding history
- Any concerns from parents or nursing/midwifery staff
- Any antenatal plans for investigation/treatment of infant, e.g. risk of haemolytic disease, hepatitis B vaccine required.

Examination

Many of the key points of the examination are available as video clips, and these are summarized in Figure 8.1.

Conventionally, examination of the newborn progresses from head to toe. It should take about 5–10 minutes, depending on the experience of the examiner and the compliance of the infant. Prepare to adapt the sequence to take advantage of settled periods (to auscultate the heart) and leave more distressing parts (e.g. examining the hips) to the end. To start the examination, the infant should be undressed down to the nappy. Observe the infant first, assessing colour, respiratory effort and any spontaneous movements. Response to handling should be noted throughout the examination. Measure the occipito-frontal head circumference with a non-distendable tape measure (occiput to brow 1 cm above the nasal bridge). Plot head circumference and weight on a centile chart, correcting for gestation.

Head and neck

- Note head shape and presence of moulding.
- Identify evidence of swelling/trauma/bleeding:
  - Caput succedaneum (oedema of presenting part)
  - Cephalohaematoma (bleeding under periosteum)
  - Subaponeurotic haemorrhage (bleeding into subaponeurotic space)

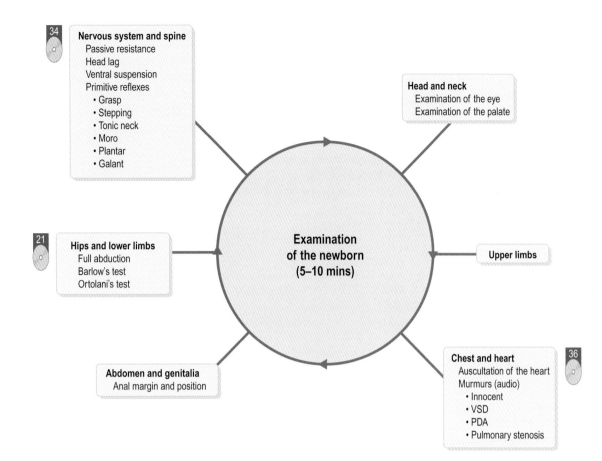

Fig. 8.1 Summary of newborn examination.
(VSD = ventricular septal defect; PDA = patent ductus arteriosus.)

- Marks from scalp electrodes, fetal blood sampling and instrumental delivery.
- Feel anterior and posterior fontanelles:
  - Normal range for anterior fontanelle 0.5–5 cm
  - Check skull sutures lines
  - Check for increased tension.
- Observe facial appearance:
  - Note any birthmarks, malformations and asymmetry
  - In newborn (obligate nose-breathers), pass nasogastric tube if any doubt about patency.
- Assess size, shape and position of ears:
  - Ensure external auditory meatus patent
  - Note any pre-auricular pits, skin tags or accessory auricles
- Assess size, dimensions, slant and position of eyes, and note:
  - Pupil size and reactivity
  - Eye movements, particularly presence of paralytic squint or nystagmus
  - Iris colour, shape and any defects
  - Evidence of corneal and lens opacities, using direct inspection/red reflex

- Evidence of conjunctival inflammation/haemorrhage
- Any discharge from eye.
- Assess size and asymmetry of mouth.
- Examine for cleft lip and palate, including soft palate.
- Assess shape, asymmetry and any swellings in neck.

Tips on clinical examination (Table 8.2)

Eyes
- A bright light (shone from the side) will reveal some cataracts and corneal opacities.
- Using the ophthalmoscope at 15–20 cm to identify the red retinal reflex will reveal most other lens and corneal opacities.
- Fundoscopy is not routine and often requires a mydriatic.

Palate
- Use a bright light (not an ophthalmoscope).
- The palate is best examined spontaneously (e.g. during crying).

73

Table 8.2 Common and important abnormalities of the head and neck in the newborn

Abnormality	Comments
Skull	
Cephalohaematoma	Common. Subperiosteal bleeding, so does not cross skull suture lines (c.f. caput succedaneum)
Subaponeurotic haemorrhage	Rare. Massive bleeding into potentially large subaponeurotic space can cause sudden collapse
Bulging fontanelle	Common in crying infant. More rarely a sign of raised intracranial pressure (e.g. hydrocephalus, meningitis)
Skull sutures	
Widened	Common in first 48 hours. More rarely indicates hydrocephalus
Overlapping	Common in association with moulding in first 48 hours
Raised	Rare. Suggests craniosynostosis
Skull fractures	Rare. Associated with prolonged labour and/or difficult deliveries. Depressed fractures can be hidden under superficial swelling
Face	
Facial nerve palsy	Uncommon
Birth marks	
Stork mark	Common. On neck and forehead. Fades
Port wine stain	Uncommon. May be associated with intracranial calcification (Sturge–Weber syndrome, rare)
Ears	
Low-set	See Figure 5.8 (p. 53) for description
Malformed	Common feature of many syndromes, from Down's to branchial arch anomalies
Eyes	
Hyper-/hypotelorism	See Figure 5.8 (p. 53) for description
Slanted palpebral fissures	Down's syndrome
Microphthalmia	Rare
Conjunctival haemorrhage	Common following delivery
Ptosis	Uncommon. Usually congenital (may be unilateral)
Coloboma (defect in iris)	Rare. Usually involves retina. May be isolated or part of syndrome (e.g. CHARGE — *c*oloboma, *h*eart defects, *a*tresia of choanae, *r*etarded growth, *g*enital hypoplasia, *e*ar anomalies)
Cataract	Uncommon. Usually inherited (autosomal dominant) but intrauterine rubella an important cause
Mouth	
Normal variants	Epstein's pearls (small white swellings along palate)
	Ranula (salivary duct cystic swelling in floor of mouth)
	Incisor teeth (usually need removal)
	Short lingual frenulum (tongue tie: rarely requires surgery)
Cleft lip/palate	Consider presence of other congenital anomalies/syndromes
Micrognathia	Uncommon. Can cause feeding or breathing difficulties, may have associated cleft palate (Pierre Robin sequence)
Neck	
Webbed	Turner syndrome
Short	Klippel–Feil syndrome
Redundant skin	Down's syndrome
Lumps and swellings	
Midline	Thyroid, thyroglossal cyst, thymic cyst, epidermoid cyst
Lateral	Cystic hygroma, branchial cyst, sternomastoid tumour (not usually present in first 2 weeks)

- Palpate the palate (using the pulp of your finger) to identify submucous clefts.
- A tongue depressor may be required to visualize the soft palate.

Upper limbs

Carefully observe for abnormality and asymmetry in:
- Bones (e.g. absent radius and associated thumb abnormalities)
- Joints (e.g. contractures or limited range of movement)
- Muscles and muscle bulk
- Posture and spontaneous movement (e.g. brachial plexus injuries)
- Fingers and thumbs:
  - Polydactyly (extra digits)
  - Syndactyly (fused/webbed digits)
  - Clinodactyly (shortened/flexed digits)
- Palmar creases:
  - Unilateral single (4% normal population)
  - Bilateral single (1% normal population).

Note any limb deformity, such as partial or complete amputations (suggestive of amniotic band injuries).

Q1. How are brachial plexus injuries assessed?

Weakness and flaccidity in one limb are highly suggestive of brachial plexus injury. It is important to exclude a fractured clavicle or humerus (they may coexist with brachial plexus injury). It is also important to look for other evidence of asymmetrical neurology, particularly in the lower limb, as this may suggest hemiplegia rather than lower motor neuron injury.

Even if the whole limb is flaccid at birth, there is often partial recovery over 48 hours, leaving the classical upper nerve root injury (C5, 6 ± 7) of Erb's palsy. The arm is internally rotated and pronated, with no abduction at the shoulder or flexion at the elbow. Occasionally, the damage extends to all the nerve roots. Rarely there is an isolated lower nerve root palsy (C8, T1), resulting in a weak claw hand (Klumpke's palsy).

Q2. What is the management plan for these injuries?

Early physiotherapy and regular reassessment are required. Infants that do not show good recovery within 3 months require specialist referral.

Heart and chest

Chest

37 Most useful signs are obtained by observation rather than auscultation:
- Colour
- Shape and asymmetry:
  - Whole chest (e.g. scoliosis)
  - Clavicles and ribs (e.g. swelling/deformity of a fractured clavicle)
  - Muscles (e.g. absent pectoralis major in Poland's sequence)

- Respiratory pattern (periodic breathing is normal)
- Respiratory rate (normal 40–60 breaths/min)
- Respiratory distress:
  - Use of accessory muscles
  - Intercostal, subcostal and suprasternal recession
  - Tachypnoea
  - Grunting
  - Stridor
- Auscultate each lung in three areas (apex, axilla and bases).

Heart

Auscultate the heart:
- Pulmonary area (and over left clavicle)
- Aortic area
- Lower left sternal edge
- Apex.

If a murmur is detected:
- Check for radiation (back, carotids and left clavicular area)
- Palpate for presence of a thrill.

Palpate the peripheral pulses:
- Radial or brachial
- Femoral (can be included during abdominal examination).

Q1. How is the distinction between innocent and pathological murmur made?

Murmurs have to have specific characteristics to be described as innocent (Box 8.1). It is important to

Q1. What cardiovascular signs suggest serious congenital heart disease?

Q2. How are duct-dependent lesions investigated and managed?

Q3. What are the important differential diagnoses?

Q4. How should asymptomatic pathological murmurs be managed?

remember that serious congenital heart disease can present without a murmur.

Q2. What causes an innocent murmur?

Innocent murmurs are often attributed to a short delay in normal closure of the ductus arteriosus. There is little evidence to confirm this, and many innocent murmurs are likely to result from blood flow in the pulmonary artery branches and to disappear before 6 months.

Q3. What investigations are necessary?

There is no evidence that chest X-ray or electrocardiography (ECG) contributes to the diagnosis if the clinical findings suggest an innocent murmur. In most UK centres, echocardiography for all these cases is not feasible, and if infants remain well without symptoms or signs, then they can be discharged with a follow-up clinical assessment. If the murmur persists, then echocardiography is indicated (Chs 41 and 47).

Q4. What advice would you give to the parents?

It is important to reassure parents that the clinical evidence points to a structurally normal heart. Before discharge, simple advice about recognizing when a baby is unwell as well as the specific symptoms of cardiac failure, colour changes and dusky spells, is required. There needs to be a clear plan for reassessment of the murmur.

Problem-orientated topic:

a cyanosed and breathless baby

A 3.5 kg male term infant delivered vaginally is noted to be 'dusky' at 6 hours of age and slow to feed. The infant has a respiratory rate of 70 breaths/min and a pansystolic murmur is clearly audible over the whole precordium. There is a 2 cm liver edge and the peripheral pulses, including femorals, are normal.

Q1. What cardiovascular signs suggest serious congenital heart disease?

Many congenital heart lesions (especially those that are complex or lethal) are diagnosed antenatally. However, a significant proportion (up to 20%) are still not detected before birth. Some of these will present with a pathological murmur identified during the newborn examination. However, the absence of a murmur does not exclude serious congenital heart disease. It is particularly important to identify congenital heart disease that has a duct-dependent pulmonary or systemic circulation. These infants may appear extremely well in the first few hours (or occasionally days) of life while the duct remains open. This means that they may present on the postnatal wards or as part of the routine evaluation of the newborn.

Lesions with a duct-dependent pulmonary circulation usually present with cyanosis (Ch. 47). This may be subtle or intermittent before becoming progressive, depending on the degree of pulmonary outflow obstruction. With transposition of the great arteries, an open duct is often essential to ensure mixing of the two circulations. Symptoms, and therefore presentation, may be delayed by additional mixing at ventricular level because of a ventricular septal defect (VSD, as in the case above).

A lesion with a duct-dependent systemic circulation presents with progressive collapse of the systemic circulation. Thus peripheral perfusion becomes poor and the peripheral pulses weak. Isolated weak femoral pulses are suggestive of coarctation of the aorta. Four-limb blood pressure and oxygen saturation differences may add to the clinical picture, but can be normal.

Duct-dependent lesions (particularly left-sided outflow obstruction) can also present with heart failure, which in the newborn presents as respiratory distress. Non-duct-dependent lesions can also present with heart failure in the early neonatal period, although these are uncommon (arrhythmias, myocardial disease or a large atrioventricular septal defect, AVSD).

Q2. How are duct-dependent lesions investigated and managed?

Chest X-ray (oligaemic/congested lung fields, cardiomegaly) and ECG (ventricular hypertrophy) may help narrow the differential diagnoses. However, urgent definitive diagnosis is required in duct-dependent lesions, and this means cardiological assessment and echocardiography (Ch. 47). The cardiological advice will include a plan for starting a prostaglandin infusion. If the infant is unwell or deteriorating, then a low-dose prostaglandin infusion should be started immediately.

Q3. What are the important differential diagnoses?

Lesions with a duct-dependent pulmonary circulation need to be differentiated from respiratory causes of cyanosis and persistent pulmonary hypertension of the newborn. Lesions with a duct-dependent systemic circulation can be indistinguishable from other causes of collapse/shock, including sepsis and hypovolaemia.

Q4. How should asymptomatic pathological murmurs be managed?

ECG and chest X-ray may help with the diagnosis of the congenital heart lesion in cases of pathological murmur, but definite diagnosis will require a plan for echocardiography and cardiological assessment. This can be done on an outpatient basis, provided there are no other cardiovascular signs (including abnormalities on ECG and chest X-ray) and the infant is healthy and feeding well. Weight gain is difficult to interpret in the first few days of life (normally there is some weight loss), but excessive gain in the first few days is suspicious.

As with innocent murmurs, parents should be advised of the symptoms and signs to look out for.

Abdomen and genitalia

Ask about:
- Vomiting (particularly if the vomit is bile-stained)
- Passage of meconium
- Passing urine (and quality of stream in boys).

Observe for:
- Asymmetry
- Abnormal pigmentation (especially genitalia)
- Umbilical flare and peri-umbilical infection
- Abdominal distension.

Palpate for:
- Organomegaly:
  - Liver edge, normally palpable up to 2 cm
  - Spleen tip, often palpable up to 1 cm
  - Kidneys, can be palpated if posterior abdominal wall supported by fingertips of your other hand: assess asymmetry and enlargement
  - Palpable bladder
  - Other masses
- Herniae in inguinal canal/scrotum.

Examine the anus with the infant in the supine position and hips flexed, checking:
- Position
- Patency
- Anal margin.

Examine the genitalia in males:
- Assessment of size of penis (measured from symphysis pubis):
  - Micropenis (< 1 cm), suggesting hypopituitarism
- Position of meatus (epispadias/hypospadias; glandular/penile/perineal)
- Palpation of testes, noting:
  - Whether undescended or ectopic
  - Any swelling or asymmetry (e.g. hydrocele)
  - Hard testicle (e.g. congenital torsion)
- Features suggesting ambiguity or virilization.

Examine the genitalia in females:
- Size of clitoris
- Partial/complete labial fusion
- Presence of vaginal discharge (clear mucus and bloody discharges normal)
- Features suggesting ambiguity or virilization.

Problem-orientated topic:

undescended testicles

A male term infant weighing 4.2 kg is born following elective caesarean section for breech presentation. A postnatal check at 24 hours reveals bilateral undescended testicles with no palpable gonads, although the genitalia appear otherwise normal. The infant is otherwise healthy.

Q1. What is the care pathway for undescended testicles?

Q2. What diagnosis is it important to consider in this case?

Q3. How would this diagnosis be excluded?

Q1. What is the care pathway for undescended testicles?

20 Careful confirmation of bilateral undescended testes is required. This means carefully examining the sites for ectopic testes (usually above the external inguinal ring but including the anterior aspect of the thigh), as well as palpating along the pathway of normal testicular descent (including the groin and internal and external inguinal rings). Do not confuse retractile with undescended testicles.

Most infants just require observation in the first year to establish whether delayed descent finally occurs. This can be done during routine child health surveillance (e.g. at 6-week and 8-month checks), following a neonatal discharge letter to the GP. Surgical management is discussed in Chapter 49.

Q2. What diagnosis is it important to consider in this case?

If there are no palpable gonads, it is essential to consider the possibility that this is a virilized female infant with congenital adrenal hyperplasia. It is important to examine the infant for other signs of virilization, especially hyperpigmentation. Female virilization includes normal scrotum and male phallus (without palpable gonads) at the extreme end of the spectrum.

Q3. How would this diagnosis be excluded?

As there are no other signs of virilization in this infant, a male infant with bilateral undescended testes is the most likely diagnosis. If there is other evidence of virilization, the case should be discussed with a paediatric endocrinologist. The investigation of an infant with ambiguous genitalia is discussed in Chapter 35.

Hips and lower limbs

Hips

Clinical examination of the hips forms a critical part of the examination of the newborn infant. It is an effective screening process for developmental dysplasia of the hip (DDH, formerly congenital dislocation of the hip). However, the sensitivity of the test is highly dependent on the clinical experience of the examiner, with up to 50% of cases missed in some case series. Even in experienced hands, it is estimated that 10–15% of cases may not be detectable at birth.

21
35 The purpose of the examination is to classify infants into three categories:

- Normal hips
- Normal hips but requiring ultrasound screening because of a high-risk history:
  - Family history of DDH
  - Breech presentation
  - Other joint deformities such as contractures or talipes equinovarus
  - Clicky hip
- Abnormal hip/hips (requiring orthopaedic assessment):
  - Dislocatable (Barlow's test positive)
  - Dislocated but reducible (Ortolani's test positive)
  - Dislocated and irreducible (reduced abduction).

The examination should be performed on a firm surface with a comforted infant and the nappy removed. The examination often upsets the infant:

- Inspect the legs/groins for asymmetry/ deformity, with the infant's hips and knees extended.
- Abduct the hips, testing for limited abduction.
- Perform Barlow's test (reducing a dislocated hip).
- Perform Ortolani's test (dislocating an unstable hip).

Lower limbs

Most lower limb deformities are positional and reflect the posture of the infant in utero. Careful assessment of the range of movement is required before diagnosing a permanent deformity. For example, 'positional talipes' is very common and can be corrected by dorsiflexion and eversion of the foot. This is not possible in true talipes equinovarus, where the combined bony and connective tissue abnormality restricts the full range of movement.

Carefully observe for abnormality and asymmetry in:

- Bones (isolated bone abnormalities very rare)
- Joints (e.g. contractures or limited range of movement)
- Muscles and muscle bulk
- Posture and spontaneous movement
- Toes:
  - Polydactyly (extra digits)
  - Syndactyly (fused/webbed digits)
  - Overlapping toes (common and of no significance).

Note any limb deformity, such as partial or complete amputations (suggestive of amniotic band injuries). The important lower limb deformities are described in Table 8.3.

Table 8.3 Lower limb deformities (all associated with developmental dysplasia of the hip)

Lower limb deformity	Comments
Talipes equinovarus	Common (1:1000). M:F > 2:1. Bilateral 50% Fixed foot held adducted, supinated and plantarflexed (equinus)
Calcaneovalgus	Spectrum of severity (20% mild, 12% very severe) Common Lax ankle with flexible foot dorsiflexed in valgus (foot may touch lower leg) Benign, usually requires physiotherapy only
Metatarsus adductus	Common. Usually bilateral Flexible deformity with forefoot curved medially and toes pointing inwards Nearly always self-correcting
Congenital vertical talus (rocker bottom foot)	Rare. 85% associated chromosome or spinal abnormalities Fixed foot, with forefoot dorsiflexed and abducted, heel in valgus and equinus. Usually requires surgical intervention

Problem-orientated topic:

talipes

A male term infant weighing 4.2 kg is born following planned caesarean section for maternal diabetes. The pregnancy was generally unremarkable, except for late polyhydramnios and right-sided talipes equinovarus. A postnatal check at 24 hours confirms bilateral talipes equinovarus, more marked on the right, but no other findings. The infant was fed early and has had no feeding problems or difficulties maintaining a normal blood glucose.

Q1. What is the care pathway for talipes equinovarus?

Q2. What other diagnoses is it important to consider in this case?

Q3. What investigations are required?

Q1. What is the care pathway for talipes equinovarus?

Clinical assessment needs to establish that the deformity is either fixed or only partially correctable. Urgent orthopaedic referral is then indicated. Physiotherapy is initiated for partly flexible deformities, with early plaster casts for severe fixed deformities.

Q2. What other diagnoses is it important to consider in this case?

The combination of polyhydramnios and bilateral talipes equinovarus should alert the paediatrician to the possibility of neuromuscular disease. A history of poor fetal movements, hypotonia and/or poor feeding would increase the likelihood of such an abnormality. However, polyhydramnios is common in diabetic mothers and this infant has an excellent feeding history with no evidence of hypotonia, making neuromuscular disease very unlikely.

Q3. What investigations are required?

All foot deformities are associated with developmental dysplasia of the hip (Table 8.3) and so require ultrasound screening of the hip.

Spine and nervous system

You will already have learned a great deal about the infant's nervous system by observing and handling the infant in the earlier part of the examination.

Lay the infant supine and review any asymmetry previously observed, especially in posture or spontaneous movements. Look for evidence of generalized hypotonia, adducted shoulders or fully abducted hips (frog-like posture).

Test resistance to passive movements by applying gentle traction to each arm, testing muscle power and tone, and repeating for the lower limbs. Gently lift the head by applying traction to both arms, testing for the degree of head lag.

Turn the infant prone, look at posture (limbs should be flexed) and observe the spine and any asymmetry. Now hold the infant in ventral suspension (hand under chest), assessing tone in the trunk, neck and limbs and the appearance of the spine. Hypotonia is suggested by an upside-down U posture, with little flexion of the limbs and no extension of the head, neck or spine. Palpate along the length of the spine for defects and asymmetry. Look for patches of pigmentation, hair or swellings, especially if in the midline. Examine any clefts or pits and determine whether the base can be visualized.

79

Table 8.4 Primitive reflexes

Reflex	Description (response to)
Grasp	Pressure in the palm or sole
Rooting	Stroking the cheek
Stepping	Lowering on a hard surface (held upright)
Tonic neck	Head being turned to one side (symmetrical start position)
Moro	Dropping head a few cm (symmetrical start position)
Plantar	Stroking sole of foot
Galant	Stroking down one side of the spine (held prone)

It is not usually necessary to elicit the primitive reflexes during a routine examination of the newborn. However, they can be useful in confirming abnormal neurological findings, especially asymmetry (Table 8.4).

Problem-orientated topic:

the jittery infant

A 2.5 kg female infant is born by emergency caesarean section for fetal distress. She was born in reasonable condition, although she needed a couple of inflation breaths before starting to breathe. You are called at 18 hours because of jittery movements. The baby is bottle-feeding well and the pre-feed blood sugar is 2.6 mmol/l. The jittery movements have stopped and nothing unusual is found on clinical examination, but you are called again at 36 hours with a history of more jittery movements intermittently over the preceding 4 hours. The last blood sugar measurement was 3.9 mmol/l.

Q1. What are jittery movements?

Q2. Are there any investigations you would perform?

Q1. What are jittery movements?

Up to half of normal newborn infants demonstrate jittery movements. Clearly, it is essential to be able to distinguish them from abnormal movements with a neurological cause, particularly convulsions (Table 8.5).

The history of the pregnancy, labour and delivery must be reviewed carefully for evidence of hypoxic–ischaemic injury, infection and congenital abnormality. The timing, severity and progression of episodes are also important.

Assess the effects of episodes on feeding or lethargy/irritability in the infant. If the history suggests fits or there are neurological signs on clinical examination, then immediate investigation is required.

Q2. Are there any investigations you would perform?

Jittery movements rarely require investigation, although it is important to exclude hypoglycaemia (essential in high-risk infants). If the movements are particularly frequent or persistent, then it is reasonable to exclude hypocalcaemia (rare, but Asian infants are at higher risk) and hypomagnesaemia. Being called back to the same infant, particularly if the parent and/or midwife are experienced, usually merits a period of observation if you have not seen the movements yourself. This has to be balanced with the problems of separation from the parents. However, direct observation of abnormal movements, together with heart rate and saturation monitoring during episodes, usually removes any doubts about diagnosis in difficult cases.

Problem-orientated topic:

the floppy infant

A 3.43 kg female infant is born in good condition following an uncomplicated pregnancy and labour. On the labour ward, 2 hours after birth, it is noted that she remains markedly hypotonic, although pink and alert with her eyes open. The midwife describes the breathing as regular, although not 'normal' in nature, and there are some unusual movements of the tongue.

Q1. What are the causes of neonatal hypotonia?

Q2. What further important features of the history and examination do you require to make a diagnosis?

Q3. How would you investigate this case?

Q1. What are the causes of neonatal hypotonia?

There are two key questions to answer when classifying neonatal hypotonia:
- Does the infant have an associated encephalopathy?
- Is there generalized muscle weakness?

Table 8.5 Comparison of jitteriness and convulsions

Feature	Jitteriness	Convulsions
Nature of movement	'Symmetrical' tremor (both phases of the tremor are of equal length)	'Asymmetrical' tremor (e.g. fast and slow phases of a tonic–clonic seizure)
Frequency	5 Hz	< 1 Hz
Stimulation	Aggravates tremor	No effect
Restraint/flexion	Stops tremor	No effect
Facial involvement	None	Sometimes involves eyes, lips or tongue
Autonomic signs	None	Apnoea, tachycardia
Neurological signs	None	Occasionally present

Neonatal encephalopathy is described in Chapter 48. Hypoxia–ischaemic brain injury is the most common cause of neonatal hypotonia in this group, but congenital malformations of the central nervous system (CNS), antenatal brain injury (e.g. congenital infection) and metabolic disease are also important. In those infants without encephalopathy the causes are classified as described below.

Hypotonia without significant weakness (neurological)

- Intellectual impairment
- Cerebral palsy
- Down's syndrome
- Prader–Willi syndrome.

Hypotonia without significant weakness (non-neurological)

- Acute infection or any severe neonatal illness
- Prematurity
- Severe growth failure
- Ligamentous laxity (e.g. Ehlers–Danlos syndrome)
- Metabolic/endocrine (e.g. hypercalcaemia, hypothyroidism).

Hypotonia with muscle weakness

- Spinal cord:
  Trauma (birth injury)
  Congenital/vascular malformation
  Spinal muscular atrophy (anterior horn cells)
- Neuromuscular junction:
  Myasthenia gravis
- Muscle:
  Congenital myotonic dystrophy
  Congenital muscular dystrophies
  Congenital myopathies
- Unknown: benign congenital hypotonia.

Q2. What further important features of the history and examination do you require to make a diagnosis?

You need to see a maternal/family history of neuromuscular conditions, and a specific history of reduced fetal movements or polyhydramnios during pregnancy. Clinical examination should focus on the observation of posture, spontaneous movement, respiratory pattern, presence of muscle fasciculation, particularly of the tongue, and the assessment of muscle weakness. The clinical history suggests the severe form of spinal muscular atrophy (SMA type I; Werdnig–Hoffmann disease, Ch. 45). The muscle weakness in these infants presents with characteristic 'jug handle' upper limb posture and a frog-like lower limb posture with a paucity of spontaneous movements, and with visible muscle fasciculations. The weak intercostal muscles lead to exaggerated diaphragmatic respiratory effort. The facial muscles are characteristically preserved.

Q3. How would you investigate this case?

Electromyography (EMG) will show fibrillation potentials at rest. Genetic analysis will confirm whether the infant is homozygous for the deletion of SMN1 on chromosome 5 in 98% of cases. This is discussed on page 96.

Skin

Jaundice

Neonatal jaundice is covered in Chapter 48. More than half of newborn infants have clinically detectable jaundice, and so recognizing physiological jaundice is an essential part of evaluating the newborn.

Problem-orientated topic:

the jaundiced infant

A 3.94 kg female infant is born at 37⁺⁵ weeks' gestation in good condition following a forceps delivery and a prolonged labour. She is slow to establish breastfeeding, passes meconium at 24 hours, and is noted to be mildly jaundiced on day 2. This is felt to be

Continued overleaf

clinically significant by day 3 (serum bilirubin 230 mmol/l) and rises further by day 4 (serum bilirubin 270 mmol/l). Thereafter, the jaundice gradually resolves, requiring no treatment.

Q1. Is this physiological jaundice?

Q2. How would you investigate this case?

Q1. Is this physiological jaundice?

The timing of onset and peak are consistent with physiological jaundice. The peak level is higher than that typical of physiological jaundice but there are a number of exacerbating factors in this case. The gestation, although term, is more likely to result in relative liver enzyme immaturity. The instrumental delivery and prolonged labour are likely to have increased bruising. Significant bruising or haemorrhage will increase red cell breakdown. Delayed passage of meconium, breastfeeding and poor intake are also exacerbating factors.

Q2. How would you investigate this case?

Investigations should be kept to a minimum if physiological jaundice is suspected. Confirmation that the hyperbilirubinaemia is unconjugated is usually sufficient. A blood group and Coombs test are appropriate if the jaundice seems too rapid in onset for physiological jaundice. The possibility of infection should always be considered.

Common neonatal skin lesions

The presence of birthmarks often provokes parental anxiety, and the nomenclature of such lesions can cause confusion, resulting in inappropriate advice (Table 8.6). There are a number of common neonatal rashes that are transient and benign, but which need to be distinguished from more serious conditions, particularly infections (Table 8.7).

Feeding advice and feeding problems

Human milk is the preferred milk for term infants, but many mothers discontinue breastfeeding. The reasons for this are discussed in Chapter 4. The paediatrician has an important role in supporting breastfeeding mothers in difficulty. As well as the medical implications of poor milk intake (dehydration and hypoglycaemia),

Table 8.6 Birthmarks

Term	Description
Pigmented	
Congenital melanocytic naevi	Raised, irregular, well demarcated, brown/blue/black, often hairy
	Giant lesions have a significant risk of malignancy
	Large lesions may be associated with CNS malformations
	Medium–large lesions over the spine may be associated with spinal abnormalities
Mongolian blue spot	Flat, irregular, poorly defined margin, blue/grey
	80% are found in Asian/black infants, 10% in Caucasian
	Usually over lumbo-sacral area, can be very large
	Fade during childhood
Vascular	
Haemangiomas (includes lesions described as strawberry, capillary and/or cavernous haemangioma)	Haemangiomas are proliferative vascular tumours
	They may grow rapidly after birth and during infancy, but then begin to resolve spontaneously
	They can obstruct airways, eyes or other vital structures
	Lesions over the face may be associated with CNS abnormalities
	Lesions over the lower spine may be associated with spinal, urogenital or rectal abnormalities
Vascular malformations	These are permanent, non-proliferative structural abnormalities, categorized according to the vascular structure involved
Capillary malformation (includes port wine stain, naevus flammeus and Sturge–Weber syndrome)	Abnormal dilated mature capillaries. Most commonly on face (can be anywhere). Responds to laser therapy in infancy
	Sturge–Weber syndrome: association between facial capillary malformation (involves 1st division of trigeminal nerve) and ipsilateral brain vascular malformation
Venous malformation	Bluish raised lump, demonstrates venous filling and emptying
Lymphatic malformation (cystic hygroma, lymphangioma)	Macrocystic, skin-covered deep lesions. Can be detected antenatally; large cervical lesions can obstruct neonatal airway
Arteriovenous malformation	Skin-coloured lump that may have a bruit. Often part of a mixed malformation
Mixed malformation	Complex lesions involving multiple vascular components can occur. Rarely the lesion may involve limb hypertrophy (e.g. Klippel–Trenaunay syndrome)

Table 8.7 Pustular/vesicular rashes in the newborn

Rash	Description
Sterile pustules/vesicles	
Toxic erythema of the newborn	Very common. Usually appears within 48 hours. On any part of body, especially trunk and face
Transient neonatal pustular dermatosis	Common. Usually appears within 24 hours. Usually on trunk and buttocks
Eosinophilic pustulosis	Relatively rare. Late neonatal period. Usually on scalp
Neonatal acne (neonatal cephalic pustulosis)	Common. First few weeks. Usually on cheeks
Infective pustules/vesicles	
Varicella	Neonatal infection, usually severe with widespread rash. Present at birth
Herpes simplex	Rash erupts at 5–8 days. Usually on presenting part (scalp) but can be localized to any area
Staphylococcal infection	Can present as pustules, bullous impetigo or scalded skin syndrome. Umbilicus important site of origin
Candida	Usually erythematous red scaly rash in nappy area. Satellite lesions can appear pustular

poor infant feeding is an important clinical sign of infant wellbeing. It is a non-specific sign of illness (e.g. infection, cardiorespiratory or neuromuscular disease) or abnormality (e.g. Down's syndrome, CNS malformation), and does not automatically imply a gastrointestinal problem. The paediatrician asked to assess a breastfed infant that is feeding poorly needs to establish whether this is due to difficulties in lactation/breastfeeding technique or neonatal illness/abnormality.

Although it is tempting in this situation to recommend complementary or supplementary feeds, these can further undermine maternal confidence and interfere with the successful latching on of the infant. Complementary or supplementary feeds can be formula or expressed breast milk and may be given from bottle, cup or even spoon/syringe. If complementary or supplementary feeds are deemed necessary, then expressed breast milk is the preferred option. There is clear evidence that the technique involved when an infant feeds from a teat is different from that required for the infant to latch on and breastfeed. Cup feeding, therefore, offers a theoretical advantage over bottle-feeding in avoiding 'nipple confusion'. Although cup feeding is recommended practice, particularly in preterm infants, the evidence base remains relatively weak.

The duty of the paediatrician, confronted with an infant that is feeding poorly, is to evaluate the infant carefully and establish that he or she is healthy with no abnormalities. Recommended intakes for term infants start at 30–60 ml/kg/day in the first 24 hours and increase by 30 ml/kg/day until 150–100 ml/kg/day. This is easy to establish in the bottle-feeding infant but requires more clinical judgment in the case of the breastfed infant. Breastfeeding mothers should be reassured if the infant appears well and given close support to continue establishing lactation. Complementary or supplementary feeds should be avoided unless the infant is high-risk (see below) or there is clinical evidence of poor intake. This includes:

- Signs of dehydration
- Hypernatraemia
- Hypoglycaemia
- Significant jaundice
- Initial weight loss > 10%
- Failure to gain any weight in first 7 days.

Sometimes lack of milk is clear from infant behaviour: persistent hunger, frequent feeding, repeatedly unsettled soon after a feed, and/or persistent crying. In these circumstances, supplementary feeding may give mothers time to rest, restore morale, and break the cycle of difficult feeding and a fractious infant.

Other newborn feeding difficulties include vomiting and choking episodes. Possetting (frequent but insignificant amounts of regurgitated milk) is normal in newborn infants. Larger vomits can be a non-specific sign of ill health, especially infection or an airway/respiratory problem. Careful assessment of the gastrointestinal system is required, from the mouth (to exclude a soft palate) to the anus (to exclude atresia). Bile-stained (green) vomit and/or abdominal distension suggest bowel obstruction and require immediate surgical assessment. Choking or dusky episodes, clearly related to a feed, are also common as isolated episodes. If the infant appears well and there are no findings on clinical examination, the parents can be reassured. However, a second episode or clinical suspicion of infection, respiratory symptoms/signs or abnormal movements requires admission, observation and investigation.

> **Problem-orientated topic:**
>
> **an infant at risk of developing hypoglycaemia**
>
> A 4.2 kg infant is born in good condition at 38 weeks, following planned caesarean section. The mother has had well-controlled insulin-dependent diabetes throughout pregnancy. The infant is noted to have some grunting and tachypnoea initially, but these
>
> *Continued overleaf*

settle in less than an hour. The infant is tried at the breast in the first hour, but the combination of the mother's post-operative condition (spinal anaesthetic) and the infant's reluctance to feed means that this is not very successful. The blood sugar at 2 hours is 2.2 mmol/l.

Q1. What infants are at risk of developing hypoglycaemia on the labour/postnatal ward?

Q2. How should this infant be managed?

Q1. What infants are at risk of developing hypoglycaemia on the labour/ postnatal ward?

Infants at risk of hypoglycaemia include:
- Infants who are born preterm
- Those of low birth weight (< 2.5 kg)
- Infants of diabetic mothers
- Those with perinatal asphyxia
- Any infant with an evolving illness
- Those with a congenital abnormality affecting feeding (e.g. cleft palate, Down's syndrome).

Some infants who are at risk of hypoglycaemia are admitted to the neonatal intensive care unit (NICU) because of the severity of the underlying problem. However, many are well enough to stay with their mothers on the postnatal ward and here their progress requires careful monitoring.

Q2. How should this infant be managed?

It is important to feed high-risk infants early, although ensuring that this is successful is sometimes difficult. Maternal and infant factors can cause delay. This infant requires a supplementary feed to allow maternal post-operative recovery and successful initiation of lactation. The volume can be gradually increased to 75 ml/kg/day (if tolerated) and 2-hourly feeds given in the first few hours. Blood glucose measurements should be taken within 4 hours, sooner if there are feeding difficulties, as in this case. Repeat pre-feed measurements should be performed at least 4-hourly until blood glucose stabilizes above 2.7 mmol/l. Bedside testing is appropriate for monitoring the trend in blood sugar, but at least one laboratory test should be performed to confirm hypoglycaemia.

Infants of diabetic mothers can be slow to establish feeds, so exacerbating the risk of hypoglycaemia. If a combination of lactation support, breast and complementary feeds does not maintain the blood glucose above 2.5mmol/l,

then nasogastric tube (NGT) feeding, hourly feeds and ultimately intravenous dextrose infusion need to be considered. Transitional care facilities (if available) enable mother and the NGT-fed infant to be kept together.

Newborn screening

Routine clinical examination of the newborn in the first 24 hours can be considered a form of screening, particularly for DDH. However, its effectiveness as a screening tool is still a matter for debate, and newborn screening is a term usually reserved for the newborn blood spot screening programme and, more recently, the newborn hearing screening programme.

Newborn blood spot screening

Newborn blood spot screening began in 1969 and has become one of the largest and most successful screening programmes in the UK. More than 99% of all newborn infants in the country are screened at 5–8 days, and approximately 250 infants with either phenylketonuria or congenital hypothyroidism are identified each year. The need to support the necessary multidisciplinary collaboration and extend the programme led to the creation of the UK Newborn Screening Programme Centre in 2002. This group has developed clear policies, standards and a quality assurance programme (p. 167).

Phenylketonuria (Ch. 34)

This was the first condition to undergo newborn screening and comes very close to fulfilling the ideal standards for a screening programme. The incidence is 1:10000. Infants are initially healthy but slowly develop irreversible neurological damage during infancy due to phenylalanine neurotoxicity. This can be prevented by an exclusion diet, if this is started in the first 2–3 weeks. The screening originally took the form of a microbiological assay but now involves direct measurement of phenylalanine levels. If a phenylalanine concentration of > 240 µmol/l is confirmed on repeat testing, then referral to a specialist phenylketonuria team, comprising consultant, dietician and specialist nurse, is indicated.

Congenital hypothyroidism (Ch. 35)

Newborn blood spot screening was extended to include congenital hypothyroidism in 1981. The incidence is 1:3500. As in phenylketonuria, infants initially appear healthy, symptoms and signs appear gradually, and neurological damage is irreversible. The treatment is thyroxine replacement therapy. The screening process measures thyroid-stimulating hormone (TSH), with levels >20 mU/l indicating a positive result and <10 mU/l a negative one. Borderline results are repeated. Some national screening programmes (notably in the USA) measure T_4 and TSH to avoid missing the rare possibility of secondary hypothyroidism.

Sickle cell disease and thalassaemia
(Ch. 43)

The newborn blood spot screening programme has recently been extended to include sickle cell screening. This has been introduced in tandem with an antenatal screening programme offering sickle cell and thalassaemia screening to all women as an integral part of early antenatal care. The form of screening will depend on the local prevalence of the condition, with high-risk areas offering universal screening, and low-risk areas offering targeted screening using an antenatal questionnaire based on ethnic origin. The rolling programme was implemented nationally in the UK in 2005/6.

Cystic fibrosis (Ch. 42)

Biochemical screening for cystic fibrosis, using a method to detect raised levels of immunoreactive trypsinogen (IRT), has been in use in parts of the UK since 1980. Currently, screening occurs in 20% of England and the whole of the rest of the UK. However, there are differing protocols and, in August 2004, the UK Newborn Screening Programme Centre initiated the rollout of a national cystic fibrosis screening programme, to be completed in April 2007.

Other inborn errors of metabolism (Ch. 34)

Tandem mass spectrometry now allows broad metabolic screening programmes detecting disorders of fatty acid or amino acid metabolism. Many centres around the world offer such a programme, but in the UK there are concerns about difficulties in interpreting findings and in counselling parents appropriately. There is a pilot programme for medium-chain acyl-coA dehydrogenase (MCAD) deficiency.

Newborn hearing screening (Ch. 32)

Congenital bilateral hearing impairment affects about 1:1000 infants. Neonatal screening can be achieved using transient evoked oto-acoustic emissions. Failures can be retested with automated threshold brainstem evoked responses. Currently, screening targets those with a family (30%) or neonatal intensive care (29%) history and those with craniofacial abnormalities (12%). This leaves 29% with no risk factors and therefore at risk of late diagnosis. There is evidence that early diagnosis (before 6 months) leads to better receptive and expressive language skills. The cost-effectiveness of universal over targeted screening has been extensively debated in the UK, and a rolling training and implementation programme was started in 2001 and completed in October 2005.

Mark Davies   Angus Clarke

9

Clinical genetics

LEARNING OUTCOMES

By the end of this chapter you should:

- Be able to recognize features suggestive of a genetic disease
- Be able to obtain a family history and draw a pedigree.
- Understand the basic science that underpins genetics
- Understand the potential advantages and difficulties of genetic testing, as well as the long-term implications
- Understand when to refer to the clinical genetics department and what genetic counselling involves.

MODULE TWO

Clinical pointers to genetic disorders

In a genetic disease the fundamental pathological problem is with the genetic material, at the level of either chromosomes or deoxyribonucleic acid (DNA). Some genetic diseases form part of the recognized differential diagnoses for relatively common presenting problems, e.g. Prader–Willi syndrome in a hypotonic child, while others are recognized by their distinctive features, e.g. the dysmorphic features of Down's syndrome.

The following features should alert you to the possibility of a genetic condition, even when the precise diagnosis is not initially apparent:

- Multiple problems in the same individual, including:
  - Congenital abnormalities
  - Growth problems (e.g. short stature, microcephaly)
  - Neurodevelopmental problems, including developmental delay or cognitive impairment, regression, seizures and focal neurological signs
  - Unusual tumours (Ch. 51), the presence of multiple tumours in an individual, or more cancers in the family history than would be expected from chance alone
- Multiple individuals in the same family being affected by the same problem(s), such as those listed above.

The history and examination in genetic disorders

There are some areas in the diagnostic process that are of particular significance in genetic conditions, in addition to the history of the presenting complaint, the past medical history and the drug history. When the presenting features do not suggest a limited differential diagnosis, then the subsequent history and examination need to be wide-ranging (Table 9.1).

The physical examination may need to be equally comprehensive, depending on the circumstances. Use of a checklist can help to ensure a systematic record of physical features (Fig. 9.1).

Many genetic conditions are associated with growth abnormalities, particularly short stature, so plot height, weight and head circumference on centile charts. Serial plots are important. Some genetic diseases, e.g. Down's

Table 9.1 Key points in the history and examination of genetic disorders

Areas within the history	Key points
Antenatal	Infections or skin rashes, exposure to teratogens (such as alcohol or anti-epileptic medication) Intrauterine growth restriction or other complication
Obstetric	Gestational age Birth weight Complications during delivery
Development	Developmental progress Evidence of regression
Family	Construct a pedigree. An adequate family history can be essential for diagnosis of a genetic condition and in determining risk to family members

Height _____ Weight _____ Head circumference _____
Head appearance _____
   Eyes _____
   Ears _____
   Nose _____
   Palpebral fissure _____
   Mouth _____
   Teeth _____
Neck _____
Chest wall _____
   Nipples _____
   Heart _____
   Lungs _____
Abdominal wall _____
Genitalia _____
Anus _____
Spine _____
Arms _____
Hands _____
   Fingers _____
   Fingernails _____
   Palmar creases _____
Legs _____
Feet _____
   Toes _____
   Toenails _____
Skin _____
Hair _____

Fig. 9.1 A checklist for the recording of physical features

syndrome and achondroplasia, have condition-specific growth charts.

Clinical photographs are useful when discussing cases with colleagues or reviewing the natural history in the future.

It is not uncommon for parents of an affected child to have mild features of a condition, of which they have been completely unaware. Examination of family members may give clues to the diagnosis, affect the estimated risk of recurrence and have health implications for those found to have a hitherto unrecognized genetic condition.

A number of concepts are relevant when interpreting family histories and the examination of family members:

• *Penetrance* refers to the proportion of individuals possessing a disease-causing alteration who show some evidence of the condition, even if this is mild. The penetrance may vary with age. If a genetic alteration is completely penetrant, all individuals who carry the alteration will show evidence of the condition; if only a proportion manifest the condition, the genetic alteration is said to be incompletely penetrant.

• *Expression* refers to the degree to which an individual is affected. Sometimes, even within a family, different individuals with the same underlying alteration may be affected by greatly varying degrees of severity and by different features of the condition.

If an affected child presents with an autosomal dominant condition, but both parents are apparently unaffected and blood tests do not show the relevant mutation in either of them, then two possibilities must be considered:

1. A new mutation may have occurred in the child.
2. One of the parents carries the mutation in a proportion of their germ cells and perhaps in other tissues too, but not in their leucocytes.

A person who carries a mutation in a proportion of their cells is said to be mosaic for the mutation. Germinal mosaicism is when the mutation affects a proportion of germ-line cells. People with mosaicism can be severely affected or may have no detectable manifestations of a

---

Skill: pedigree construction

Drawing a family tree or pedigree is a key skill in genetics. A pedigree synthesizes a large amount of genetic information and presents it in a clear manner that can aid interpretation. Possible mechanisms of inheritance or links between conditions in family members can be clarified, allowing the differential diagnosis to be refined. Understanding the position of a person in the family tree is also essential for risk estimation.

A pedigree should encompass at least three generations and be drawn using conventional symbols (Fig. 9.2). Start with the person you are seeing (known as the consultand) and place that person on the pedigree sheet, positioning him or her according to anticipated place in the family structure. The person through whom the family was brought to attention, or 'ascertained', is known as the proband and should be marked with an arrow. The pedigree should be structured into tiers, with every member of a generation being on the same tier.

When drawing a pedigree it is good practice to:

• Ask about miscarriages, abortions, stillbirths and infant deaths
• Take details about both sides of the family
• Ask about consanguinity, specifically but tactfully
• Record dates of birth rather than ages.

The degree of information required about each family member will vary depending on the nature of condition, the person's position within a family and whether he or she is potentially affected or not. Obtaining a family history, like taking the history of a presenting complaint, should be focused and driven by clear ideas of what information is required and what use is going to be made of that information, bearing in mind that the information required may often be wide-ranging.

Pedigrees can be complicated, particularly in large families or where there is multiple consanguinity. Whilst accuracy is more important than aesthetics, one of the skills of pedigree drawing is to maintain clarity of presentation in such complex families. Even the most experienced pedigree drawer will sometimes have to redraw a pedigree taken in a clinic, particularly when a suddenly remembered uncle with multiple offspring has to be introduced, at the last minute, into what was until then a model of pedigree design.

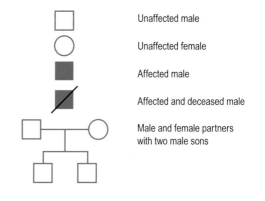

Unaffected male

Unaffected female

Affected male

Affected and deceased male

Male and female partners with two male sons

Fig. 9.2 **Symbols used in pedigrees**

condition. Even those with no signs of being affected may have a high risk of the condition recurring in future children, if a high proportion of germ-line cells carry the mutation. If the child of someone who is mosaic inherits the mutation, that child will carry the mutation in every cell in the body and is, therefore, likely to be more severely affected than the parent.

Clinical genetics and genetic counselling

When a referral is made for a clinical genetics assessment, the family may be addressed on more than one level. While a clinical genetic consultation will sometimes have a very clinical or technical focus, with the clinician attempting to understand the cause of a disease or transmitting detailed information about this to the family, at other times it may address deep emotional issues or family strategies for coping with the difficult practical problems of life with disease or disability. It is hoped that this range of issues will be dealt with in an integrated, holistic manner that is experienced by the family as supportive. Clinical genetics services often take pride in being led by their clients; it is therefore difficult to produce standardized measures of outcomes or effectiveness, because the goals differ from one consultation and family to the next.

One of the key tasks of genetic counselling is providing information. However, this process must begin by listening to find out what the concerns and questions of the clients are. (People attending a genetic counselling clinic are generally referred to as clients rather than patients to avoid the implication that they are suffering from a disease when often they are not.) The information sought may encompass diagnosis, likely prognosis and management of the condition, inheritance, risks that other relatives, including future children, may be affected, and options available to deal with these risks.

It is important to establish the diagnosis as clearly as possible. This can involve taking a history and examining affected individuals, performing investigations, obtaining a family history and reviewing the notes of other family members. If the counsellor is unfamiliar with the condition, it may be necessary to seek out information from the medical literature or from colleagues. A risk estimation can be calculated, based on knowledge of the condition and its inheritance, and the position of the clients within their family.

The information sought by the clients must then be communicated to them, in a manner sensitive to their ability to understand it. If clients are then faced with decisions, e.g. regarding prenatal or predictive testing, they can be offered support in the decision-making process. One approach is to discuss the various scenarios that could arise and to encourage them to consider their anticipated responses to the different scenarios and also the possible responses of their partner, family and others. The clients should feel supported, whatever their decision. Once decisions have been made, it may be necessary to make the practical arrangements required to implement them.

One of the long-standing tenets of genetic counselling is that the process should be non-directive, i.e. that a person should not be led to make particular decisions but be helped to make decisions that seem most appropriate from their perspective. This reflects the importance attached to autonomy in the current view of medical ethics.

However, the context in which genetic counselling takes place makes it reasonable to ask if truly non-directive counselling is possible. Choices and beliefs will be clouded by the options made available and by perceived societal values, and the counsellor is not immune from these influences. It is not always necessary to try to maintain a position of strict neutrality when presenting options. For example, when a person is undergoing presymptomatic testing for a condition for which an effective medical intervention is available, then it may be appropriate for the counsellor to favour testing whilst allowing the client to make his or her own informed decision.

Genetic testing

A genetic test can be considered to be any investigation that may reveal evidence of genetic disease. However, genetic testing is generally considered to refer to investigations where DNA or chromosomes are directly analysed, or where a specific genetic condition is tested for by another means (such as abdominal ultrasound for polycystic kidney disease or serum creatine kinase for Xp21 muscular dystrophy).

Types of genetic test include:
- *Diagnostic genetic test.* A person with signs or symptoms of a genetic disease is tested to confirm or exclude the diagnosis.
- *Predictive or presymptomatic test.* This establishes whether an otherwise healthy person carries a genetic alteration that may lead to a particular genetic disease in the future.

This distinction is particularly important in children. Genetic investigations are often essential in establishing the diagnosis in a sick child. Genetic testing of healthy (so far unaffected) children may also be warranted in those at increased risk of a condition likely to develop in childhood. Otherwise, uncertainty over a child's risk may lead to serious distress within a family, with over-interpretation of minor problems. If a condition can be prevented or ameliorated by treatment, then genetic testing will be worth while. However, it is not always beneficial to carry out presymptomatic testing in children, particularly for adult-onset conditions for which no treatment is available. Children tested for Huntington's disease lose their opportunity to decide for themselves whether to be tested as adults (bearing in mind that only 15–20% of adults at risk of Huntington's disease decide to be tested). Adults retain control of the confidentiality over a test result and how this information is used, whilst this control is generally forfeited when a child is tested. Knowledge of the test result could lead to emotional and social problems in the child, altering both relationships within a family and expectation for the future in a variety of areas such as education, employment and relationships.

The nature of genetic disorders, our incomplete understanding of their complexities and the limitations of the techniques used to carry out genetic testing mean that care must be taken when interpreting test results and explaining their implications to children and their families.

For many types of genetic analysis, a negative test result must be interpreted with caution in case it is a false negative, i.e. a genetic abnormality is actually present but was not detected by the test.

The pathological significance of a detected genetic alteration may be unclear. For example, a missense mutation may not always lead to an alteration in a protein's function and may not lead to disease. Even when a person is shown to carry a genetic alteration known to cause disease, it can be difficult to predict just how the person will be affected because of variable penetrance and expression.

When performing genetic testing, it is important to be aware that the diagnosis of a genetic disease will not only have implications for the affected individual but may have ramifications for other family members, who may be at risk of being affected or of being carriers for the condition.

Screening (see also Ch. 15)

Genetic screening involves testing apparently unaffected individuals in order to detect unrecognized genetic disease, its precursors or carrier status, when there is no particular reason to suspect that the individual is at increased risk compared to other members of the group being targeted for screening. Screening programmes may include the whole population or large subgroups, e.g. all pregnant women or all newborn babies (Box 9.1).

Screening programmes can be evaluated against well-recognized criteria (Box 9.2). Screening programmes for genetic conditions do not always fulfil these criteria, as with newborn screening for Duchenne muscular

---

BOX 9.1 Conditions screened for in newborn babies in the UK

In all areas
- Phenylketonuria
- Congenital hypothyroidism

In some areas, but being introduced in all areas within the UK
- Cystic fibrosis
- Sickle cell disease

In some areas only and/or under evaluation
- Medium-chain acyl-coA dehydrogenase (MCAD) deficiency
- Duchenne muscular dystrophy
- Galactosaemia

BOX 9.2 Abbreviated criteria for a screening programme*

- The condition being screened for is an important health problem despite optimal use of treatments and of other attempts to make an early diagnosis
- Early intervention before affected individuals would otherwise present leads to improved outcome
- The screening test is simple, safe and precise
- The test is acceptable to those screened and to health professionals
- The test is introduced with adequate resources, monitoring and management

* Adapted from National Screening Committee.

---

dystrophy. Screening for this condition has been advocated on the basis that it enables families to make informed reproductive decisions in the future and spares them from the distress of an often delayed and protracted diagnostic process.

There are four major categories of population genetic screening programme:

1. *Newborn screening* — as for phenylketonuria and congenital hypothyroidism
2. *Antenatal screening* — the use of maternal blood samples and fetal ultrasound screening to identify those pregnancies in which the fetus has a structural malformation or a chromosomal anomaly
3. *Carrier screening* — which may take place in the antenatal clinic or elsewhere
4. *Disease susceptibility screening* — as with cholesterol screening for evidence of familial hyperlipidaemia or DNA-based screening for haemochromatosis.

The word 'screening' has three other related meanings in this context:

- 'Cascade screening' — the relatives of those carrying a genetic disorder are approached to see if they wish to be tested for that condition.
- A search for mutations within a gene may be described as 'screening' of the gene — this use is probably best avoided.
- The ongoing monitoring of a patient at risk of complications from the family's condition.

Whenever we use the word 'screening', we should strive to keep its meaning clear.

Prenatal testing and the selective termination of pregnancies

Prenatal testing is offered for some but not all genetic conditions. Factors that influence this provision include the severity of the condition, the effectiveness of treatment available and the accuracy of the prenatal test. When prenatal testing is available, then in any individual case several factors need to be taken into account, including the genetic risk to that pregnancy, the couple's wish to proceed with testing and their attitude to the risks involved and to a possible termination of pregnancy. Given the risk to the fetus associated with invasive diagnostic procedures, some consider it unethical to carry them out if the couple would continue with the pregnancy anyway; others accept that parents may wish to prepare themselves for an affected child. It is important to note that promoting the termination of affected pregnancies is not the primary goal of prenatal testing; it is rather to promote informed reproductive decisions and to reduce suffering in those affected by genetic conditions.

Commonly used techniques available for prenatal diagnosis and screening

Maternal serum screening is used to look for evidence of neural tube defects and trisomy 21 (p. 165). Neural tube defects result in elevated serum alpha-fetoprotein levels. Risk of trisomy 21 is assessed using combinations of alpha-fetoprotein, oestriol human chorionic gonadotrophin, inhibin or pregnancy-associated plasma protein-A (PAPP-A). Alpha-fetoprotein, PAPP-A and oestriol are reduced in trisomy 21 pregnancies; human chorionic gonadotrophin and inhibin are raised.

Ultrasound is similarly non-invasive. It can detect a wide range of abnormalities. Some of these, termed 'soft markers', indicate abnormality only in a proportion of cases, e.g. nuchal oedema, which is associated with trisomy 21. A 'fetal anomaly scan' is usually made available to women at 18–20 weeks' gestation, and ultrasound assessment of nuchal translucency is increasingly being performed in the first trimester to identify pregnancies at risk of chromosomal aneuploidy.

Amniocentesis involves the aspiration of amniotic fluid that contains a suspension of cells of fetal origin. It is usually performed at 15–16 weeks and is associated with a 0.5–1% risk of miscarriage. Once obtained, the sample is centrifuged; the supernatant can be used for alpha-fetoprotein estimation and the cells are cultured. Biochemical, molecular and chromosomal studies can be carried out on these cells. The time delay before a result is available depends on the particular test, and is partly due to the time needed to culture sufficient cells. Typically, chromosomal analysis now takes < 10 days.

Chorionic villus sampling (CVS) involves obtaining a sample of the fetal-derived chorionic villus by ultrasound-guided transcervical or transabdominal aspiration. The procedure can be carried out from ~11 weeks and carries a 1–2% risk of miscarriage. Direct chromosomal analysis of uncultured chorionic villus cells often allows a provisional result to be obtained in 24 hours but detailed chromosomal analysis requires cultured cells. Most DNA and biochemical studies can be performed on uncultured cells.

Counselling issues in genetic laboratory prenatal diagnosis

When counselling a woman or couple regarding prenatal testing, it is important to discuss a number of issues:

- The nature of the condition being tested for
- The risks of the fetus having the condition
- The different options of testing available, including the risks of the procedures
- The fact that results may not be obtained, or may be ambiguous or unexpected
- How the information gained from testing may alter their plans with regard to continuing the pregnancy.

Problems complicating prenatal diagnosis

Failure to obtain a result

Sometimes it can prove impossible to obtain a suitable sample or the cells fail to grow. For CVS and amniocentesis, the risk of either of these events occurring is under 1%.

Unanticipated results

Most invasive prenatal diagnostic procedures are carried out because of concern about the increased risk of trisomy 21, but testing will sometimes reveal unexpected chromosomal abnormalities, e.g. trisomy 18 or Klinefelter's syndrome.

Results of uncertain significance

For example, an apparently balanced translocation may be seen in the fetus. If either of the parents carries the same arrangement, then there is only a very small chance that the fetus will be affected. However, if the translocation is a new event, then the risk is higher.

Apparent mosaicism

This is seen in 1% of CVS. It may arise as an artefact of culture or as a result of sample contamination with maternal cells when it has no implications for the fetus. Sometimes it is restricted to the placenta and may have no implications for the fetus. An amniocentesis will often be chosen by the parents to try to clarify the situation if CVS has indicated mosaicism. However, even if the fetus is confirmed as a mosaic, there may well still be uncertainty as to the likely effects of this on the child.

Basic science

DNA

Genetic information is encoded by molecules of DNA, which is a polymer made up of nucleotide units. Each nucleotide consists of a deoxyribose sugar molecule, a phosphate group and a nitrogenous base. There are four different types of base:

- Adenine and guanine (which are based on purine rings)
- Thymine and cytosine (which are based on pyridimine rings).

Two linear but antiparallel and complementary strands of DNA wrap around each other, giving rise to an interlocked double helix. The sugar and phosphate groups form the linear backbone of the strands with the bases projecting inwards towards their partners, forming hydrogen bonds with the complementary base in the opposing strand. Adenine bonds with thymine and guanine with cytosine.

RNA

Ribonucleic acid (RNA) differs from DNA in that it is single-stranded, uracil is found in place of thymine, and the sugar group is ribose. RNA has a number of functions in the cell, including:

- Transfer of information from chromosome to ribosome during protein synthesis
- Bringing the appropriate amino acids to the ribosomes during protein synthesis
- Catalytic activities
- Structural role in macromolecules, such as ribosomes
- Control of gene expression.

Genes

A gene is a unit of DNA containing information that determines the composition of an RNA molecule and is most often translated into protein.

Genotype and phenotype

The genotype refers to a specific version of a gene (alleles at a particular position or locus) or more widely to the genetic constitution of an individual organism. The phenotype refers to the observable characteristics or clinical features arising from a particular genotype.

Genes and the environment

The phenotype arises as a result of an interaction between the genotype and the environment from conception and throughout life. This interaction can account for the phenotypic variation sometimes seen between individuals with the same mutation in a given gene. For some phenotypic features the genetic influence is predominant; for others there is a much larger environmental influence.

A phenocopy is an environmentally induced phenotype that mimics the phenotype produced by a mutation. For example, autosomal recessive tubular dysgenesis, which is characterized by fetal anuria, perinatal death, skull ossification defects and absent or scarce renal proximal tubules, is caused by mutations in genes encoding components of the renin–angiotensin system. A similar phenotype results from in utero exposure to angiotensin-converting enzyme (ACE) inhibitors or angiotensin II receptor antagonists.

From gene to protein

Protein synthesis requires a number of steps.

Transcription

An RNA copy of one strand of the gene sequence (used as a template) is synthesized by the enzyme,

RNA polymerase. The raw transcript is then edited to produce the messenger RNA (mRNA) molecule. Each nucleotide in the mRNA is complementary to one in the DNA template.

Post-transcriptional processing

Most mammalian genes consist of exons, which are units of coding sequence, and introns, the intervening non-coding sequences. The initial transcript is edited to splice out the introns from the RNA and the exons are ligated together.

Translation

Protein synthesis occurs at cytoplasmic structures called ribosomes (consisting of ribosomal RNA and proteins). At the ribosome the mRNA forms a template for the synthesis of a specific sequence of amino acids, giving rise to a polypeptide chain. This process is mediated by transfer RNA (tRNA). A transfer RNA bound to a specific amino acid recognizes a sequence of three bases (termed a codon) in the mRNA. This correlation between codons and amino acids is the basis of the genetic code. There are 20 essential amino acids but, as there are four different types of base, there are 64 possible combinations of three bases. Some of the codons represent stop signals that terminate protein synthesis. Some amino acids are coded for by more than one triplet.

Post-translational modification

Many proteins undergo some form of post-translational modification, e.g. cleavage of the polypeptide chain or addition of sugar groups.

Chromosomes

Chromosomes consist of DNA and proteins with structural or functional roles. Most human cells are diploid; they contain two copies of the genome. There are 22 pairs of autosomal chromosomes and one pair of sex chromosomes, giving a total of 46 chromosomes per somatic (i.e. non-germ line) cell. The normal male karyotype is 46,XY and the normal female karyotype is 46,XX.

Chromosomes are identified under a microscope by their size, by their pattern of banding when stained, and by the position of a region known as the centromere that plays a key role in cell division. The centromere divides chromosomes into short (termed p) and long (termed q) arms. If the centromere is located centrally, the chromosomes are designated metacentric; if it is located peripherally, the chromosome is acrocentric.

The end of each chromosome arm is termed the telomere. This is a specialized structure thought to play an important role in maintaining the integrity of chromosomes. The chromosomal regions adjacent to telomeres, the subtelomeric regions, are particularly gene-rich.

Mitosis and meiosis

There are two different types of cell division: mitosis and meiosis. During the interphase before cell division, there is a round of DNA synthesis leading to duplication of the genome. Each replicated chromosome consists of two sister chromatids, joined at the centromere. Mitosis is the mechanism by which most cells replicate and results in the production of two genetically identical daughter cells, both with a diploid genome. During mitosis there is one cell division, with sister chromatids being split and partitioned into the daughter cells. Meiosis is the type of cell division that gives rise to spermatogonia and öogonia. This involves two successive cell divisions, giving rise to daughter cells with a haploid genome, i.e. only one copy of each chromosome. In the parent cell, one copy of each chromosome was maternally derived, the other paternally derived. As the daughter cells only contain one copy of each chromosome (either the original paternally or maternally derived chromosome), they are not genetically identical. Further genetic diversity results from the exchange of material between homologous chromosome pairs during meiosis.

Chromosomal abnormalities and mutations

A mutation is both the process of alteration of DNA and the altered DNA sequence that results. Mutations range from structural chromosome changes that are visible microscopically to single nucleotide alterations. Mutations may result in disease (pathogenic mutations) or not (non-pathogenic mutations).

A polymorphism is traditionally said to exist when there are at least two variants at a site (at least two alleles at a locus), with the least common variant accounting for at least 1% of the alleles in the population. A polymorphism generally does not result in overt disease, although it may influence factors such as susceptibility to disease or risk of side-effects from a drug. A single nucleotide polymorphism (SNP) is an alteration of a single nucleotide.

Chromosomal abnormalities

These can be classified as either numerical or structural.

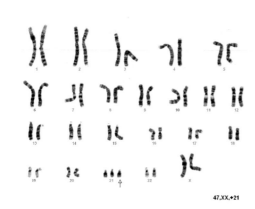

47,XX,+21

Fig. 9.3 Karyotype showing trisomy 21

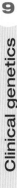

Numerical abnormalities (Fig. 9.3)

- *Polyploidy* is the presence of additional sets of 23 chromosomes, e.g. triploidy.
- *Aneuploidy* is the presence or absence of one or more individual chromosomes.
- *Trisomy* is the presence of three copies of a chromosome, e.g. trisomy 21 in Down's syndrome. Box 9.3 shows early clinical findings in trisomies.
- *Monosomy* is the presence of only one member of the relevant chromosome pair, e.g. monosomy X in Turner's syndrome.

Structural abnormalities (Fig. 9.4)

- A *translocation* involves the transfer of material from one chromosome to another. A balanced translocation results in no loss of genetic material. A reciprocal translocation involves breaks in two chromosomes and exchange between them, giving rise to two derivative chromosomes. A Robertsonian translocation arises from breaks at or close to the centromeres of acrocentric chromosomes, leading to the fusion of two acrocentric chromosomes and the loss of their short arm sequences.
- An *insertion* is the insertion of a chromosomal segment into another position on a chromosome.
- A *deletion* is loss of part of a chromosome.
- A *duplication* is the duplication of part of a chromosome.
- An *inversion* involves the position of a segment of chromosome being rotated by 180°.
- A *ring chromosome* arises when a break occurs in both arms of a chromosome and the two ends then join to form a ring.

Sex chromosome abnormalities

Turner's syndrome (p. 241)

There is loss of part or all of one of the sex chromosomes. About 50% of affected individuals have the

a) **Reciprocal chromosomal translocation**

b) **Insertion**

c) **Deletion**

d) **Inversion**

e) **Duplication**

f) **Ring chromosome**

Fig. 9.4 Chromosome rearrangements

karyotype 45,X; the remainder have a variety of abnormalities of one of the sex chromosomes. (About 5–10% will have some Y chromosome material.)

Klinefelter's syndrome

People affected by Klinefelter's syndrome have an additional X chromosome (47,XXY) or occasionally 46,XX chromosomes, with one X carrying the *SRY* gene.

Clinical features include:

- Infertility
- Hypogonadism
- Tall stature
- Gynaecomastia

Trisomy 13 (Patau's syndrome)
- Cleft lip
- Brain malformations
- Hypotelorism
- Small eyes
- Scalp defects
- Polydactyly
- Cardiac and other organ abnormalities

Trisomy 18 (Edwards' syndrome)
- Microcephaly
- Micrognathia
- Clinodactyly
- Rocker bottom feet
- Cognitive impairment
- Cardiac and renal abnormalities

Trisomy 21 (Down's syndrome)
- Hypotonia
- Epicanthic folds and upward-slanted palpebral fissures
- Protruding tongue
- Brushfield spots in iris
- Abnormal palmar and plantar skin creases
- Duodenal atresia
- Cardiac abnormalities

- Normal cognitive function usually (but can have learning and psychological difficulties).

Submicroscopic mutations

These can be classified as:
- *Substitutions*: the replacement of one nucleotide by another
- *Insertions*: the addition of one or more nucleotide
- *Deletions*: the loss of one or more nucleotide.

Additionally, mutations in the coding regions of genes can be classified depending on their effect on the amino acid sequence:
- *Synonymous mutations*: these do not alter the polypeptide sequence, e.g. the conversion of one codon to another coding for the same amino acid.
- *Non-synonymous mutations*: these do lead to an alteration in the polypeptide sequence. There are different types of non-synonymous mutation:
  - *Missense mutations* are single-base pair changes that result in the substitution of one amino acid for another.

  - *Nonsense mutations* are changes that result in the formation of a stop codon and lead to premature termination of protein synthesis.
  - *Frameshift mutations* are insertions or deletions of nucleotides that are not a multiple of three. This shifts the reading frame, leading to totally different codons downstream from the mutation, usually arriving before very far at a nonsense triplet and therefore to chain termination.

Patterns of inheritance

Autosomal dominant

The disorder is expressed either largely or completely in the heterozygote. All offspring of an affected person will have a 50% chance of inheriting the mutation, giving rise to vertical transmission in a pedigree. Variable expression and incomplete penetrance can complicate recognition of autosomal dominant inheritance. Examples of autosomal dominant conditions are given in Box 9.4.

Autosomal recessive

The disorder is expressed largely or completely in the affected homozygote. Often this presents as an isolated case within a pedigree or as affected siblings. Where both parents are carriers, each of their offspring has a 25% risk of being homozygous and a 50% risk of being a heterozygous carrier. Examples of autosomal recessive disorders are given in Box 9.5.

Sex-linked (X chromosome) disease

These conditions result from mutations in a gene carried on the X chromosome. Males will usually be affected, as they will only have one copy of the gene.

- Achondroplasia
- Facioscapulohumeral dystrophy
- Hereditary elliptocytosis
- Hereditary spherocytosis
- Huntington's disease
- Marfan's syndrome
- Myotonic dystrophy
- Neurofibromatosis types 1 and 2
- Noonan's syndrome
- Tuberous sclerosis complex
- von Willebrand's disease

BOX 9.5 Examples of autosomal recessive conditions

- Alpha$_1$-antitrypsin deficiency
- Ataxia telangiectasia
- Beta-thalassaemia
- Congenital adrenal hyperplasia
- Cystic fibrosis
- Fanconi anaemia
- Galactosaemia
- Glycogen storage disorders
- Haemochromatosis
- Homocystinura
- Mucopolysaccharidoses (except Hunter's syndrome)
- Oculocutaneous albinism
- Phenylketonuria
- Sickle cell disease
- Spinal muscular atrophy
- Wilson's disease
- Zellweger's syndrome

BOX 9.6 Examples of X-linked disorders

- Becker muscular dystrophy
- Duchenne muscular dystrophy
- Fabry's disease
- Glucose-6-phosphate dehydrogenase deficiency
- Haemophilias A and B
- Hunter's syndrome (mucopolysaccharidosis type II)
- Hypohidrotic ectodermal dysplasia
- Incontinentia pigmenti (usually in females only)
- Lesch–Nyhan syndrome
- Ocular albinism
- Rett's syndrome (very largely restricted to females)
- Wiskott–Aldrich syndrome

In females one of the X chromosomes is inactivated. This occurs at around day 15 of gestation. Which X chromosome is inactivated is a random event, but once inactivated, the X chromosome remains inactivated in all daughter cells. Not all the genes on an inactivated X chromosome are silent; some are expressed (which is why XO women exhibit the Turner phenotype). Female carriers of sex-linked conditions are usually unaffected but may show some features of the disease, depending upon the pattern of X chromosome inactivation in the woman's tissues and the biology of the gene product. A woman will tend to manifest such conditions rather less severely than an affected male. Features of this sex-linked form of inheritance are:

- There is no male-to-male transmission.
- All daughters of an affected male will be carriers.
- The risk to sons of women who are carriers is 50%.
- The risk that daughters of female carriers will themselves be carriers is 50%.

There has been a tendency to separate X chromosome gene disorders into X-linked recessive, which tend not to manifest much in females, and X-linked dominant, in which females are commonly affected and males may be so severely affected as to die in utero or in infancy (X-linked dominant, male-lethal). This demarcation is useful in looking at patterns of inheritance in a family, but is not very helpful in understanding how some women but not others come to show signs of the condition. Examples of X-linked disorders are given in Box 9.6.

Duchenne muscular dystrophy (Ch. 28)

This condition results from mutations in the dystrophin gene on Xp21. About 65% of mutations are deletions of one or more exons in the *DMD* gene, with another 5% or so being duplications and most of the rest being point mutations.

Female carriers of DMD mutations can develop problems such as muscle weakness (20%) and dilated cardiomyopathy (8%). About 50% have a raised serum creatine kinase. Rarely, females can have a more severe phenotype like that of affected males, due to chromosomal arrangement involving the *DMD* locus, non-random inactivation of the X chromosome due to problems with the inactivation process, or because they have coexistent Turner's syndrome.

Trinucleotide repeat disorders

Trinucleotide repeats are sequences in which a set of three nucleotides is repeated a variable number of times within a gene. Several disorders are associated with the abnormal expansion of trinucleotide repeats. Generally, the severity of the phenotype in these conditions is related to the number of repeats. The number of repeats can increase in successive generations, giving rise to the phenomenon of anticipation where there is an earlier age of onset and/or more severe manifestations in succeeding generations.

Important trinucleotide repeat disorders in paediatrics include the congenital form of myotonic dystrophy, the juvenile-onset form of Huntington's disease, Friedreich's ataxia and fragile X syndrome.

Fragile X syndrome

Fragile X (Ch. 29) is a common cause of cognitive impairment. It is associated with abnormal tri-

Table 9.2 Repeat lengths and expression in fragile X syndrome

Repeat length	Category
5–44	Normal
45–54	Intermediate
55–200	Premutation
> 200	Full mutation

nucleotide repeats in the *FMR1* gene. The size of the repeat and the sex of the affected person influence the phenotype (Table 9.2).

The repeat length of a premutation allele can increase during transmission, so the child of a premutation carrier could have a full mutation.

Males with a premutation do not have childhood cognitive impairment but can develop late-onset ataxia/tremor and cognitive deficits: fragile X-associated tremor/ataxia syndrome (FXTAS). Males with a full mutation have cognitive impairment (often moderate, but varies from mild to severe), a distinctive facial appearance (large head, prominent ears and chin) and post-pubertally large testes.

Females with a premutation are at risk of premature ovarian failure and, to a lesser degree than premutation males, late-onset ataxia. Females with a full mutation can exhibit the same physical and cognitive features as full mutation males but usually to a lesser extent.

Problem-orientated topic:

genetic counselling

Jack, a 4-year-old boy, has moderate cognitive impairment. You have received a report from the laboratory, which says he has a full mutation in *FMR1*, the gene responsible for fragile X syndrome. When you see the parents to give the result, they ask about the risk of this condition recurring in future pregnancies. The boy's mother, who is in her mid-30s, says they have been trying to conceive for the past 2 years without success. When reviewing the family history, you note that Jack's maternal grandfather developed a tremor and unsteady gait in later life that was attributed to Parkinson's disease.

Q1. What do you tell the parents about the risk of this recurring in another pregnancy?

Q2. Does this diagnosis have health implications for other family members?

Q1. What do you tell the parents about the risk of this recurring in another pregnancy?

There are a number of different possible explanations for this family history that have different implications for the risk to future offspring. It is possible that Jack's mother carries a full mutation but is unaffected or, more likely, is a premutation carrier. If she carries a full mutation, there will be a 50% risk of transmitting the mutated allele to each future child. If she is a premutation carrier, the risk of having an affected child depends on the premutation size in her and the sex of the child. For a repeat of 60–69, the risk that a son will be severely affected will be around 10%; for a repeat of 90–99, that risk will be around 47%. Analysis of the *FMR1* gene in Jack's mother would help to establish the likely risk for future pregnancies.

Q2. Does this diagnosis have health implications for other family members?

Other family members, who may not have any cognitive problems, may be at risk of having affected offspring, of FXTAS or of premature ovarian failure, and should be counselled accordingly.

Mitochondrial disorders

Each mitochondrion in a cell contains a circular DNA molecule that encodes components of the respiratory chain, ribosomal RNA and tRNA. The mitochondrial DNA is compact, contains little repetitive DNA and has no introns. The genetic code of mitochondrial DNA differs from nuclear DNA using some different amino acid codons.

Mitochondrial disorders can result from mutations in mitochondrial DNA or in nuclear genes coding for proteins that are transported into mitochondria. The nuclear gene abnormalities are inherited in an autosomal dominant or autosomal recessive manner. Mitochondrial DNA mutations are transmitted by maternal inheritance, i.e. they are passed down from mother to child but not from father to child. In most people all mitochondria contain identical copies of the mitochondrial genome at birth (i.e. are homoplastic), but in those with mitochondrial disorders there may be a variable mix of mitochondria with normal (wild-type) and mutated DNA within each cell (heteroplasmy).

Some affected individuals display a cluster of features suggestive of a particular syndrome (Table 9.3 and Box 9.7). However, many display symptoms that do not fit into a specific pattern.

Table 9.3 **Examples of some mitochondrial disorders**

Disorder	Primary features
Mitochondrial encephalomyopathy with lactic acidosis and stroke-like episodes (MELAS)	Stroke-like episodes, seizures, dementia, lactic acidosis
Leber hereditary optic neuropathy	Subacute painless visual loss, cardiac pre-excitation
Leigh's syndrome (not always caused by mutations in mitochondrial DNA)	Subacute relapsing encephalopathy, cerebellar and brainstem signs

BOX 9.7 Features associated with mitochondrial disorders

- Myopathy (especially ptosis and cardiomyopathy)
- Sensorineural deafness
- Diabetes mellitus
- Pigmentary retinopathy
- Lactic acidosis
- Seizures
- Ataxia
- Dementia
- Stroke-like episodes
- Spasticity
- Fluctuating encephalopathy

Where clinical features are suggestive of a particular mitochondrial syndrome, then specific clinical investigations can be used to define the phenotype and diagnostic testing of specific genes can be performed. A family history can be invaluable in suggesting the pattern of inheritance and the diagnosis. When a mitochondrial disorder is suspected but the diagnosis is not so clear, the following can be helpful: blood and/or cerebrospinal fluid lactate levels; genetic testing on blood for homoplasmic mutations; muscle biopsy (for histological/histochemical evidence of mitochondrial disease and for DNA analysis for heteroplasmic deletions); neuroimaging; and cardiac assessment.

Imprinting

For most autosomal genes, both alleles are expressed in a cell. However, for some genes only one allele is expressed, while the other is switched off. Whether an allele is expressed or not is determined by the sex of the parent that contributed it. This phenomenon is termed 'imprinting' (Fig. 9.5). In a maternally imprinted gene the maternally derived allele is inactivated. In a paternally imprinted gene the paternally derived allele is inactivated. Examples of conditions associated with imprinted genes are:

- Prader–Willi syndrome (PWS)
- Angelman's syndrome
- Beckwith–Wiedemann syndrome
- Silver–Russell syndrome (some cases only).

PWS is caused by a lack of *paternal* contribution at 15q11–13. This can arise:

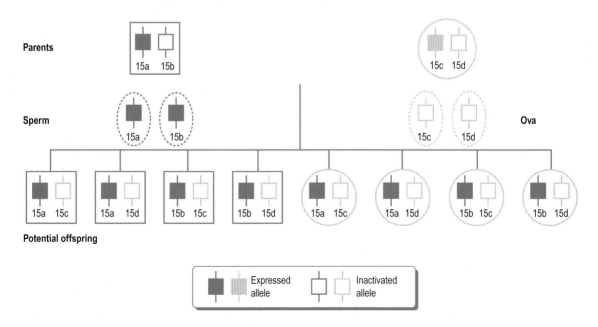

Fig. 9.5 The inheritance of a maternally imprinted gene.
Father represented in blue, mother in mauve. In the parents, only the paternally derived copies are expressed. In the ova, imprinting inactivates all maternally derived copies of the allele.

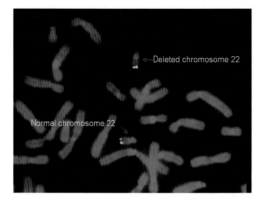

Fig. 9.6 Fluorescent in situ hybridization (FISH) with probes that hybridize to regions of chromosome 22.
 The region that the red probe binds to has been deleted in one chromosome 22.

- By deletion of this region in the paternally derived chromosome 15
- By uniparental disomy (where both copies of a chromosome are derived from one parent) — in this case, two copies of maternally derived chromosome 15
- Very uncommonly, by an imprinting centre mutation.

Angelman's syndrome, in which the degree of cognitive and motor problems is rather greater than for PWS, is caused by a lack of *maternal* contribution at part of 15q11–13 that is paternally imprinted. There are often deletions in the same chromosomal region as for PWS or, occasionally, paternal uniparental disomy for chromosome 15, or point mutations in the *UBE3A* gene or in the imprinting control region.

Applications of DNA technology

Examining chromosomes, stained to demonstrate their characteristic bands, under a microscope remains a mainstay of genetic diagnosis. However, techniques are available to demonstrate chromosomal abnormalities too small to be seen by this technique. Fluorescent in situ hybridization (FISH) involves the use of a fluorescently labelled probe to bind to a specific DNA sequence (Fig. 9.6). If that sequence is present in both copies of a chromosome, then under fluorescent microscopy the probe can be visualized binding to both. If it is absent in one copy, the probe will only bind to the chromosome homologue retaining the target sequence.

In the subtelomeric regions, which are gene-rich, small rearrangements can have profound phenotypic consequences. A number of techniques can be used to look for such subtelomeric rearrangements. One of the most commonly applied is multiprobe FISH, in which fluorescently labelled telomere-specific probes for all

chromosomes are used. Subtelomeric rearrangements have been found to account for approximately 6% of cases of mental retardation. Thus, analysis of the subtelomeric region has become an important second-line investigation in affected individuals when conventional cytogenetic techniques have revealed apparently normal chromosomes.

Comparative genomic hybridization (CGH) can be used to look at submicroscopic abnormalities along the length of chromosomes. Different colour fluorescent markers are used to label the patient's DNA (green) and reference DNA (red). These are then applied to a slide covered with normal human chromosomes and allowed to hybridize. The amount of green and red fluorescence is then compared, and will be 1:1 throughout if the patient's DNA is normal. More green means the patient has extra DNA in that area (because more copies of green-labelled patient DNA have 'stuck'). More red indicates that the patient is missing DNA in that area.

Several techniques are available to look for mutations at the DNA level. There is a trade-off between cost in resources needed for a given technique and accuracy. Because of this, one approach is to screen the gene in question using a high-throughput technique and to confirm any abnormalities detected using a resource-intensive but more accurate method. An alternative, useful for genes in which a small number of different mutations account for most cases, is to use the resource-intensive but more accurate methods just to look for those mutations and not to screen the rest of the gene.

Recombinant DNA technology

Recombinant DNA can be defined as DNA molecules constructed outside living cells by joining natural or synthetic DNA segments to DNA molecules that can replicate in living cells, or the molecules that result from their replication.

Recombinant DNA techniques can be used to isolate, characterize or alter genes and to insert genes into cells, allowing their product to be studied or commercially utilized.

Gene cloning refers to the production of multiple identical copies of a gene. One strategy for cloning a mammalian gene is to introduce that gene into bacteria. This strategy requires a number of steps:

1. Prepare complementary DNA (cDNA) from mRNA extracted from the mammalian cells. The total complement of mRNA represents all the genes that are transcribed. The mRNA does not contain any intronic material, as this has been spliced out. Complementary DNA can be prepared from the mRNA using a reverse transcriptase.

2. Amplify the cDNA of the target gene by polymerase chain reaction (PCR).
3. Insert the target gene into a cloning vector, a DNA molecule that carries the foreign DNA into a host cell where the vector with the inserted gene can replicate. A typical vector is a bacterial plasmid that has been constructed to carry a selectable marker, e.g. a gene that confirms resistance to an antibiotic.
4. Insert the plasmid into bacterial cells. Culturing the bacteria in media containing the antibiotic to which the plasmid confers resistance will select the bacteria that have taken up the plasmid, as only these will grow.

The successfully transformed bacteria, those that contain the plasmid with the target gene, will express the gene product and can be easily grown in the laboratory or, if necessary, on an industrial scale to provide supplies of biomolecules too complex to synthesize commercially using conventional chemical techniques, such as human factor 8 or insulin.

Imti Choonara

Pharmacology and therapeutics

LEARNING OUTCOMES

By the end of this chapter you should:

- Know and understand the principles of pharmacokinetics in children
- Know and understand the major pathways of drug metabolism in paediatric patients of different ages
- Know and understand some of the major adverse drug reactions that have occurred in paediatric patients
- Know and understand the mechanisms by which adverse drug reactions may occur in paediatric patients
- Know how to prescribe medicines safely
- Be aware of the most frequent types of medication error associated with drug prescribing for children
- Know and understand the principles of the use of antimicrobials
- Know how to assess pain in paediatric patients of different ages
- Understand how to manage pain in children.

MODULE TWO

Introduction

To prescribe medicines safely, one needs to understand how the human body handles different medicines. In order to do this, one needs to have a basic understanding of clinical pharmacology. It is important to recognize that children handle medicines differently to adults, and therefore one needs to understand the interaction between age and clinical pharmacology; this is described below.

Pharmacokinetics

Pharmacokinetics is the relationship between the dose of a drug and its concentration in different parts of the body (usually plasma) in relation to time, and is defined numerically in a quantitative manner. Mathematical formulae are available that describe the interrelationship between clearance, volume of distribution and elimination half-life. These terms are described below.

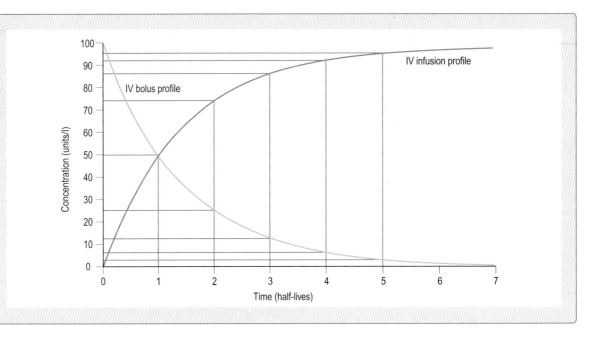

Fig. 10.1 Concentration–time profiles following a single intravenous bolus dose and during a constant rate infusion. Time is shown in half-lives. A total of 97% of the drug is eliminated and 97% of steady state is achieved in five half-lives.
(Reproduced from Thomson 2000, with permission.)

Absorption

If a drug is given intravenously, then 100% of the dose enters the blood stream. If a drug is given orally, then usually only a fraction is absorbed; the term 'bioavailability' is used to describe the percentage of the drug administered that reaches the systemic circulation. Absorption is often reduced following oral administration in the neonatal period.

Volume of distribution (V)

This is not a physiological volume, but rather an apparent volume into which the drug would have to distribute to achieve the measured concentration. Water-soluble drugs, such as gentamicin, have a V that is similar to the extracellular fluid volume. Drugs that are highly bound to plasma proteins have a low V. Differences between paediatric and adult patients stem mainly from the fact that neonates and young children have a higher proportion of body water and lower concentrations of plasma proteins.

Clearance

Clearance describes the removal of a drug from the body and is defined as the volume (usually of plasma) that is completely cleared of drug in a given time period. In adults, clearance is therefore described in relation to volume/time (ml/min). In paediatric patients, clearance is also described in relation to body weight (ml/min/kg).

Elimination half-life

The elimination half-life is inversely related to the clearance. The elimination half-life is the time it takes for the concentration of a drug (usually in plasma) to fall to half its original value. By definition, therefore, 50% of the dose will be eliminated in one half-life. Five half-lives is the time required for 97% of the drug to be eliminated (Fig. 10.1). This is also the time required for steady state to be achieved following initial administration of the drug.

Therapeutic drug monitoring

Therapeutic drug monitoring (TDM) consists of measuring plasma concentrations of the drug in order to improve efficacy and reduce toxicity (Box 10.1). It is useful if there is a clear relationship between the plasma concentration and the clinical effect. A specific, precise and accurate analytical technique is required to measure plasma concentrations of a drug. TDM is recommended for aminoglycosides in order to reduce toxicity (p. 106). It may be beneficial in patients with poorly controlled epilepsy who are receiving carbamazepine, phenytoin or phenobarbital (Chs 24 and 28). It is also clinically useful with a variety of other medications. Interpretation of the plasma concentration of a drug requires details of the time of administration of the drug and time of collection of the blood sample, as well as an understanding of why TDM has been requested.

Key points

- Clearance is usually reduced in the neonatal period.
- The half-life is usually longer in the neonatal period.

Drug metabolism

The major pathways involved in drug metabolism are divided into phase 1 (oxidation, reduction, hydrolysis and hydration) and phase 2 (glucuronidation, sulphation, methylation and acetylation) reactions. As a general rule, the clearance of drugs in the neonatal period is reduced. For many drugs, adult clearance values are reached by the age of 2 years (Table 10.1).

The major pathway in phase 1 is oxidation, which involves the cytochrome P450 enzymes (CYP) that are present mainly in the liver. The major CYP enzymes are CYP3A4 and CYP1A2. CYP3A4 is responsible for the metabolism of many drugs such as midazolam, ciclosporin, fentanyl and nifedipine. CYP3A4 activity is reduced in the neonatal period and early infancy. There is considerable inter-individual variation in enzyme activity, and this results in considerable variation in plasma concentrations of drugs such as midazolam, despite usage

Table 10.1 Age and morphine clearance

Age group	Number of patients	Mean or median plasma clearance (ml/min/kg)	Range
Preterm neonates	72	3.5	0.5–9.6
Term neonates	44	6.3	0.6–39
Infants 1–24 months	11	13.9	8.3–24.1
Children 2–11 years	18	37.4	20.1–48.5
Adolescents 12–17 years	6	25.4	9–53.4

(Reproduced from de Wildt, Johnson & Choonara 2003, with permission.)

of similar doses. CYP1A2 accounts for 13% of total enzyme activity in the liver. Caffeine and theophylline are metabolized via the CYP1A2 pathway. Enzyme activity is reduced in the neonatal period but increases rapidly such that, by the age of 6 months, activity is approaching that of older children and adults.

Glucuronidation and sulphation are the two major phase 2 pathways. Glucuronidation is reduced in the neonatal period and there is compensatory sulphation. The development of glucuronidation varies, in that children who are 2 years old have rates of glucuronidation for morphine similar to that in adults (Table 10.1). In the case of paracetamol, however, adult rates of glucuronidation are not reached until puberty.

Drug toxicity

Almost 1 in 10 children in hospital will experience an adverse drug reaction (ADR), of which 1 in 8 will be severe. About 2% of children in hospital are admitted following an ADR. Children can experience a wide variety of ADRs.

Children are at risk of specific ADRs that do not affect adults, as growth and development are not an issue in adult patients. Differences in drug metabolism make certain ADRs a greater problem in children (e.g. valproate hepatotoxicity in young children, where toxic metabolites are more likely to be produced) or less of a problem (e.g. paracetamol hepatotoxicity following an overdose). There is a greater capacity for the sulphation of paracetamol in prepubertal children, which reduces the formation of toxic metabolites. The mechanisms of ADRs specifically affecting children are illustrated in Table 10.2.

Percutaneous absorption

The newborn infant has a higher surface area to weight ratio than both adults and children. Percutaneous toxicity can therefore be a significant problem in the neonatal period. Examples of this include the use of antiseptic agents such as hexachlorophene, which have been associated with neurotoxicity.

Protein-displacing effect on bilirubin

The sulphonamide, sulphisoxazole, was used as an antibiotic in neonates in the 1950s. It was associated with increased mortality due to the development of kernicterus. Sulphonamides have a higher binding affinity to albumin than bilirubin. Thus, the administration of sulphonamides results in an increase in the free fraction of bilirubin, which crosses the blood–brain barrier and causes kernicterus if the neonate is ill

Table 10.2 Major adverse drug reactions (ADRs) in paediatric patients

Year	Drug/compound	Age group	ADR	Mechanism
1886	Aniline dye	Neonates	Methaemoglobinaemia	Percutaneous absorption
1956	Sulphisoxazole	Neonates	Kernicterus	Protein-displacing effect on bilirubin
1959	Chloramphenicol	Neonates	Grey baby syndrome	Impaired metabolism
1979	Sodium valproate	Young children (< 3 years)	Hepatic failure	Abnormal metabolism?
1980	Salicylate	Children	Reye's syndrome	Unknown
1990	Propofol	Children	Metabolic acidosis	Unknown Dose-related?
1996	Lamotrigine	Children	Skin reactions	Unknown Associated with co-medication with sodium valproate

(Reproduced from Choonara & Rieder 2002, with permission.)

and jaundiced. In most areas of paediatrics, protein binding is not a significant issue.

Impaired drug metabolism

Chloramphenicol was associated with the development of the grey baby syndrome in neonates. Infants developed vomiting, cyanosis and cardiovascular collapse, and in some cases died. The newborn infant metabolizes chloramphenicol more slowly than adults and therefore requires a lower dose. Reduction in the dosage prevents the development of the grey baby syndrome.

Altered drug metabolism

Paediatric patients may have reduced activity of the major enzymes associated with drug metabolism in the liver. To compensate for this, they may have increased pathways of other enzymes. This is thought to be one of the factors contributing to the increased risk of hepatotoxicity in children under the age of 3 years who receive sodium valproate. This increased risk is raised by the use of additional anticonvulsants alongside the sodium valproate, which may result in enzyme induction of certain metabolic pathways.

Drug interactions

Skin reactions to the anticonvulsant, lamotrigine, are more likely to occur in children than in infants. The incidence is significantly increased by co-medication with sodium valproate alongside the lamotrigine. The mechanism of this drug interaction is unknown.

Unknown

There are several examples of major ADRs that occur in children for which we do not understand the mechanism. Salicylate given during the presence of a viral illness will predispose children of all ages to develop Reye's syndrome. By avoiding the use of salicylates in children with viral infections, the incidence of Reye's syndrome has been dramatically reduced. Propofol is a parenteral anaesthetic agent with minimal toxicity when used to induce general anaesthesia. Used as a sedative in critically ill children, however, it has been associated with the death of over 10 children in the UK alone. The propofol infusion syndrome is thought to be related to the total dose of propofol infused, i.e. high dose or prolonged duration is more likely to cause problems.

Fetal toxicity

The majority of medicines used during pregnancy do not result in harm to the fetus. Both health professionals and pregnant women usually over-estimate the risk of drug toxicity associated with the use of medicines during pregnancy. Thalidomide, however, is an example of how a drug that is relatively safe in adults can result in significant harm to the fetus (phocomelia) when it is given during a critical stage in pregnancy (24–27 days). The drug that is most likely to be associated with fetal toxicity at present is alcohol, which may result in the fetal alcohol syndrome. With the increasing use of recreational drugs by young women, it is highly likely that the major cause of fetal toxicity in the future will be associated with recreational drug use rather than prescribed medicines.

Key points

- Percutaneous toxicity can occur in newborn infants.
- The protein-displacing effect of medicines should be considered in sick preterm neonates.
- Paediatric patients, and neonates in particular, are more likely to have a reduced capacity to metabolize drugs than adults. Therefore lower doses are usually required.

- Sodium valproate should not be used as a first-line anticonvulsant in children under the age of 3 years.
- Drug interactions may increase the risk of an ADR.
- Propofol should not be used as a sedative in critically ill children.

One should always consider the possibility of an ADR being responsible for a child's symptoms. Recognizing which patients are at greater risk of ADRs can help reduce the overall incidence. Health professionals should try to follow guidelines. Suspected ADRs should be reported to the regulatory authorities: for example, by using the yellow forms at the back of the *British National Formulary (BNF) for Children*. This book contains further advice on reporting, with which you should be familiar.

Prescribing for children

Many medicines used in children are not licensed for such use. This is usually because the pharmaceutical company has not asked for a licence from the regulatory authorities. Additionally, many medicines given to children are off-label, i.e. used at a different dose or route than specified within the product licence or for a different age or different indication. The Royal College of Paediatrics and Child Health recommends using the medicines for which there is the greatest amount of evidence to justify its usage. In certain circumstances, this may involve off-label use.

The metabolism of some drugs may be affected by one or a number of the following mechanisms:
- Certain illnesses, e.g. cystic fibrosis
- Clinical conditions, e.g. shock, which may affect the metabolism of drugs
- Liver and renal failure, which will delay the elimination of drugs and hence dictates reduced dosages.

One needs to recognize that not all medicines are prescribed, i.e. they can be obtained over the counter from a pharmacy either by a parent or, in the case of adolescents, by children themselves. Parents may not always be aware of the active ingredient present in over-the-counter medicines and therefore a full history needs to be obtained before prescribing medicines such as paracetamol or ibuprofen. In adolescent girls, one also needs to be aware of the possibility of any possible teratogenic effects of medicines if they become pregnant.

Most medicines can be taken by a breastfeeding mother and will not cause a significant problem to the breastfed infant. One should not discourage mothers from breastfeeding because they are uncertain of possible toxic effects. Formularies such as the *BNF for Children* give detailed information regarding which medicines to avoid during breastfeeding.

Table 10.3 **Types of medication error**

Type of medication error	Number	Fatal
Incorrect dose	32	13
Incorrect drug	16	5
Incorrect strength	3	1
Omitted in error	4	1
Incorrect patient	4	–
Duplicate dose	3	–
Expired drugs	3	–
Incorrect route	3	3
Incorrect container	2	1
Incorrect label	2	–
Incorrect rate	2	2
Miscellaneous	6	3
TOTAL	80*	29

* Six children experienced more than one error each.
(Reproduced from Cousins et al 2002, with permission.)

BOX 10.2 In the event of a medication error
- Inform the parents (and the child if old enough and if this is appropriate)
- Inform all relevant health professionals directly involved with the patient
- Discuss with the pharmacy/poison centre
- At a later stage, discuss with all relevant parties what lessons can be learnt from the medication error and whether a similar error can be prevented in the future

Medication errors are a significant problem in paediatric patients. A review of press reports of medication errors described 29 deaths of paediatric patients in the UK over a period of 8 years (Cousins et al 2002). The types of medication error are illustrated in Table 10.3. All health professionals will commit a medication error at some stage in their career. Systems need to be introduced to try to minimize the impact of these errors.

Incorrect dose is the most frequent type of medication error and is also the type of error most likely to be associated with a fatality. One therefore needs to have an accurate note of the child's weight, and dose calculations, especially on the neonatal unit and when using parenteral medicines, require careful checking. Tenfold errors are a particular problem in both neonates and children.

Incorrect drug is the second most common type of medication error and is also associated with significant fatalities. Incorrect route is a particular problem with intrathecal drugs and great care is required for medicines administered via this route (Box 10.2).

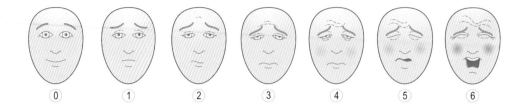

Fig. 10.2 Faces pain scale.
'These faces show how much something can hurt. This face [point to the left-most face] shows no pain. The faces show more and more pain [point to each one from left to right] up to this one [point to the right-most face]. It shows very much pain. Point to the pain that shows how much you hurt (right now).'
(Reproduced from Bieri et al 1990, with permission.)

Key points

- Incorrect dose is the most frequent medication error.
- Tenfold errors are a significant problem in paediatric patients.
- Incorrect drug is a common type of medication error.

Use of antimicrobials

The choice of antimicrobial agent needs to be made in conjunction with the local microbiologist, who will be aware of local resistance patterns. A broad-spectrum antimicrobial is of value where the organism is unknown, but is not recommended if the organism is known and sensitive to more specific antibiotics. Benzylpenicillin remains the drug of choice for streptococcal lobar pneumonia and both pneumococcal and meningococcal meningitis in the vast majority of cases. In general, one should aim to use the lowest effective dose of an antimicrobial agent, as drug toxicity is more likely to be associated with higher doses. This is especially the case with aminoglycosides. The preterm neonate handles drugs differently to the term neonate and therefore the frequency of administration of many antibiotics needs to be reduced in premature infants.

The duration of antibiotic therapy needs to be carefully considered. Certain organisms, such as the meningococcus, are extremely sensitive and in the vast majority of cases 5 days' treatment is more than sufficient. Most hospitals have local antibiotic guidelines that should be followed.

The cost of medicines is usually an important factor in the choice of antibiotic. If there are two equally effective and safe drugs, then one would normally choose the cheaper medicine. In certain cases, however, the increased cost of the drug may be compensated by savings in nursing expenditure by allowing reduced frequency of administration of intravenous antibiotics.

Pain assessment and management (see also p. 284)

One always needs to consider the possibility of a child being in pain, as a result either of the disease process or of the interventions. The assessment of pain requires an age-appropriate, validated pain assessment scale. Self-reporting is the ideal, but the child needs to have the cognitive ability to do this and therefore needs to be at least 3 years old. It is also important that a pain scale that has been validated for an acute painful response is not used for children with chronic pain.

Self-report scales usually involve the child pointing to a photograph (the Oucher Scale) or a diagram of a child in pain (Bieri Faces Pain Scale, Fig. 10.2). The Oucher Scale has been validated in children as young as 3 years of age and the Bieri Faces Pain Scale for children aged 6 years and over. The Wong–Baker Faces Pain Scale is more reliable in children aged 8–12 years than in the 3–7-year age group. The Adolescent Paediatric Pain Tool is for children between the ages of 8 and 17 years.

Behavioural pain scales are used for preverbal children and include the Toddler–Preschooler Post-operative Pain Scale (TPPPS) and the Children's Hospital of Eastern Ontario Pain Scale (CHEOPS). These pain scales rely on assessment of the child's behaviour and have been validated for children aged 1–5 years. The Faces, Legs, Activity, Cry and Consolability (FLACC) Scale has been validated for children aged 2 months–7 years.

There are numerous pain assessment tools for use in neonates (Bieri et al 1990). These rely on behavioural observation and, in some of the pain scales, measurements of pulse, blood pressure and oxygen saturation. For preterm neonates, it is important to use a scale that has been validated in preterm neonates (van Dijk et al, 2004).

Management involves the use of techniques such as distraction as well as analgesia. Paracetamol is the safest analgesic available and is the first-line drug to be used for paediatric patients of all ages with mild pain. Children who either do not respond to paracetamol or are unlikely to respond to paracetamol should receive a non-steroidal anti-inflammatory drug (NSAID) such as ibuprofen or diclofenac. Alternatively, codeine or dihydrocodeine can be administered orally. Patients with severe pain require opiates, and morphine remains the drug of choice. It can be administered intravenously, intranasally or orally. For certain painful conditions, e.g. change of dressings in burns patients, it may be more appropriate to use inhaled entonox. This is an effective and safe analgesic with a short duration of action, which children can control themselves.

www.rcn.org.uk/resources/guidelines.php

The recognition and assessment of acute pain in children

References

Bieri D et al 1990 The faces pain scale for the self-assessment of the severity of pain experienced by children: development, initial validation, and preliminary investigation for ratio scale properties. Pain 41:139–150

Choonara I, Rieder MJ 2002 Drug toxicity and adverse drug reactions in children — a brief historical review. Paediatric and Perinatal Drug Therapy 5:12–18

Cousins D et al 2002 Medication errors in children — an eight-year review using press reports. Paediatric and Perinatal Drug Therapy 5:52–58

De Wildt SN, Johnson TN, Choonara J 2003 The effect of age on drug metabolism. Paediatric and Perinatal Drug Therapy 5:101–106

Thomson AH 2000 Introduction to clinical pharmacokinetics. Paediatric and Perinatal Drug Therapy 4: 3–11

van Dijk M, Simons S, Tibboel D 2004 Pain assessment in neonates. Paediatric and Perinatal Drug Therapy 6:97–103

MODULE TWO

Julie-Clare Becher   Neil McIntosh

11

Ethics and children's rights

MODULE TWO

LEARNING OUTCOMES

By the end of this chapter you should:

● Understand a parent's responsibility for his or her child
● Appreciate the rights of a child and how you can ensure them
● Understand confidentiality issues pertaining to children
● Know about the issues surrounding considerations of care reorientation
● Understand the importance of autopsy and the issues surrounding authorization
● Understand the importance of research for the future of children.

Introduction

The increasing availability of sophisticated medical technology has raised ethical and legal questions about the appropriateness of provision of care for children who may ultimately die or survive with severe disability. At the same time, society is demanding greater personal involvement in decision-making. The expertise of doctors and nurses in their field may not extend to the skills required to deal with problems of parental dissent, decisions about whether a severely damaged baby should be allowed to die or the extent to which parents should be involved in their child's management. Expertise in moral and legal argument is fundamental to such issues. This chapter aims to provide the reader with an understanding of how ethical and legal issues interact with clinical practice in paediatrics.

Children's rights and parental responsibilities

Rights may be defined as the entitlement for all individuals to have their worth and dignity respected.

The United Nations Convention on the Rights of the Child (UNCRC) declares that children are entitled to special consideration and care due to their immaturity and vulnerability. The Convention was ratified by the UK government in 1991. The articles of this convention state that the primary consideration of actions affecting children should be the 'best interests of the child' (Article 3), and that it is every child's right to enjoy the highest attainable standard of health and to be able to access facilities for the treatment of illness and the rehabilitation of health (Article 24), subject to the resources available (Article 4). The Convention also recognizes the right of a child to 'freedom of expression, freedom to seek, receive and impart information and ideas of all kinds, regardless of frontiers' (Article 13), and states that the 'child who is capable of forming his or her own views has the right to express those views freely on all matters. The views of the child will be given due weight in accordance with the age and maturation' (Article 12). In addition, in 2000, following the Human Rights Act 1998, rights acknowledged in the European Convention of Human Rights became incorporated into UK law. These rights, also pertaining to children, include the right to life, the right not to be subjected to degrading or inhuman treatment, and the right to private and family life.

www.childrenslawcentre.org/UNCRC_
international.htm
www.pfc.org.uk/legal/echrtext.htm

European Convention on Human Rights

A child has autonomy and a separate identity to that of his or her parents, and respect for this is fundamental to trust and communication, even in the smallest child. Healthcare professionals have an important role in sharing information with children and listening to their needs, empowering them to make confident decisions with their parents about treatment. Support of parents, who may express different needs and desires to those of their child or those of staff, is also crucial in this process.

Both the Children Act 1989, which applies to England, Wales and Northern Ireland, and the Children (Scotland) Act 1995 emphasize that the principal role of parenthood is to provide care for a child and to raise him or her in emotional, moral and physical health. Parents can generally be expected to protect the interests of their child to a greater degree than anyone else, but parental rights do not equate to ownership and it is essential that these rights be exercised for the benefit of the child and not for the benefit of the parent. Currently, biological parents are the legal parents unless the child has been adopted. The mother has parental responsibility, and so does the father if he is married to the mother at the time of birth or marries her thereafter (Box 11.1).

BOX 11.1 Unmarried fathers

Unmarried fathers can obtain parental responsibility by entering into a voluntary parental responsibility agreement with the mother or this can be granted by a court. Recent legislation in England and Wales grants the father parental rights if he registers the child's birth jointly with the mother.

Adoptive parents have parental responsibility, as do others such as guardians or local authorities when granted these by the courts. The court itself may consent to treatment on behalf of a child or may limit parental responsibility in certain circumstances.

Consent, dissent and competency

The right to autonomy declares that each individual can decide what happens to his or her body. This applies to any act of touching, including medical treatment. Without consent, such violation of this right may constitute assault. Consent makes the act of touching or medical treatment lawful and such consent may be 'implied', as in the rolling up of a sleeve for a venepuncture, or 'expressed', as in verbal or written assent. Exceptions to the requirement for consent arise in the situation of an unconscious patient, where to delay until a patient is conscious would result in unreasonable treatment delays, and in the context of mental illness where, under the Mental Health Act (England and Wales 1983, Scotland 2003), non-consensual treatment may be instituted.

All healthcare decisions involve choices and, in the case of children, the question arises 'by whom?' Consent requires competence. In England and Wales a child of 16 or over is deemed legally able and competent to make decisions about his or her own medical treatment. However, case law has undermined the ability of such young people to refuse consent to a procedure or treatment where refusal might result in significant harm; this they can only do at 18. Under the age of 16, if competency is not present, consent is generally obtained on the child's behalf from a parent or other person exercising parental powers. However, if a child is deemed 'competent', that child is able to give consent or assent with the parental consent. Competency is difficult to define and assess (Box 11.2).

If the child is considered competent, encouragement should be given to that child to involve the parents in the decision-making. However, this is not mandatory and the consent of a competent child to treatment cannot be overruled by the dissent of parent. Such competency of a 'mature minor' is often termed 'Gillick

> **BOX 11.2 Competency**
>
> This involves a capacity to retain and comprehend information, and an ability to weigh up the risks and benefits to arrive at a choice and to understand the consequences of not consenting. It depends not only on the mental age of the child, but also on the complexity of the procedure or treatment and the experience of that child to date.

competence' and has been established legally in the case of a minor who won her right to be prescribed contraception without her parent's knowledge. Good practice takes account of children's views irrespective of their minimum legal age, and good standards of communication, such as informing, listening and respecting a child's views, are central to informed and ethical decision-making. In Scotland, competency must be assumed from the age of 12 years unless it is clearly not present. Careful documentation would be necessary if one were to act against the young person's wishes.

www.gpnotebook.co.uk/simplepage.cfm?ID
=-1254817788

Gillick competency and consent in children

Dissent or difference in opinion may arise between the healthcare team and parents, or between the members of the team, or between parents. When such disagreement arises, the reasons must be discussed. Parents may have a different understanding of the complex issues involved, and cultural and language barriers may compound the problem. Good-quality communication over time may result in consensus. It may be necessary to involve other specialists or to consider extended investigations to help resolve any uncertainty about prognosis. An opportunity should be allowed for parents to consult religious advisers or others of their choice. If they and the medical team disagree about which management strategy is in the child's best interests and this cannot be resolved through local means (such as involving another colleague), it is advisable to seek involvement from the courts. Legal support is always available for such matters and parents should be notified immediately about such a move so they can seek representation, and put forward their views and seek alternative opinions.

Dissent within the healthcare team may also occur and, although unanimity is not essential, consensus should be sought. If individuals express dissent, it is important to record such opinion in the notes and attribute to it weight in proportion with that member's experience or status. Such members may be given an opportunity to ask for a second opinion.

Clinical ethics committees have been encouraged by professional bodies in the United States and may be useful in developing policies or dealing with individual cases. Very few such committees exist in the UK. Although recommendations made by such committees may be more palatable to parents than those made by clinicians, the doctor remains legally and professionally responsible for any decision made.

Confidentiality

Doctors have a duty of confidentiality to all patients, including children. A child who is deemed legally competent has the right to expect that information about him or her will not be disclosed to a third party, including a parent, without the child's consent. However, such children should be encouraged to involve their parents wherever possible, if it is in their best interests to do so. It is only justified to disclose confidential information to a third party if it is thought a child may suffer or come to harm through non-disclosure. In such a case, the child should be informed of this decision prior to the third party being informed. Similarly, confidentiality with regard to a non-competent child should incur the same respect, and disclosure of any information pertaining to that child and should first be discussed with the parent. Clinicians have a statutory duty under the Children Act 2004 and the Children (Scotland) Act 1995 to safeguard children by sharing information with relevant agencies when there is manifest evidence of child abuse. All clinicians should be aware of recent data protection legislation that allows all individuals the right to access their medical records.

Sanctity of life and quality of life

Traditional Hippocratic medical ethics advocates respect for the sanctity of all human life, combined with a medical duty of care and a duty to act in the sole interest of the patient. However, some modern philosophy challenges this perspective as outdated and argues that 'personhood' with its attendant rights and obligations is dependent on the presence of consciousness and self-awareness, as well as an ability to reason and to have control over one's existence. In this view, newborn infants and those children with severe brain damage are not regarded as persons. However, the concept of the sanctity of life, although originating in religious tradition, is a central tenet in our society, where murder is perceived as wrong, vulnerability is protected and resources are provided to treat the sick and save lives where possible. Guidelines published by the General Medical Council (GMC) emphasize that the care of the patient should be a doctor's primary responsibility and that doctors should strive to protect their patients from risk. This moral commitment to the preservation and protection of human life is also supported by the Royal College of Paediatrics and Child Health document (RCPCH 2004) on the withdrawal of life-saving treatment and by the British Medical Association (BMA 2003), both of which support the illegality of euthanasia in the United Kingdom.

However, as neonatal and paediatric intensive care has advanced, it has become apparent that saving life may cause harm. Survival of an infant at all costs may lead to unbearable suffering or a bleak life of severe disability. Such individuals may be unable to have any meaningful interaction with the environment and lack ability to reason, both measures of quality of life. Despite the primary motivation of preservation of life in these situations, many clinicians find such 'therapeutic successes' at odds with the concept of 'the sanctity of life'. It is not always in a child's best interests to prolong life at all costs. Decisions not to provide or to withdraw life-sustaining treatment in the face of intolerable suffering are increasingly accepted as morally appropriate, and guidelines have been produced by the RCPCH as a framework for such practice (RCPCH 2004).

www.gmc-uk.org/guidance/good_medical_practice/index.asp

GMC, 'Good Medical Practice'

Withdrawal and withholding of life-prolonging treatment in children

The healthcare team has a duty of care, with the principle goal of sustaining life and restoring health. However, technological advances have led to an increasing ability to sustain life in infants and children who would otherwise have died. As a result, ethical dilemmas have arisen as to whether all attempts to prolong life are sensible or in the best interests of the child. In particular, concern has arisen as to the justification of continuing pointless treatment in patients who are not dying and to the prolongation of life in those who are dying or destined for severe disability.

In the consideration of the withholding or withdrawal of curative life-saving medical treatment, the RCPCH (2004) has defined five situations in which prolongation or initiation of active treatment may be considered unjustified (Box 11.3):

- The brain-dead child, where criteria of brain-stem death are confirmed by two practitioners in accordance with accepted medical standards

> **BOX 11.3 Five situations where the withholding or withdrawal of curative medical treatment might be considered**
>
> - The brain-dead child
> - The persistent vegetative state
> - The 'no-chance' situation
> - The 'no-purpose' situation
> - The 'unbearable' situation

- The permanent vegetative state, in which a child is reliant on others for all care and shows no interaction with his/her environment
- The no-chance situation, where a child will die despite treatment and where continuation of such treatment may simply delay death without significant alleviation of suffering
- The no-purpose situation, where survival is possible with treatment but results in such severe physical or mental impairment that it is unfair to expect the child to bear it
- The unbearable situation, where the child or family feels that further treatment in the face of an incurable and relentless disease is intolerable.

These situations rely on a degree of certainty about death, cure or outcomes between the two, and if there is doubt about either of these extremes, the motivation should always be to protect life until a value judgment based on outcome can be ascertained. In such instances, advice from specialist colleagues or more detailed investigations may be warranted. It is essential that enough time be allowed to gather and disseminate information and to allow opinions to be expressed by all involved.

Historically, end-of-life decisions were taken by medical staff with or without involvement of the parents. Nowadays, parents increasingly want to share this responsibility. Doctors must help guide parents towards a decision that is medically appropriate and within the law and, in doing so, need to respect the fact that parents may have their own values, beliefs, priorities and resources. In addition, parents will have to live with the consequences of any decision made. Siblings must not be forgotten in the decision-making process; they may have important insights into the feelings of their brother or sister and may have differing views to those of their parents.

All members of the healthcare team should be involved in such decision-making and, although the final responsibility lies with the consultant in charge of the child, such decisions are virtually always taken by a multidisciplinary group involving nurses, social workers, family members and specialist medical staff who together form the 'moral community' within a paediatric unit.

It is important to remember that withholding or withdrawing life-prolonging treatment is not withdrawal of care. All dying children should receive warmth, loving human contact and feeds as tolerated, and should be assured of freedom from distress or pain by the use of sedation or analgesics. There should be a commitment to the family as a whole with the opportunity for parents to maintain close contact and participate in their child's care until death.

Omission, commission and the principle of double effect

Commission in this context refers to an act that has the certain result of death, and such deliberate killing of any individual is prohibited. However, the withdrawal of life-prolonging treatment in appropriate circumstances is accepted by the courts and is not regarded as a breach of the right to life. Omission refers to the withholding of treatment.

Ensuring that a dying child is free from distress is a sensitive matter that has attracted much debate. Legally, any treatment given to hasten death is murder but administration of medication to alleviate suffering is permissible, even if a side-effect may be to hasten death. This principle of 'double effect' is seen in the administration of opiates to prevent pain or distress where the drug may also have the effect of depressing respiration. Such a prescription is regarded as being for the benefit of the patient during life and not intended to cause or hasten death.

Refusal of blood products by Jehovah's Witnesses

The position of Jehovah's Witnesses in refusing donor blood transfusions in view of their personal deeply held religious beliefs is well known. This position includes the refusal of whole blood and red cells, white cells, platelets and plasma. Members who wilfully accept prohibited blood components have historically been disfellowshipped by their church and are considered outcasts. However, recent significant changes in policy mean that members can now remain silent about the medical treatment they receive and avoid punishment. Blood transfusions in the children of Jehovah's Witnesses have often raised medical dilemmas and ultimately involved the jurisdiction of the courts. Previously, decisions in favour of the clinician may have meant risking the subsequent ostracization of that child or family from the religious community. Although Jehovah's Witnesses are an increasingly diverse group, this recent policy change may mean that conflict in

such cases will be less common. As this change may be interpreted differently by various members of the group, the clinician must explore the personal preference and conviction of parents before treatment and remember that breaches in patient confidentiality may result in significant punishment for the family.

Resource allocation

Decisions about funding experimental and expensive treatments raise ethical and practical dilemmas. A clinician has a duty of care to an individual patient. However, in a world where resources are scarce, clinicians and managers have an ethical duty to consider cost in rationing healthcare. Treatments or procedures must be justified in terms of cost-effectiveness, medical efficacy and maximum benefit to the community. A decision to offer one patient a particular treatment may deny treatment to another.

The principle of health gain maximization ranks procedures or treatments so that those that generate more gains to health for every unit of resource take priority over those that generate fewer. Gains to health may be measured by life expectancy, lives saved, 'quality-adjusted life years' (QALYs) or other outcomes. All individuals are regarded as equal in health gain maximization. Any departure from this ranking involves a loss of efficiency and a judgment that the value of one life is more important then the value of another. However, high-profile cases in the media have demonstrated the difficulties of weighing the needs of an individual and the interests of the community, and there may be situations where 'rescue' treatment may be justified for an individual, even when this may be at conflict with the priorities of the community as a whole (Ham 1999).

To address problems of inequality in the delivery of healthcare provision highlighted in the Health Act of 1999, the Government has established the National Institute for Clinical Excellence (NICE) in England and Wales and the Health Technology Board for Scotland.

Post-mortem and organ retention

The usefulness of post-mortem in establishing cause of death, determining unrelated diagnoses and assisting grieving is well documented. In infants and children information may also be provided for genetic counselling. The post-mortem rate has been falling throughout the developed world over the last three decades, and this has been particularly so since well-publicized criticisms of post-mortem standards appeared in the media over the last decade. In particular, the practice of retention of organs from individuals without the knowledge or consent of relatives has led to a crisis in public confidence and a subsequent overhaul of the post-mortem consent and examination process.

Information, communication and knowledge are fundamental in rebuilding the public's trust in the post-mortem examination. As a result, the consent process is now unambiguous and explicit. Parents need to be assured that examination will only be carried out with their authorization and that any examination of their child will be with the utmost dignity and respect. The extent of the examination and retention of organs and the purposes for such retention must be fully explained to parents, and high-quality written information provided in order to aid their decision. The extent of examination and retention must correspond to the level of consent given. Any breach of such authorization now results in legal penalty. Recommendations for post-mortems, as specified by the Human Tissue Bill 2004, are that the examination be carried out by a paediatric pathologist within 2 working days, and that all retention of tissue blocks, slides and whole organs requires authorization by next of kin and will be subsequently regarded as part of the medical record. Although historically it was common for doctors to withhold post-mortem results from parents in the belief that these details would result in distress, information from the examination should now be freely available. This information is best provided and discussed at a meeting between the clinician, parents and involved support staff in the weeks following bereavement.

In specific instances, the coroner or procurator fiscal may ask for a post-mortem examination to ascertain cause of death, irrespective of parental consent. Such a requirement follows sudden, suspicious or accidental deaths or where death may have occurred due to medical mishap or the result of a medical treatment or surgical procedure. In this situation, tissue retention is not authorized unless specific consent has been obtained.

Research in babies and children

Medical research is essential for advancing child health and wellbeing. Many disease processes in children have no close analogies in adults. Moreover, children have different physiology to adults and as a result drugs may have different pharmacokinetics (p. 103). Many disorders can only be understood in the context of a child's growth and development. Research in children can also advance our understanding of some adult diseases that are thought to have their origins in childhood.

Both the Medical Research Council and the RCPCH recognize that children require special protection in research, as they are less likely to be able to communicate their needs or protect their interests compared to adult subjects (McIntosh et al 2000). Both bodies recommend certain ethical considerations in research involving children:

- All proposed research should be approved by a research ethics committee.
- Entry into a study should be preceded by witnessed written informed consent from a parent following the provision of high-quality information and the opportunity to discuss the research with another member of staff. All language used should be appropriate to the intellectual level of the parent and supported with written information.
- Many parents will be under significant stress, particularly following labour and delivery or the diagnosis of significant morbidity. This may affect their ability to listen, comprehend and retain information.
- All risks involved in study participation should be shared with the parent.
- Parents should be assured that their child will receive the best possible medical care, irrespective of their participation in the study.
- Parents should understand that they are free to withdraw their child from the study at any time and that this will not affect the care their child will receive.
- Where parents give consent, agreement should also be sought from school-age children. A child's refusal to participate or continue in a study should always be respected.
- The researcher has an ongoing obligation to monitor the risks to each child and inform both the parents and the data monitoring committee of the progress of the study and any adverse effects.
- A data monitoring committee should be active in monitoring for significant side-effects and interim analysis.

Both bodies recognize that good-quality research is essential for improving the efficacy and safety of clinical practice, and should be actively encouraged (Box 11.4).

www.mrc.ac.uk/pdf-ethics_guide_children.pdf
MRC Ethics Guide

Neonatal issues
Viability and outcome

For extremely preterm infants there is a close relationship between gestational age and mortality/morbidity,

BOX 11.4 Six principles about research with children

- Research involving children is important for the benefit of all children and should be supported, encouraged and conducted in an ethical manner
- Children are not small adults; they have an additional, unique set of interests
- Research should only be done on children if comparable research on adults could not answer the same question
- A research procedure that is not intended to benefit the child subject directly is not necessarily either unethical or illegal
- All proposals involving medical research on children should be submitted to the local research ethics committee
- Legally valid consent should be obtained from the child, parent or guardian as appropriate. When parental consent is obtained, the agreement of school-age children who take part in research should also be requested by researchers

with significant decreases in mortality for each week of prolonged intrauterine survival. The decision to attempt to prolong a pregnancy may have to be balanced against considerable ongoing risk for both the mother and the fetus. Moderate to severe disability affects over a third of extreme preterm survivors, many of whom have needed prolonged intensive care. The emotional and financial burden of disability and handicap means that families require accurate information about the survival and prognosis for such infants. There are no randomized trials to advise clinicians facing such complex medical, emotional and social challenges about whether or not to resuscitate the extreme preterm infant. Recent statistics on short-term survival and long-term sequelae may already be outdated. The United Kingdom EPICURE study (Wood et al 2000) and a similar study of extremely preterm infants born in the United States in the mid-1990s found a survival rate of 11–30% at 23 weeks' gestation, increasing to 34–76% by 25 weeks' gestation. Moderate to severe disability affected around 50% of survivors, but this data is now 10 years old. There is also a relationship of mortality and morbidity with birth weight but outcome studies seldom explore the variable influences of growth restriction or gender. There is a well-described poorer outcome for multiple pregnancies.

In practice, accurate estimation of gestational age may be problematic in the absence of first trimester ultrasound, and fetal weight estimates are notoriously inaccurate. Obstetricians have more pessimistic views than paediatricians about survival in very early gestation

deliveries, and all clinicians who are involved in counselling parents should be familiar with both national and local statistics for survival and long-term outcome. Counselling should be sensitive to ethnic and cultural diversity, and input from clergy, social workers or translators may be important.

The delivery of extremely premature infants and infants with severe congenital abnormalities raises issues about the initiation of resuscitation. Practices include the resuscitation of all infants, resuscitation according to previously defined parameters or application of an individualized risk assessment approach. Although absolute rules are inappropriate for such difficult issues, guidelines can provide a framework for acceptable practice but without prescriptive guidance. Current international guidelines advise that resuscitation is inappropriate where an infant has a condition or characteristic unlikely to result in survival or survival without extreme disability (Niermeyer et al 2000). This includes infants with a confirmed gestation of less than 23 weeks, a birth weight below 400 g, anencephaly or confirmed trisomy 13 or 18. The guidelines recognize that it may be difficult to obtain reliable or accurate information prior to delivery, and a trial of therapy may be instituted while full assessment of the infant is undertaken. Withdrawal of full support may follow ascertainment of status. Discussions with parents and obstetricians in the antenatal period are valuable and enable repeated communication with time for reflection and questions. It is important to develop a plan that has consensus for the family and clinician. Both parties should agree that in the face of uncertainty, evaluation and further investigations may be needed. Where the situation is complex or where there is irreconcilable disagreement, it is useful to involve other colleagues.

In all cases, the final decision not to initiate resuscitation should be made by a senior clinician; when one is not present, a junior doctor should initiate treatment until a more experienced doctor arrives. This approach allows time to gather information, counsel parents and allow parents some time to cherish their baby. The disadvantage is the danger that in some instances subsequent withdrawal of life-sustaining treatment may not result in death but in an infant with severe disability.

All treatment strategies have benefits and risks, and their availability does not necessarily justify their use. The provision of intensive care when there is evidence of severe neurological damage is ethically unjust. All centres offering intensive care should have a comprehensive and standardized method of follow-up ascertainment, and outcome data should be available for public consumption and for benchmarking with other centres.

References and further reading

British Medical Association Ethics Department 2003 Medical ethics today. BMJ Books, London

Ham C 1999 Tragic choices in health care: lessons from the child B case. British Medical Journal 319(7219):1258–1261

McIntosh N, Bates P, Brykczynska G et al and Royal College of Paediatrics and Child Health Ethics Advisory Committee 2000 Guidelines for the ethical conduct of medical research involving children. Arch Dis Child 82(2):177–182

Niermeyer S, Kattwinkel J, Van Reempts P et al, International Consensus on Science and Contributors and Reviewers for the Neonatal Resuscitation Guidelines 2000 International guidelines for neonatal resuscitation: an excerpt from the guidelines 2000 for cardiopulmonary resuscitation and emergency cardiovascular care. Pediatrics 106(3):E29

Royal College of Paediatrics and Child Health Ethics Advisory Committee 2004 A framework for practice in relation to the withholding and withdrawing of life-saving treatment in children, 2nd edn. RCPCH, London

Wood NS, Marlow N, Costeloe K et al and EPICURE Study Group 2000 Neurologic and developmental disability after extremely preterm birth. New England Journal of Medicine 343(6):378–384

MODULE TWO

Practical procedures and investigations

LEARNING OUTCOMES

By the end of this chapter you should:
- Have reviewed your approach to learning and performing practical procedures
- Be able to perform specific common procedures
- Be able to discuss interpretation of investigations, particularly with regard to common X-rays.

Investigations in children

Procedures and investigations in children are often more difficult than those in adults. The smaller size of the child may make the technical aspects more challenging; the child may be less cooperative (or refuse outright!); and the distress caused may be greater — both to the child and the parents. Although investigations should not be done without good reason in any branch of medicine, this is particularly the case in paediatrics. Consider the test characteristics, the potential contribution to diagnosis and management, and the risks and costs of doing the test (p. 56).

Approach to practical procedures

You need to become competent in performing common practical procedures. The best way to achieve this is to be taught and supervised by an experienced practitioner. Many investigations will be explained in more detail in later chapters. The notes below are not meant to be a comprehensive manual, but practical tips to help you achieve success and avoid common problems.

Learning a new practical procedure

Only learn a procedure when you can practise it regularly with appropriate supervision and support near at hand. Make sure you know any relevant background physiology and anatomy, and any associated risks and how to minimize these. Watch experienced practitioners perform the procedure a number of times and take time to review it with them afterwards until you are sure you know what to do.

Perform the procedure (or part of the procedure) under close supervision by an experienced colleague. If you fail, do not make repeated attempts, as this is unfair to the child. Let the experienced colleague take over and complete the test, and then review afterwards with him or her how you can complete the procedure successfully next time.

You need to learn not only the technical aspects of performing the procedure but also how best to communicate to parents and children about what you are going to do before, during and after the procedure. This 'communication competence' is just as important as the technical competence that you need (Box 12.1).

If at first you don't succeed …

Even the best operators have occasions where they fail to complete a procedure that they are usually good at. This is more likely when you are tired or relatively inexperienced. Do not keep repeating the procedure until you achieve success, since this is like to be a fruitless exercise and may only lead to a fraught child and parents. Do not be embarrassed to ask somebody else to try.

Minimizing distress

For every procedure you perform, make it your goal to minimize any distress to the child and parents. Remember the golden rules of *p*reparation, *p*arents present and *p*ain control.

Preparation

This includes having everything ready so that you look proficient and minimize anxious waiting. It also includes explanation to child and parent of what is involved, and arranging for other appropriate staff to be present to help you. For most procedures the presence of an experienced children's nurse can make a huge difference.

Parents present?

Decide together with the parents whether they will be present in the room for the procedure, and what part they will play. In general it is best to have at least one parent present, although often parents decline to watch a lumbar puncture in a younger child but wait nearby to cuddle and comfort the child afterwards.

Pain control

This is important (p. 106).

Distraction

Distraction can be a powerful tool in children. You will see many examples of it in use on paediatric wards and in clinics. Aim to build up your own repertoire of useful distractions, which may include funny toys, funny faces, flashing lights, projected images and blowing bubbles. For the younger infant, a feed may be all that is needed. Well-judged distractions like these can make an unpleasant procedure almost a happy occasion, and acquiring a good repertoire is an important part of your toolkit.

Local anaesthesia

Many procedures carried out without pain control in adults require local anaesthesia at the least in children. Make sure you are familiar with local anaesthetic creams and the procedures for their use in your hospital, and offer these in all but the most grown-up adolescents (and even these patients might appreciate them). For more painful procedures, or where a greater depth of anaesthesia is needed, infiltrate the area with up to 0.4 ml/kg of 1% lidocaine solution. Make sure that you allow time for it to take effect.

Analgesia

Prescribe at least paracetamol following any procedure where the child is likely to continue to experience pain afterwards.

Venepuncture and cannulation

Although many ask an experienced helper to squeeze the limb being cannulated to produce appropriate venous engorgement, it is worth buying a good quality tourniquet and learning to adjust it to get exactly the right degree of compression each time. The problem with using a helper (particularly if it is a different person each time) is that the compression may vary considerably and you have little control over it. Learn a reliable method to secure any cannula you insert and try to ensure that it is easy to check for 'tissuing' of the cannula (e.g. by having a clear adhesive dressing over the tip), particularly if you are using irritant solutions containing calcium or high concentrations (> 10%) of glucose. Wherever possible, these should go through a central line; if they do have to go through a peripheral line, great care must be taken, with frequent monitoring (every 15 minutes or so) according to an agreed protocol with good documentation. Otherwise the child is at risk of unpleasant burn scars.

Capillary sampling

Capillary sampling is a useful technique and can be employed for nearly all samples, except those that

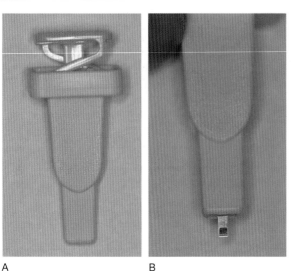

A   B

Fig. 12.1 Capillary sampling safety flow lancet.
(A) Sheathed before use; (B) lancet activated with blade protruding.

need to be sterile or require a large volume of blood. Use a capillary sampling safety device (Fig. 12.1) or an automated device wherever possible. If an automated lancet is chosen and the puncture depth is less than 2.2 mm, then this device can be used safely anywhere over the plantar surface of the heel, except the posterior heel in preterms < 33 weeks' gestation. Make sure the heel (infants under 2 years) or finger (older children) is warm before you start. If a large sample is needed, wrap the target area in a warm wet towel for 5 minutes to induce hyperaemia.

Lumbar puncture

Positioning is key for this investigation, and having an experienced assistant hold the baby or child will greatly increase your chances of success. Lay the infant on his or her side, held by your assistant, such that the head and hips are flexed and the spine is curved with the convexity towards you. The plane of the spine should be horizontal (Figs 12.2 and 12.3).

An imaginary line joining the highest points of the iliac crests passes just above the fourth lumbar spine. You should insert the lumbar puncture needle in either the L3–L4 space or the space below (L4–L5).

In children over a year, use local anaesthesia, with a combination of topical anaesthetic cream, followed by local infiltration with lidocaine 1%, aspirating before each injection (to check you are not in the spinal canal or a blood vessel), and waiting a minute or so for each injection to take effect.

Aim towards the umbilicus through the flexed spine and make sure your needle entry point is in the plane of the spinous processes. Firmly advance the needle with the stylet in place. You may feel a faint 'popping' sensation as you pierce the dura, in which case stop and remove the stylet. The distance to advance in cm is 0.03 × height (in cm), which is about 1.5 cm in a baby and up to around 5 cm in an adult. In a baby, stop after 1.5 cm, remove the stylet and gently rotate the needle. If no cerebrospinal fluid (CSF) appears, then reinsert the stylet and advance the needle a little further. Repeat this until you are in the CSF space.

Take three sterile bottles (6 drops in each) labelled ready for microscopy, and then one for protein and a fluoride container for glucose. Do not forget to send blood for glucose measurement at the time of the lumbar puncture to allow comparison of blood and CSF glucose.

Contraindications to lumbar puncture

- Signs of raised intracranial pressure: altered pupillary responses, absent Doll's eye reflex, decerebrate or decorticate posturing, abnormal

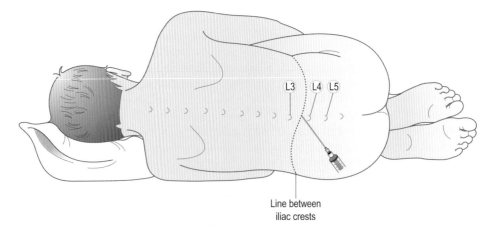

Line between
iliac crests

Fig. 12.2 Recumbent position for lumbar puncture showing correct site

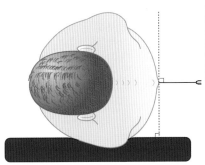

a) **Correct position.** The LP needle is at right angles to the plane of the back, which is perpendicular, at right angles to the plane of the couch, and near the edge of the couch. The LP needle is in line with the spinous processes.

Fig. 12.3 Lumbar puncture — achieving success.
Schematic representation of a view of the curled child, looking from the head (black oval) down the back.

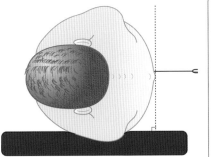

b) **Incorrect entry point.** The LP needle is not in line with the spinous processes. This can occur when
- the overlying skin is stretched while inserting the needle, so that skin recoil pulls the needle point out of line
- the spinous processes are difficult to feel due to overlying fat
- the child is moving at the time of insertion.

Remedy: *Take time to feel the processes, avoid skin stretch, and ensure your assistant can hold the child still.*

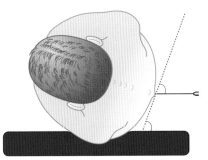

c) **Body roll.** The child's body has rolled so that the plane of the back is no longer perpendicular and at right angles to the couch. This is a common reason for a failed LP.

Remedy: *Have a second assistant view down the spine as shown in these pictures, or stop periodically and check yourself.*
Roll back to the correct position.
If this is difficult, adjust the plane of the needle to be at right angles to the plane of the back.

respiratory pattern, papilloedema, hypertension and bradycardia
- Recent (within 30 minutes) or prolonged (over 30 minutes) convulsive seizures
- Focal or tonic seizures
- Other focal neurological signs: hemiparesis/ monoparesis, extensor plantar responses, ocular palsies
- Glasgow Coma Score < 13 or deteriorating level of consciousness
- Strong suspicion of meningococcal infection (typical purpuric rash in an ill child) or state of shock (but perform lumbar puncture once the child is stable)
- Local superficial infection
- Coagulation disorder.

Injection

Intramuscular injection is used for most immunizations, and is occasionally used for intramuscular antibiotics if access is difficult and only a short course is required. For immunization, check that the expiry date has not been reached, that it is the correct immunization for the child, and that appropriate consent and explanation have been given. Ensure that any powder is fully dissolved and then, using a sterile technique, draw up the full amount into the syringe. Use a 25G (green) needle and pinch a large fold of skin, either on the upper arm (around the insertion of the deltoid muscle) or in the anterolateral aspect of the thigh; in older children, skin in the upper outer quadrant of the buttocks may be chosen (to avoid the risk of sciatic nerve damage). Insert the needle into the muscle, exert

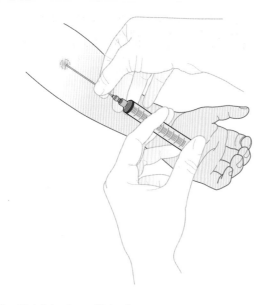

Fig. 12.4 Intradermal injection

some brief gentle suction to check you are not in a blood vessel, and then inject the contents. Remove the needle promptly and apply a dressing if needed.

Intradermal injections (Fig. 12.4)

BCG (bacille Calmette-Guérin) vaccine is always given intradermally. Use a 26G needle (or smaller), stretch the skin between the thumb and forefinger of one hand, and with the other hand slowly insert the needle (bevel upwards) for about 2 mm into the superficial layer of dermis. Keep the tip of the needle almost parallel with the surface. Slowly inject the vaccine. You should feel considerable resistance and see a blanched, raised bleb appear, showing the tips of hair follicles. If not, the needle is likely to be too deep. Reinsert before further vaccine is given. A vaccine amount of 0.1 ml should produce a bleb of about 7 mm in diameter. BCG vaccine is usually given over the insertion of the deltoid muscle. The tip of the shoulder should be avoided because of the increased risk of keloid formation at this site.

Suprapubic aspiration of urine

(Fig. 12.5)

This procedure is useful in infants where there is doubt about the presence of a urine infection or a specimen is needed promptly before antibiotics are started (e.g. in suspected sepsis). Portable ultrasound to check for a full bladder before proceeding increases the success rate from about 50% to 80%. There is no point performing this procedure if the child has just passed urine. Use a sterile technique, take a 5 ml syringe and attach a 25G (green) needle. Ask an assistant to hold the child's legs straight and hold the hands or arms with the

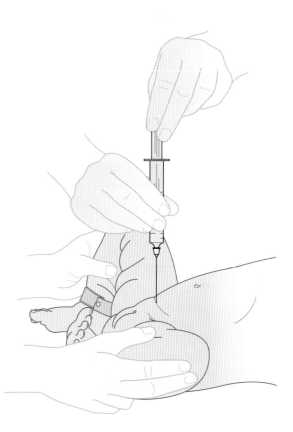

Fig. 12.5 Suprapubic aspiration of urine

other hand. Insert the needle downwards just above the pubic bone to a distance of about 2 cm. Gently aspirate urine into the syringe, then withdraw the needle and apply a small sticking plaster. *Any* bacterial growth from a suprapubic aspirate is significant, even if less than 10^5 organisms per ml.

Pulse oximetry

This measures the percentage of haemoglobin that is saturated with oxygen. It is based on the fact that deoxyhaemoglobin and oxyhaemoglobin absorb red and infrared light differently. The change in the amount of light of both frequencies passing through a digit or earlobe with each pulse is measured. This allows calculation of the relative amounts of oxygenated and deoxygenated haemoglobin in arterial blood. Accuracy is affected by peripheral vasoconstriction, venous congestion, movement, bright or flickering ambient light, different forms of haemoglobin and severe anaemia. Oxygen saturation has a non-linear correlation with partial pressure of oxygen (PaO_2). It is usually above 96% in children, and below 92% is considered to be hypoxia with a need for oxygen.

Intraosseus access

Learn this technique as soon as you start looking after sick children, since it gives you rapid vascular access

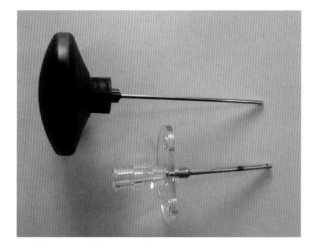

Fig. 12.6 **Intraosseous needle**

even in a very shut-down child. It is taught on paediatric advanced resuscitation courses. Use the specially designed needle (Fig. 12.6) with the handle cupped in your palm. With a firm rotating action, insert it at 90° to the skin into the anteromedial aspect of the tibia about 2 cm below and medial to the tibial tuberosity. (This avoids the growth plate.) Once correctly inserted, the needle should feel solid in the bone. Remove the trochar and aspirate for blood samples, then push in fluid with a syringe.

Long lines

Fine, flexible central catheters inserted through a peripheral vein (usually antecubital or saphenous) are used especially in neonatal patients who will need total parenteral nutrition (TPN) for several days, to minimize the handling and trauma of repeated peripheral lines. A butterfly needle is inserted into a peripheral vein, through which the line is passed until the length inserted matches that measured externally prior to the procedure. The needle is then slid out of the vein and either passed over the line or pulled into two parts to allow removal. Place the catheter tip in the superior or inferior vena cava well outside the heart to avoid the risk of tamponade, and use radio-opaque catheters or contrast injection to check the position regularly on X-ray (beware of migration).

Interpretation of investigations

General principles

1. Check the basics (e.g. name, units, orientation of a film, normal ranges for the lab used).

2. Never assume that normal ranges in children are the same as for adults. Many are different and vary across age range (Box 12.2).
3. Consider repeating unexpectedly abnormal results. They may be due to artefact or sampling error.
4. List differentials and use a logical approach: for example, listing all categories of aetiology (sometimes called a 'surgical sieve') to ensure you consider all possibilities.
5. Take all the available information into account when interpreting results, including salient features from the history, examination and other investigations. Aim to find a diagnosis that will explain all if possible.

See page 57 for a discussion of interpretation of common investigations. Other investigations are discussed later in the text.

Reference ranges

Most hospital laboratories make their own reference ranges available through a Trust intranet system or in published form. It is best to use these whenever possible, since ranges (and the units used) can vary between laboratories.

 www.labtestonline.org.uk
Information on investigations

 www.prodigy.nhs.uk
Search 'investigation' or by topic

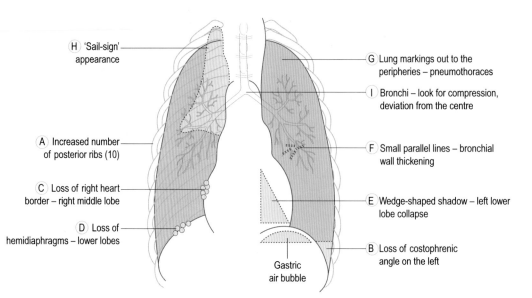

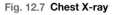

H 'Sail-sign' appearance

G Lung markings out to the peripheries – pneumothoraces

I Bronchi – look for compression, deviation from the centre

A Increased number of posterior ribs (10)

F Small parallel lines – bronchial wall thickening

C Loss of right heart border – right middle lobe

E Wedge-shaped shadow – left lower lobe collapse

D Loss of hemidiaphragms – lower lobes

B Loss of costophrenic angle on the left

Gastric air bubble

Fig. 12.7 **Chest X-ray**

Interpretation of X-rays

Develop a system for looking at X-rays that ensures you go through them logically without missing any important features. Always start with the basics: name and patient details, and orientation of both film and patient. Review films regularly with more experienced colleagues to help you improve your interpretation skills.

Chest X-rays (Fig. 12.7)

Basics (as above)
- Is the patient rotated (check symmetry of clavicles and ribs)?
- Was the film shot as postero-anterior (PA, usual) or antero-posterior (AP, may magnify the cardiac shadow)?

Lung fields
- Volume? (N.B. The number of posterior ribs above the diaphragm should be 8 or 9.)
  - Inadequate inspiration?
  - Hyperinflation: increased number of posterior ribs (10 in Fig. 12.7 — A), flattened diaphragm, ribs more horizontal.
- Collapse, consolidation, effusion:
  - Check for clarity of heart borders and both hemidiaphragms (including costophrenic angles — B on Fig. 12.7 shows loss of the angle on the left).
  - Clues to site of consolidation: loss of right heart border — right middle lobe (C), loss of left heart border — lingula; loss of hemidiaphragms — lower lobes (D).

- Look carefully behind the cardiac shadow; e.g. left lower lobe collapse may show as a wedge-shaped shadow (E), often accompanied by increased lucency of the left lung field compared to the right.
- Bronchial wall thickening:
  - Common in viral infections, especially in the perihilar regions (look for small parallel lines, F).
- Pneumothoraces:
  - Use bright light if in doubt to check for lung markings out to the peripheries (G).
- Lucency:
  - Is this symmetrical? Compare upper middle and lower zones. If uncertain, try covering the cardiac shadow with your hand.
  - Asymmetry if large collapse or foreign body.
- Other lung field changes:
  - Cystic (as in cystic fibrosis)
  - Ground glass (respiratory distress syndrome).

Heart and mediastinum
- Cardiac size and shape:
  - Cardiothoracic ratio (PA) < 0.55 under 2 years, < 0.50 above 2 years.
- Thymus:
  - May be quite large in small children, and have a flat lower border due to it resting on the horizontal fissure. This gives it the 'sail-sign' appearance (H).
- Trachea, carina (at the level of the 6th posterior rib) and bronchi (I):
  - Compression, deviation from centre, other signs of mediastinal shift?

Table 12.1 Guide to investigations you should have seen and/or performed

System/type	Investigation	Reference in *Master Course*
Biochemistry	Urea and electrolytes (U&Es), creatinine	Ch. 40
	Glucose	Ch. 35
	Liver function tests (LFTs)	Ch. 39
	C-reactive protein (CRP)	Ch. 44
	Calcium and phosphate	Ch. 33
	Magnesium	Ch. 44
Microbiology and virology	Microscopy and culture	Ch. 44
	Viral culture	Ch. 44
	Polymerase chain reaction (PCR)	Ch. 44
	Respiratory syncytial virus (RSV) immunofluorescence	Ch. 44
	Bordetella pertussis culture	Ch. 44
	Viral titres	Ch. 44
	Hepatitis serology	Ch. 44
Haematology	Full blood count (FBC) and film	Ch. 43
	Erythrocyte sedimentation rate (ESR)	Ch. 43
	Plasma viscosity	Ch. 43
	Clotting screen	Ch. 43
	Sickle test	Ch. 43
	Advanced tests of clotting and platelet function	Ch. 43
	Platelet antibodies	Ch. 43
Immunology, infections, and allergy	Total and specific IgE	Ch. 44
	Functional antibodies	Ch. 44
	Coeliac screen	Ch. 44
	Immunoglobulins	Ch. 44
	IgG subclasses	Ch. 44
	Neutrophil function tests	Ch. 44
	Cell markers	Ch. 44
	Human immunodeficiency virus (HIV) testing	Ch. 44
	Autoantibodies	Ch. 44
	Immune complexes and complement	Ch. 44
	Human leucocyte antigen (HLA) typing	Ch. 44
Cardiology	Electrocardiography (ECG)	Ch. 41
	Echo	Ch. 41
Respiratory and ear, nose and throat	Peak flow	Chs 23 and 42
	Respiratory function tests	Chs 23 and 42
	Sweat test	Chs 23 and 42
Gastrointestinal and hepatobiliary	Test feed	Chs 25 and 39
	Endoscopy	Chs 25 and 39
	White cell scan	Chs 25 and 39
Renal, fluid and electrolyte balance	Plasma and urine osmolality	Ch. 40
	Urine electrolytes	Ch. 40
	Renal ultrasound	Ch. 40
	DMSA	Ch. 40
	MCUG	Ch. 40
	MAG3	Ch. 40
	Glomerular filtration rate (GFR)	Ch. 40
Neurology	Lumbar puncture	Chs 24 and 28
	Ultrasound head	Chs 24 and 28
	Computed tomography (CT) head	Chs 24 and 28
	Magnetic resonance imaging (MRI) head	Chs 24 and 28
	Electroencephalogram (EEG)	Chs 24 and 28
	Nerve conduction	Chs 24 and 28
	Creatine kinase	Chs 24 and 28
	Muscle biopsy	Chs 24 and 28
Oncology	Tumour markers	Ch. 51

Table 12.1 Guide to investigations you should have seen and/or performed (*cont'd*)

System/type	Investigation	Reference in *Master Course*
Endocrine and metabolic	Thyroid function	Ch. 35
	HbA₁C	Ch. 35
	Glucose tolerance test	Ch. 35
	Metabolic screen	Ch. 35
	Tandem mass spectrometry	Ch. 35
	Follicle-stimulating hormone (FSH) and luteinizing hormone (LH)	Ch. 35
	Sex steroids	Ch. 35
	Cortisol	Ch. 35
	Growth hormone	Ch. 35
	Vitamin D	Ch. 35
Child protection	Skeletal survey	Chs 21 and 37
Rheumatology and orthopaedics	Tissue biopsy	Ch. 33
	Synovial fluid analysis	Ch. 33
	Athroscopy	Ch. 33
Genetic	Karyotype	Ch. 9
	Fluorescent in situ hybridization (FISH) testing for mutations	Ch. 9

Bones

- Check all carefully for fractures (especially ribs and clavicles) or other abnormality.

Other

- Look at other features visible on the film: upper abdomen, arms, neck, upper airway, soft tissues, and tubes and lines.

Abdominal X-rays

These are useful for the acute abdomen, especially when obstruction or perforation is suspected. For the latter, combine with an erect chest X-ray to look for gas under the diaphragm (and also for pneumonia). Some units advise an erect abdominal film too. Check for pattern and amount of bowel gas, any fluid levels and bowel distension. A gasless abdomen is suggestive of obstruction, as are fluid levels on an erect film. Abdominal X-rays are generally not useful in constipation.

Skull X-rays

These are not now routinely done in children with head injuries since they do not reliably identify child-ren who need a computed tomography (CT) head scan. They may be indicated in certain situations; for example, in suspected non-accidental head injury it is helpful to know whether a fracture is present. You need to be familiar with the appearance of normal vascular markings and sutures lines, so that you can distinguish these from fractures. Fractures tend to be blacker than vascular markings (because both tables of the skull are involved), and may have less-defined edges. If there are any branches, they do not taper uniformly as do vascular markings. Depressed fractures appear denser (whiter) on a radiograph.

 **www.rch.org.au/clinicalguide/index.cfm?
doc_id=5033**

The Royal Children's Hospital Melbourne has an excellent Clinical Practice Guidelines section with guidelines and further information (including videos) on most practical procedures

Table 12.1 indicates the procedures that you should have either performed or seen.

David Evans   Alison Pike

CHAPTER

13

Evidence-based paediatrics and audit

LEARNING OUTCOMES

By the end of this chapter you should:

- Be able to describe the structure used to formulate a clinical question
- Be able to identify the advantages of using the Cochrane Library as a starting point for searching evidence on the effectiveness of interventions
- Know how to compare and contrast bias and chance as sources of error
- Be able to critically appraise a randomized controlled trial
- Be able to interpret the commonly used measures of treatment efficacy and understand the utility of confidence intervals
- Be able to describe the purpose of clinical audit
- Be able to identify the steps required in formulating a clinical audit project.

MODULE TWO

What is evidence-based medicine?

Evidence-based medicine (EBM) involves the 'integration of best available external evidence with individual clinical expertise. In other words, it means applying relevant, up-to-date research findings to the management of your patients.

There are many reasons why familiarity with the techniques of EBM has become increasingly necessary. Firstly, we now require evidence of efficacy from the results of randomized control trials (RCTs) reporting clinically relevant outcomes, whereas in the past, an understanding of the pathophysiological process was deemed sufficient. Secondly, evidence changes with the growth of our knowledge base through continued research, so that it is crucial that we develop techniques that search out the latest evidence. Thirdly, traditional medical education has evolved from the handing down of knowledge and skills from expert practitioners to apprentices. In the past, this may have placed too much reliance on believing the experts, thus inhibiting questioning behaviour.

What EBM is not!

EBM is not 'cookbook' medicine, threatening to take away individual clinicians' judgment (honed over years of experience). Clinical expertise and experience are

125

very much required. It is still essential to make a correct diagnosis! Communication skills, enabling appreciation of your patient's values, are important in selecting whether a particular treatment choice would be in your patient's best interests.

It is not the primary function of EBM to ration or deny patient choice. Rather, it provides a framework by which healthcare interventions can be judged or compared, in terms of important patient outcomes. Whether achieving these outcomes is worth the financial expenditure is largely a political decision.

EBM is not restricted to RCTs and meta-analyses. We need to be just as stringent when considering non-therapeutic interventions.

The five steps of EBM

- Formulating an answerable clinical question
- Searching for the evidence
- Critical appraisal of the evidence
- Applying the evidence to help your patient
- Evaluation of your performance.

Step 1: Posing the question

It is all too easy to practise without asking questions, as these have the annoying habit of exposing gaps in knowledge which then require time and effort to plug! When we do have questions about current practice, however, they often appear unstructured, too vague or too complex. Good questions should be focused on the medical problem and concentrated on outcomes of interest. The framework most commonly used to formulate clinical questions has four components:

- P The *patient* with the pathology
- I The *intervention*, diagnostic test or exposure of interest
- C The *comparison* (if relevant)
- O The *outcomes* of interest.

Questions clearly focused in this way (PICO) have the greatest chance of being answerable (see example, Box 13.1).

Step 2: Searching for the evidence

What to search for?

We are looking for high-quality contemporary studies that address our clinical question. Textbooks are unlikely to be sufficiently up to date and, despite their claims, expert colleagues may not be aware of all the relevant literature. When looking for evidence about the effectiveness of

---

BOX 13.1 Example of PICO

Would preterm infants at risk of respiratory distress syndrome (< 30 weeks' gestation) [*patient and pathology*] benefit from early treatment (< 15 minutes) with an animal-derived surfactant [*intervention*], as opposed to delayed treatment for established respiratory disease [*comparison*], in terms of mortality, length of respiratory support, days in oxygen, pneumothorax and intraventricular haemorrhage [*outcomes*]?

---

clinical interventions (such as surfactant), we require data from RCTs. However, searching a bibliographical database, such as Medline or Pubmed, can be an unrewarding exercise unless a focused search strategy is employed.

How to search

Electronic searching of databases allows combinations of search keywords, most often combined with either 'AND' or 'OR' Boolean operators. For example, a search to address the surfactant question might have the following structure (PICO):

- P Infant, preterm *OR* Respiratory distress syndrome
  AND
- I Surfactant
  AND
- O Mortality *OR* Pneumothorax *OR* Chronic lung disease *OR* Intraventricular haemorrhage.

The combination of terms 'Infant, preterm *OR* Respiratory distress syndrome' will result in the search returning articles containing either of the terms. The combination of 'Infant, preterm *AND* Surfactant' will return only those containing both terms. There are many refinements to searching, such as using a combination of text word and medical subheadings, or using wildcard characters (useful for North American spelling, e.g. an?emia — for anaemia or anemia) and truncated words (e.g. neonat* — for neonate, neonates, neonatal, neonatology etc).

Medical librarians can offer expert tips and advice on how to make a search either more sensitive, which is useful when the initial strategy results in few articles, or more specific, which is useful when the initial strategy results in too many articles, some of which are not useful. Many of the search engines, such as Medline or Pubmed, have the ability to restrict the publication type (e.g. only retrieve reports of RCTs).

www.ncbi.nlm.nih.gov

The Cochrane Library

It would be great if every search found a definitive study that addressed our clinical question. More usually, search results fall into two categories. Either we fail to find a single relevant article or we find too many.

Let us consider the first situation. One reason for not finding a study is that, unfortunately, not all studies can be found by searching Medline. This is because they may be published elsewhere: in journals that are not listed on Medline (which favours English language journals) or in what is known as the 'grey literature' (abstracts, proceedings of meetings, university theses etc.). Fortunately, the Cochrane Collaboration employs trained searchers to look through all the literature in its differing types and languages. From this search, any RCTs are picked out and listed in a separate database, known as CENTRAL/Cochrane Controlled Trials Register, a component of the Cochrane Library. This can be searched in the same way as Medline and is probably the best place to start when looking for RCTs.

> www.cochrane.org
> www.thecochranelibrary.com

The Cochrane Library also offers a solution to the second problem (i.e. the need to synthesize information from many studies). The library contains a database of systematic reviews; these are a summary of the literature relating to the effectiveness of an intervention. By preparing and publishing reviews, the Cochrane Collaboration aims to help clinicians by undertaking a lot of the background work required to answer common clinical questions about the effectiveness of interventions. The preparation of a review involves conducting a comprehensive search of the literature, followed by critical appraisal of any retrieved studies. The results are presented in a purposeful format, which might or might not include a meta-analysis of trial data.

The Cochrane Library is restricted to information about healthcare *interventions* but there are an increasing number of other secondary publications that address diagnosis, prognosis, harm, cost-effectiveness etc. A list of these can be found on the Public Health Resource Unit website.

> www.phru.nhs.uk/casp/sources_of_evidence.
> htm

Search strategies

The Centre for Evidence-Based Medicine gives very useful guidance on 'how to get the right stuff and avoid getting the wrong stuff'! This includes methods of altering the sensitivity and specificity of your searches and also strategies to pick out the most relevant publication types (RCTs, cohort studies etc.) in order to answer the different types of question (interventions, prognosis, harm, diagnosis etc.).

> www.cebm.net/searching.asp

Step 3: Critical appraisal of the evidence

There are four main stages to appraising any evidence:
1. *Relevance*. This stage is largely intuitive (i.e. you are not going to waste time reading a paper if it is not relevant!), although using the PICO formulation helps you focus your attention and quickly decide whether the study is assessing the relevant intervention in the appropriate patients and reporting the important outcomes.
2. *Validity*. Can I believe the results? A dictionary definition of validity might include 'based upon or borne out by truth'. Why do we need to appraise validity? Surely, if evidence is published it must be correct? Although research fraud does exist, no one is suggesting that the majority of authors are trying to falsify claims, but there might be many reasons why the evidence you have just found will not be as valid as you hoped. Despite all the best intentions, a research study might not produce results that are 'based upon truth' as far as the researchers had anticipated (see below).
3. *Significance*. Are the results likely to result in an important improvement? We will consider this in more detail in the section on assessing significance.
4. *Applicability*. Can I apply the results so that my patients receive similar benefits to the study participants?

The importance of validity

Box 13.2 represents an analogy of a research experiment.

There are a number of reasons why the results obtained do not match those anticipated. These can be grouped into three categories:
- *Wrong hypothesis*. Perhaps the object was a tetrahedron, not a dice.
- *Random error (chance)*. Confidence intervals (CIs) give an indication of variation in results attributable by chance (see later section). In this example, the 95% CIs include the possibilities that the object could have between three and seven sides. Performing a larger study (e.g. 600 throws) will reduce this variation and narrow the 95% CIs.
- *Systematic error (bias)*. Was the dice weighted? Was your friend lying? Is your friend also visually impaired? Is he innumerate? Do you also have a

You are given a solid object and your task is to determine how many surfaces it has. You have been told that the object has a number of flat surfaces of equal area. Each surface has a number of dots but only one surface has one dot.

You suspect from your prior knowledge that the object is a dice (hypothesis). Unfortunately, you cannot see or feel the object well enough to determine this by inspection (because of a visual impairment and peripheral neuropathy). Thus, you test your hypothesis by throwing the object and asking your friend to call out each time the surface with the single dot is uppermost. You throw the object 60 times, expecting your friend to call out on 10 occasions but, in fact, he calls out 15 times.

Think of the reasons why the result was not what you expected.

hearing impairment? In contrast to random error, statistics or CIs are not helpful with these sources of bias; performing a larger study would just compound the error. The sources of bias need to be minimized by improving study design. In the vignette, one might want to test your friend's vision against a known standard beforehand (e.g. Snellen chart). Other ways of assessing the outcome might be to use two independent observers, who separately record their observations, or by filming the throws for validation purposes etc.

How is this analogous to a research study? Well, in real life the truth is only ever *inferred through observation*. If we wish to study the effectiveness of surfactant therapy on the delivery suite, we cannot actually see the surfactant molecules benefiting the infant. We have to make observations on outcomes that we can measure, such as mortality or chronic lung disease. Unfortunately, these outcomes are not necessarily easy to define and are subject to both random effects and systematic influences (gestation, presence of infection etc.). Statistics help us assess random error, but good study design is essential and constitutes the only way of minimizing systematic error or bias.

The validity of a study is therefore determined by its design; good study design ensures validity by minimizing bias. Thus, the most appropriate place in an article to assess validity is in the description of methods. Unfortunately, this is often the least-read section of an article. Many of the teachings of EBM and critical appraisal courses are intended to equip readers with the skills to interpret the methods of the more commonly employed study designs in clinical medicine.

Randomized controlled trials

One of the most important study designs used to assess the effectiveness of an intervention is the RCT. When assessing whether an RCT has reported valid claims, it is important to know what aspects of this design make it such a powerful methodology and hence which aspects of design must, where possible, be strictly adhered to in order to minimize bias.

Randomization method

Randomization refers to the method of treatment allocation. It is an extremely powerful technique because it controls for both known and unknown confounding variables. For example, a known confounding variable influencing survival of preterm infants is the infant's sex. It would be possible to match for sex by simply allocating the early surfactant treatment to equal numbers of boys and girls without randomizing; this would indeed control for this known confounding variable. However, let us suppose that you run a (non-randomized) study in this way, confident that you have matched for the infant's sex. Just before you are due to receive the accolades of your colleagues, someone discovers that high maternal body fat composition is associated with improved perinatal survival and you realize that the early surfactant group had mothers with more body fat, effectively ruining your results. Random allocation would have protected you from the confounding influence of maternal body fat, even though, at the time, you did not know of its significance.

Allocation should be truly random (e.g. computer-generated random number lists). Other methods, such as allocation by alternating assignment, hospital number, dates of birth etc., are known as quasi-randomization and are prone to selection bias.

Randomization is frequently stratified. This is because, although randomization should balance all the confounding variables, in trials with relatively small numbers all the variables may not be equally balanced. A common situation in which stratification is used is where an RCT evaluates the effectiveness of a treatment for a rare disorder, with many participating centres. Each centre will only recruit a modest number and stratifying randomization for each centre (i.e. each centre having its own random number list) will ensure that any centre-specific differences in treatment are balanced within the trial. It is also common to stratify for disease severity (if reliable markers of severity can be determined before trial entry), so that the groups contain patients of a similar prognostic profile.

Allocation concealment

This technique prevents prior knowledge of the treatment allocation before patient entry into a trial. It is particularly important in RCTs where the treatment is complex and resource-intensive, and cannot be blinded. An example would be extra-corporeal membranous oxygenation (ECMO) for severe respiratory failure in infants. The treatment might require the very sick infant to be transferred to a referral centre for the procedure, whereas the control might involve standard respiratory care at the original hospital. If the clinicians responsible for entering patients into the trial were to know what the allocated treatment would be before they enrolled the infant, this could bias selection for the study. For example, if the infant were extremely unstable and the clinicians were worried that the infant might not survive transfer, they would be more willing to enter the infant into the study if they knew that the allocated treatment was standard respiratory care at the original hospital. Selection bias in this way would result in the control group having a higher proportion of sicker infants than the intervention group.

The best method of concealing the allocation is to require the clinician entering a patient into an RCT to telephone and register the pre-randomization details (including any markers of disease severity used for stratification). The patient is then entered into the trial before the clinician is told the allocated treatment. Less robust methods include using opaque-sealed envelopes, although eager clinicians have been known to attempt transillumination or steam treatment in an effort to find out the allocated treatment!

Intention-to-treat analysis

There are many reasons why patients' treatments deviate from what was allocated at randomization: misdiagnosis, being given the wrong treatment by mistake (it happens!), not complying with the treatment, withdrawal of consent, loss to follow-up etc. Despite all these mishaps, the patients' data should always be analysed according to the group allocated at randomization (intention-to-treat analysis). Randomization is the point in the study when patient characteristics (and confounding variables) are matched. There may be a systematic reason (connected to the treatment) why certain patients cannot comply with the protocol. Using the ECMO example, if infants do not survive transfer to the ECMO treatment centre, it would be misleading to disregard their data (the excuse being 'they did not receive ECMO') and, worse still, to analyse their data with the control group ('because they received standard care'). This is because the transfer is a necessary part of ECMO and ignoring data from patients allocated

ECMO but not surviving leads to a misleading over-estimation of any beneficial ECMO treatment effect.

The three techniques described above are mandatory for an RCT to be valid; there can be little excuse for not carrying out true randomization with allocation concealment and intention-to-treat analysis.

Blinding

This is an important technique in RCT methodology but there may be pragmatic constraints on researchers' abilities to blind various aspects of a study. Blinding is useful when the outcome of interest is subjective (think about the 'placebo effect') or the definition is open to interpretation. The use of a placebo, indistinguishable from the active treatment, controls the natural tendency in carers and parents to believe that new treatments confer benefit. However, it is not always possible or ethical to use a placebo or to blind caregivers (think of surgical procedures, injections etc.). In these cases, it is important to try to blind the outcome assessment. For example, if the outcome is to be a severity score of lung disease on chest radiographs, the radiographs should be interpreted by someone who is unaware of the treatment allocation.

The Public Health Resource Unit publishes a useful appraisal checklist comprising ten questions, which encompass appraisal of the techniques described above.

www.phru.nhs.uk/casp/critical_appraisal_tools.htm#rct

Systematic review and meta-analysis

As outlined previously, a systematic review aims to summarize all the available evidence relating to studies addressing a defined clinical question. Systematic reviews that address questions about the effectiveness of interventions follow a rigorous methodology. They should comprise a comprehensive search for RCTs (that address a focused question), selection with the use of explicit predetermined criteria, critical appraisal of each study and synthesis of results. The review lists the characteristics of each RCT (which patients, which intervention compared with which control, and which outcomes are reported). A review will also draw the reader's attention to whether or not the trial employed sufficient methodology to protect against bias (allocation concealment, intention-to-treat analysis etc.).

Strictly speaking, meta-analysis refers to the statistical technique of combining the results of a number of RCTs, unearthed by the systematic review (although, confusingly, North Americans often use the term synonymously with the term systematic review). It is only appropriate to combine results from RCTs if: (a) the definitions of outcomes are sufficiently similar, and (b) the trials are of sufficient methodological standard. We will look at how to interpret the results of a meta-analysis in the section on assessment of significance.

Other study designs

Two other study designs deserve mention: cohort and case-control studies. These designs are frequently used in clinical epidemiological work to determine the answers to questions about prognosis, risks, harm and diagnosis.

Cohort study

This is useful for examining what happens to a selected sample of patients exposed to a risk factor over time, compared to a non-exposed population — the comparison being in the form of relative risk. Cohort studies are able to measure more than one outcome. For example, in children whose risk was that they were born prematurely, the outcomes might be death, cerebral palsy and cognitive impairment. Cohort studies also allow temporal relationships to be observed. They are relatively expensive if run over a long timescale. The main sources of bias are:

- *Selection bias*. The population should be established at a common (early) point in their disease following exposure to the risk factor.
- *Loss to follow-up*. This needs to be minimized.
- *Diagnostic (ascertainment, surveillance) bias*. If the exposed group are being followed up more closely (e.g. with more frequent examinations) than controls, there is a greater chance of detecting an outcome (and at an earlier stage).
- *Recall bias*, if retrospective.

Case-control study

In this study design, cases are sought with the outcome of interest (e.g. autism) and controls are picked from the population who do not have this outcome. The prevalence of exposure to a number of risk factors is determined retrospectively and compared between the two groups (e.g. maternal infections, measles/mumps/rubella (MMR) vaccinations), in the form of odds ratios. The advantage of a case-control study is that it allows study of the impact of multiple risk factors on a rare outcome, in contrast to a cohort study, which examines the effect of a rare risk factor on multiple outcomes. The disadvantage is that any temporal relationship between risk and outcome is difficult to identify.

The main sources of bias are:
- *Selection bias*, particularly in the selection of controls. Ideally, it should be a random sample from the population, but often hospital-based controls are used because they are easily identified.
- *Information (recall) bias*. Exposure information is reported differently in cases and controls (e.g. parents with autistic children are more likely to recall a reaction to MMR vaccination, particularly if they are aware of the hypothesis).
- *Information (observation) bias*. The investigator, who may be aware of the hypothesis, interprets the information differently.

The major confounding variables (that are known) can be controlled for in the design of both cohort and case-control studies by matching. The results have to be adjusted for other known confounders by use of complex statistical techniques in the analysis, such as logistic regression. (In comparison, the statistical techniques for analysing the results of RCTs are relatively straightforward.) Unknown confounders remain unknown and cannot be controlled for in study design (unlike randomization).

The Public Health Resource Unit also publishes appraisal checklists for systematic reviews, cohort and case-control studies, as well as other study designs.

www.phru.nhs.uk/casp/critical_appraisal_tools.htm

A note of caution

There is no such thing as a perfect clinical research study; this is because there are usually practical constraints upon clinicians (ethical, financial, time, wilful patients! etc.). The skill in appraising a study is not simply to 'pick holes' in someone else's endeavour but, rather, to determine whether or not the problems you have noted compromise the study to the extent that the results are no longer reliable. Think to yourself, 'Could I have improved the design?' and also 'Are these improvements actually feasible?'

Assessment of significance
Measurements of efficacy

Box 13.3 gives the definitions of some of the common measurements of efficacy derived from the results of RCTs. Conventionally, events are considered to be adverse outcomes (e.g. death, cerebral palsy etc.) and therefore we are hoping for a reduction in the odds and risks of such events in the treatment group, compared to the control group. Thus, an odds ratio or a relative risk of less than 1 indicates that the treatment is associated with a lower risk of adverse outcome. If the odds ratio or relative risk is greater than 1, the treatment is associated with increased risk. If the ratios are equal to 1, the treatment is neither effective nor harmful.

P-values and 95% confidence intervals

If any experiment or study were repeated, it would be unlikely to produce exactly the same results each time because of the random variation that occurs each time a differing patient population is sampled. Therefore, there is a risk that the result yielded by a single study does not represent a true treatment effect in the population at large but, rather, a chance effect. The p-value is the probability that the observed result has arisen purely by chance. It can be seen that if the p-value is small, then the result is unlikely to be a chance effect and, hence, more likely to be a treatment effect. Conventionally, a p-value of < 0.05 is taken as a low enough risk of a random effect (< 5%) for the result to be 'statistically significant'.

Whilst the p-value gives us a good idea of the risk of random error or chance effects, CIs give more useful information. A CI is a range of values that is likely to include the true treatment effect in the population, the estimated range being calculated from the sample studied in the RCT. The confidence level (usually 95%) describes how confident we are that the true effect falls within that range. A 95% CI means that if the study were repeated 100 times, 95 of the studies would give a result within that range. Choosing a higher confidence level, such as 99%, would make us even more confident that the range included the true result.

In the case of the odds ratio or relative risk, if the 95% CI includes the value 1, it means that we cannot confidently exclude the possibility that the treatment has no effect (and therefore the result is not statistically significant, with p > 0.05). An example of such a study is Egberts 1993 in Figure 13.1. If the whole of the 95% CI for the relative risk or the odds ratio is less than 1, the treatment effect is statistically significant (p < 0.05) (e.g. Bevilacqua 1996 in Fig. 13.1).

The width of the CI gives us some idea about how uncertain we are about the treatment effect. A very wide interval may indicate that more data should be collected before anything very definite can be construed.

Meta-analysis

The results from a number of RCTs may be combined to give a more precise estimate of the treatment effect, as long as: (a) the definitions of outcomes are sufficiently similar, and (b) the trials are of sufficient methodological standard. The results can be displayed in the form of a forest plot. An example is given in Figure 13.1, which comes from a Cochrane review of RCTs evaluating the effects of early prophylactic surfactant therapy versus delayed surfactant treatment for respiratory distress syndrome on death or chronic lung disease (Yost & Soll 1999). The studies that report a statistically significant beneficial treatment effect can be clearly seen due to the fact that their point estimates and 95% CIs all fall to the left of the line on the graphical representation. Non-significant studies have 95% CIs that cross the line.

The results are combined in a meta-analysis, giving greatest weight to those studies that report results with higher precision (narrower 95% CIs). An advantage of a meta-analysis is that many small studies, each with equivocal results, may be combined to produce a more precise overall estimate of treatment effect. Also, if a treatment effect is seen to be consistent across all the studies (with varying, albeit similar, populations), one might be more confident that the treatment will

	Expt	Ctrl	RR (95% CI)	
Bevilacqua 1996	40/136	63/132	0.62 (0.45–0.85)	
Dunn 1991	31/62	16/60	1.88 (1.15–3.05)	
Egberts 1993	30/75	31/72	0.97 (0.66–1.43)	
Kattwinkel 1993	32/627	54/621	0.59 (0.39–0.90)	
Kendig 1991	108/235	129/244	0.87 (0.72–1.04)	
Merrit 1991	35/102	29/101	1.20 (0.80–1.80)	
Walti 1995	53/134	66/122	0.73 (0.56–0.95)	
Combined relative risk (RR)			**0.85 (0.76–0.95)**	

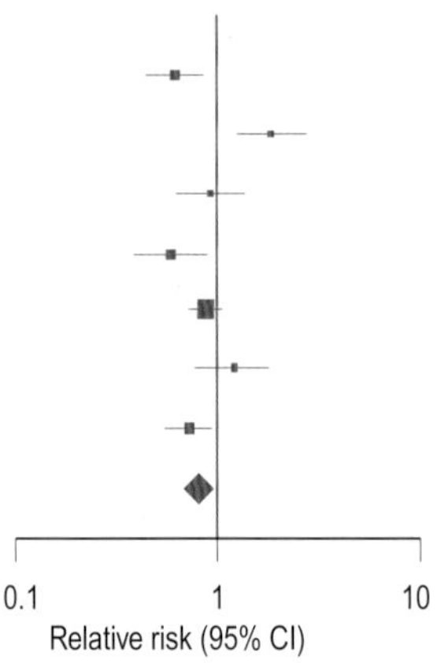

Relative risk (95% CI)

Fig. 13.1 Forest plot: meta-analysis of randomized controlled trials comparing prophylactic surfactant therapy (Expt) with later surfactant treatment (Ctrl) for respiratory distress syndrome.
  Outcome: death or chronic lung disease.

be beneficial when applied outside the strict confines of a research study.

Sample size

A sample size calculation is performed before the study to provide an estimate of how many patients will be required to generate meaningful data. The sample size for an RCT is dependent upon four factors:
1. *Event rates*. If the outcome of interest is rare (e.g. death from acute asthma), the sample size will be greater than for studies with more common outcomes (e.g. death following leukaemia).
2. *Treatment effect*. Studies looking for small treatment effects will need to be larger than studies that are looking for larger, more obvious effects.
3. *Significance* (α). This is the level of probability below which you would accept that the results would not have occurred by chance (i.e. p-value $< \alpha$). The smaller the p-value with which you need to convince yourself the observed effect is real, the larger the study required.
4. *Power (1-β)*. This is the ability of a study to detect a true treatment effect. RCTs are often powered to detect a true treatment effect 80% of the time; this means there is a 20% risk ($\beta=0.2$) that the RCT will produce an equivocal result, despite the treatment being effective. Hence, one needs to be cautious about stating that a treatment is not effective, based upon the results of a small RCT of low power, since there is a fair chance that the RCT might have missed an unequivocal result. Studies that are designed to have more power require more patients.

Clinical versus statistical significance

Although the results may be statistically significant, the treatment effect may not necessarily be clinically significant. For example, a bronchodilator is found to produce a 10% increase in peak expiratory flow rates in asthma (95% CIs 8–12%), but this statistically significant result might not result in a clinically significant improvement in symptoms.

Determining whether the results from a study are clinically significant requires clinical judgment and depends upon the values of your patient, which brings us to the penultimate step in EBM.

Step 4: Applying the evidence to help your patient

If we have determined that the results of a study are valid and significant, we then have to decide whether applying the evidence will benefit our patient. The following questions are useful when coming to such decisions:
1. *Is my patient similar to those patients studied?* Look at the eligibility or selection criteria. Was the frequency of outcome in the study what I would expect in my practice? For example, if the death rates were much higher than I would expect, perhaps the studied population might be more severely affected by the disease than my patient.
2. *Do the potential side-effects of treatment outweigh the benefits?* Did the study report all the side-effects that would be important to my patient? Does the benefit/risk ratio accord with my patient's expectations and values? Will my patient comply with the regimen?

3. *Can I offer the treatment?* Do I have the facilities to ensure the treatment is administered safely (e.g. technology, trained staff)? Do I have the required resources (e.g. time, money)?

Step 5: Evaluation of your performance

We need to learn from the process of practising EBM. Firstly, are we challenging our current practice and asking questions in an appropriately formulated manner? Can we find good evidence using searches with the right balance of sensitivity and specificity? Are we critically appraising papers relevant to our practice (both individually and in 'journal clubs')? Has the application of evidence led to an improvement in patient outcomes? This final step shares many of the concepts and techniques with clinical audit.

Clinical audit

What is clinical audit?

Clinical audit is the systematic process by which we assess, evaluate and improve the quality of healthcare of our patients. As doctors, clinical audit provides us with a powerful tool for improving patient care and ensuring that we are performing effective evidence-based practice.

The Healthcare Commission (2004) states that:

The overall aim of clinical audit is to improve patient outcomes by improving professional practice and the general quality of services delivered. This is achieved through a continuous process where healthcare professionals review patient care against agreed standards and make changes, where necessary, to meet those standards. The audit is then repeated to see if the changes have been made and the quality of patient care improved.

 ww.healthcarecommission.org. uk/serviceproviderinformation/ nationalclinicalaudit/aboutclinicalaudit. cfm?cit_id=306

Why should we take clinical audit seriously?

Clinical audit is an essential part of our professional practice. As juniors working within National Health Service (NHS) departments, it is sometimes difficult to visualize the important role our small contribution to clinical audit projects or other activities plays. Pursuit of the highest quality of care based on the best evidence within the available resources must be the goal of all medical practitioners. Clinical audit provides us with a tool for reviewing and confirming our quality of patient care and outcome and enables us to highlight and plan strategies for improvement.

The concept of audit or performance review as part of good medical practice is not new. Medical audit performed by doctors has now evolved into clinical audit, where ownership lies with each and every healthcare professional assessing all aspects of care. Patients themselves may be included. Importantly, with the formal introduction of clinical audit to the NHS over the past decade has come the allocation of resources.

Currently, regular or indeed compulsory participation in clinical audit is endorsed by government NHS policies and our Royal Colleges. It is integral to guidelines for best medical practice (General Medical Council) and is stated as a professional requirement by recommendations from public enquiries.

It is therefore vital that we understand the principles behind successful clinical audit and ensure that our working environment provides the necessary level of support and culture for achieving it.

What aspects of healthcare can be audited?

The three main areas of practice that clinical audit focuses on are:
1. *Structure.* What resources are available and how are they organized?
2. *Process.* How are the resources used and what activities or interventions are undertaken?
3. *Outcome.* What is the effect of the activities or interventions on the health and wellbeing of the patient?

The most common audits are usually those involved with processes, i.e. if evidence-based practice tells us that intervention A is best for our patient, is this what we are doing?

If problems within the structure of healthcare are identified, the solution usually has financial implications and needs to be part of a managerial plan.

Audits of outcome look at whether our care and interventions are producing the right results. Has the patient, having received the proven intervention A, had the anticipated outcome? This sort of project can be complicated if it involves comparisons of outcome between different case mixes or population groups. Monitoring of outcomes per se cannot be classified as audit unless the data are used as the driver for change in practice.

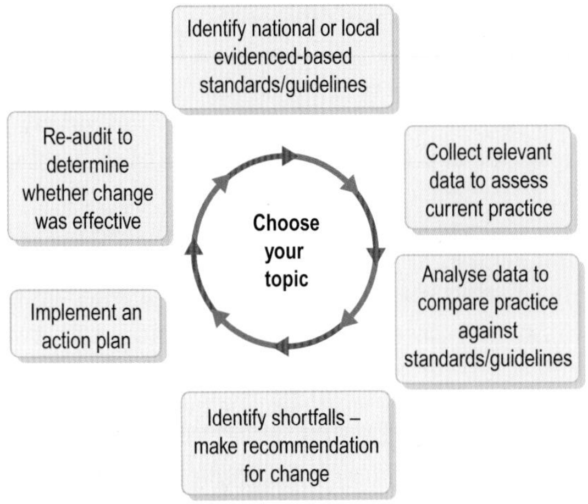

Fig. 13.2 The clinical audit cycle.
As each cycle is successfully completed, the process spirals upwards towards a higher level of quality.

The clinical audit cycle

The most frequently used clinical audit method is the standards-based or criterion-based clinical audit cycle (Fig. 13.2). The method involves completing a number of stages and activities in a systematic process. Whether the audit is being carried out as part of a national objective or to address local issues, the principles are the same:

- Identify best practice.
- Collect relevant data to assess current practice.
- Analyse data to compare practice against selected criteria.
- Identify actions to recommend change and improve care.
- Implement an action plan.
- Re-audit to determine change was effective ('closing the loop').

Other related activities

There are other activities occurring within NHS departments that, although not classical standards-based audit, help to provide useful information that can link into the planning and execution of successful audit:

- Monitoring outcome by data collection is not audit unless the intention is for the data to be used to set standards (pre-audit).
- Morbidity and mortality meetings involve peer review of the care of a selected group of patients with adverse outcomes.
- Critical incident reporting and monitoring within NHS departments have the prime intention to minimize risk.
- Patient feedback and surveys are productive methods of monitoring consumer views and

satisfaction with their quality of care. If the focus of the feedback involves whether standards have been met, then this activity can be included as audit.

The interaction between clinical audit and clinical governance

Clinical governance was introduced into the NHS in the 1997 White Paper, 'The New NHS: Modern, Dependable' (Department of Health 1997). The aim is to ensure that patients receive the highest quality of care. Existing quality assurance activities, such as research and development, education and training and risk management, were incorporated under its framework. As clinical audit is central to healthcare improvement, it forms one of the core components.

Two other components of clinical governance that audit is most frequently confused with are clinical effectiveness and research. Their relationship is shown in Figure 13.3.

Clinical effectiveness

Clinical effectiveness concerns the extent to which a healthcare intervention works and whether the greatest health gain is being provided from the available resource. Its purpose is to:

- Inform practitioners of the best available clinical and cost-effective evidence
- Change clinical and managerial practice if necessary
- Monitor changes that occur and result in real improvements in quality of healthcare.

The role of audit within clinical effectiveness is to confirm that clinically effective practice is being undertaken.

Audit or research?

The principles behind clinical audit and research are also similar but distinct. It is important that there is differentiation between the two because of the consequences and actions that by necessity follow both. Research is about creating new knowledge and defining what is 'best practice'. Clinical audit is about using that knowledge to ensure that we are 'carrying out the agreed best practice'.

How to be successful with audit

Good preparation is crucial before undertaking any project. The National Institute for Clinical Excellence (NICE) outlines five steps to create the right environment for success.

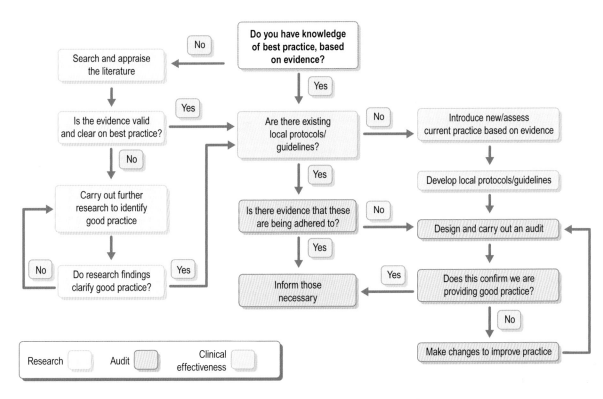

Fig. 13.3 The relationship between research, clinical effectiveness and clinical audit.
(Acknowledgements to North Bristol NHS Trust Clinical Audit & Effectiveness Department.)

Step 1: Preparation

First choose your topic. Priorities for audit are often directed by clinical effectiveness or governance teams and are driven by national or local targets. They can be prioritized, depending on frequency, risk and level of concern. At a national level NICE provides advice on best practice and cost-effective care with existing and new treatments. The Healthcare Commission has responsibility for the national audit plan. Standards for children's health, social services and the interface with education were published in the Children's National Service Framework (NSF) in 2004.

Local projects are usually dictated by clinician interest or service-users' concern. The following questions should be considered:

- Is there good evidence to set standards, e.g. professional or national guidelines?
- Is change achievable?
- Is sustained improvement possible?
- Does it address a serious quality problem?
- Is the subject high-volume and high-cost?

The aims of the project must be clearly defined in a broad statement of intent. Useful phrases to include are 'to provide', 'to ensure' and 'to improve'. The objectives must be defined measurable components. Useful phrases here are 'to determine', to assess' and 'to identify'.

www.nice.org.uk
www.dh.gov.uk/PolicyAndGuidance/
HealthAndSocialCareTopics/Children
Services

Step 2: Selecting criteria

Criteria, as far as possible, should be derived from evidence. The objective criteria should be 'SMART' (*s*pecific, *m*easurable, *a*chievable, *r*elevant to local requirements and practice, and *t*heoretically sound, based on current evidence). The criteria can be based on research findings, consensus of experienced clinicians or guidelines.

Step 3: Measuring level of performance

This is often the most labour-intensive step. To use resources efficiently, data must be precise and address the criteria statement. All too frequently, projects fail because data are too difficult to collect, are inaccessible or are not relevant measures of clinical quality. An important step is to pilot data collection forms. There are many sources from which data can be collected (medical records, databases, questionnaires, interviews and surveys). Issues of confidentiality must be considered when data are collected.

135

Step 4: Making improvements

Implementing change is often difficult. Improvements are based upon the results and conclusions of each objective. It is important to gain consensus for an action plan from the professionals involved, which is more likely if there is ownership of the process and people are kept informed of progress. The action plan must define what is to change, how change is to happen, who is responsible for change and over what time period it should occur.

Step 5: Sustaining improvement

Finally, a target for re-audit should be agreed. The aim should be to demonstrate that the action plan has been implemented successfully. It should also highlight further improvements required for the cyclical and spiralling process to continue. There is no doubt that sustained improvement is more likely to occur if it is part of a planned strategy within a supportive environment.

Data information systems

Monitoring of data for statistical and clinical purposes is one of the continuing objectives of the NHS Information Strategy. Data from these information systems can also be used for audit.

Patient Administration System (PAS) is the principal system of computerized data for storage, analysis and recording of information. It processes the administrative information associated with a patient's contact with the hospital, e.g. referrals, admissions and discharges.

Clinical coding is the process of translating medical terminology written by a clinician into an easily tabulated and accurate form. To ensure uniformity, standard classifications must be agreed nationally. Classifications for use in the NHS are the World Health Organization's International Statistical Classification of Diseases — 10th revision (ICD–10) and the Office of Population, Censuses and Surveys' Classification and Surgical Operations and Procedures — 4th revision (OPCS–4). Clinical coded data can be used in the healthcare planning of the aetiology and incidence of diseases and allows comparison of patient care and outcome. The data play a major role in the development of national policies and service frameworks.

References

Department of Health 1997 The new NHS: modern, dependable. The Stationery Office, London

Yost CC, Soll RF 1999 Early versus delayed selective surfactant treatment for neonatal respiratory distress syndrome. Cochrane Database of Systematic Reviews 4:CD001456; DOI 10.1002/14651858.CD001456

Edited by Mitch Blair, Mary Rudolf

Child public health

MODULE

THREE

Rachel Crowther

CHAPTER

Epidemiology

14

LEARNING OUTCOMES

By the end of this chapter you should:

- Understand what child public health is and why it is important
- Be familiar with the broad characteristics of the child population in the UK — and the world
- Know about the key factors that affect the health of children, including wider determinants of health
- Recognize the main causes of mortality and morbidity in children
- Know about different types and structures of health, education and social care services for children
- Understand how to assess health and health needs in a population, including key data sources
- Know about different types of health inequality and how they affect children
- Understand the impact of poverty, stigma and social exclusion on child health
- Know about current UK government targets for tackling health inequalities
- Be familiar with key methods for measuring social deprivation
- Understand the particular health needs of certain vulnerable groups, including at-risk children, children from black and minority ethnic groups and children with disabilities.

MODULE THREE

Child public health

Doctors frequently see children out of their everyday context, and gain a sense of their family and social background largely at second hand. The children who pass through the doors of the hospital, GP's surgery or clinic are part of a wider population of children whose characteristics can be difficult to grasp from the perspective of a clinician. Child public health is concerned with this wider population — with children's daily lives, and what

139

goes on before and after encounters with healthcare professionals; with how to assess and measure the health and health needs of children; with how to improve their health and wellbeing, in the broadest sense, and tackle health inequality (Box 14.1). The size and nature of the 'population' varies enormously; child public health practitioners are involved in everything from large-scale international projects through the World Health Organization (WHO) to local community projects such as 'Sure Start'.

The child population

In 2001, there were 13.5 million children aged under 18 in the UK, of whom 11.7 million were 'dependent' (under 16, or aged 16–18 and still in full-time education) and 3.4 million were under 5. However, the number of children and young people in the UK has fallen by nearly 2 million in the last 30 years, and the proportion of children in the population has changed quite significantly over this period (Table 14.1). There are now — for the first time in history — more people aged over 60 than under 16 in Great Britain.

Look at Box 14.2 and consider the questions about the child population in the UK before checking the answers below. Do the answers surprise you?

In 2001 there were 2.1 billion children worldwide aged under 18 and 613 million under 5. The world's child population is concentrated in the poorest countries, where child and infant mortality rates are highest. The life expectancy from birth in the world's poorest countries is only 51 years. The infant mortality rate for these countries is 16 times higher than in the UK and the under-5 mortality rate is 22 times that of the UK.

Determinants of health in children

Children's health is affected by a wide range of factors that operate at many different 'levels', from within

Table 14.1 Changes in child population in the UK

Year	Proportion of population aged under 16
1971	25%
2001	20%
2031 (projected)	17%

the child (e.g. genetic factors) to across the globe (e.g. international agreements such as the United Nations Convention on the Rights of the Child). Socioeconomic and environmental factors, especially poverty, play a very significant part and account for much of the variation between different children's experience of life and of health.

A commonly used framework for understanding the interaction of determinants and the various 'levels' is the Dahlgren and Whitehead model (Fig. 14.1). This places the individual in the centre and explores the influences on the child — see the boxes on the figure for details of each 'layer'.

Health inequalities

Introduction

Health inequalities can be defined as differences between the experience of health and wellbeing of different groups that result in an unfair distribution of morbidity and mortality in the population. The population in question might be that of the whole world or of a much smaller area or community. The extent of health inequality in the child population in the UK is considerable, even in the first year of life, and is continuing to increase. In the last quarter of the 20th century, as average levels of health improved, health inequalities grew wider. A large proportion of this inequality is socially determined: that is to say, it reflects differences in children's environments, circumstances, opportunities and resources. Children themselves have almost no control over these factors, but the remedies for this inequality lie within the power of society. We cannot avoid a collective responsibility for the experience of children who are less well off, in health terms, than others.

Types of health inequality

Differences in health, and in the distribution of determinants of health, can be identified between many different kinds of children. Factors include:

- *Gender*: e.g. the rise in smoking and binge drinking among young women in the UK
- *Geography*: e.g. differences in the prevalence of childhood obesity between regions in England
- *Socioeconomic status*: e.g. differences in infant mortality between those born into families from manual and non-manual groups in the UK
- *Ethnicity*: e.g. greater rise in prevalence of and mortality from asthma among black children in the USA
- *Disability*: e.g. greater risk of child abuse among children with disabilities
- *Age*: e.g. differences in the type and overall risk of injury in children of different ages.

Causes of health inequalities

A complex web of factors contribute to the existence of health inequalities, and lead to differences in health status and outcome that can be clearly observed at a collective level. Some of the most important causes include:

- Socioeconomic factors
- Stigma and social exclusion
- Family circumstances and parenting
- The wider social and physical environment
- Lifestyle and behaviour (e.g. smoking, diet and physical activity, substance misuse, sexual behaviour)
- Access to services (e.g. the 'inverse care law', a term coined by Tudor Hart in 1971: those most in need are least likely to access and benefit from health services).

These factors are closely interrelated. Poverty and deprivation are more common among socially excluded groups, and social exclusion makes it harder to find a job (or to get a decent education) in order to climb out of poverty. Effective and empathetic parenting is much more of a challenge when living in poverty, and the impact of poor parenting can put children at a disadvantage in educational (and later employment) terms, as well as emotional and health terms. The quality of the built environment is very often poorer in areas where many of the residents are poor, and promotes crime and social fragmentation. Unhealthy lifestyles are substantially affected by social and environmental constraints, such as the lack of availability of affordable fresh food in deprived areas. Most clinicians will have seen children whose lives tragically illustrate the clustering of disadvantageous circumstances, with inevitable consequences for their health and wellbeing both now and in later life, and often for the next generation too.

Key contributors to health inequality in children are described below.

Socioeconomic inequalities

A substantial proportion of health inequality is directly related to socioeconomic inequality. There is a clear social class gradient for most of the leading causes of morbidity and mortality in children, and poverty and social deprivation remain the most significant determinants of child health, even in prosperous 21st century Britain. The Joseph Rowntree Foundation has estimated that 1400 children's lives would be saved each year in the UK if child poverty were eradicated, an objective that the UK government has taken on board. Both *absolute poverty* and *relative poverty* are important,

Age, sex and constitutional factors
- Some conditions have a clear **genetic** cause or predisposition — e.g. sickle cell disease, cystic fibrosis, Huntington's chorea, Down's syndrome.
- There is growing evidence of the impact of prenatal life on later health — e.g. Barker hypothesis (p. 6); specific insults such as rubella virus
- **Gestational age and birth weight** affect the incidence of cerebral palsy and other conditions. Preterm birth and low birth weight are significant causes of infant mortality
- There are gender differences in the pattern of mortality from many diseases in children.

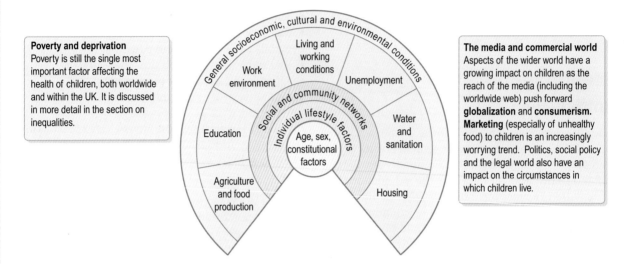

Poverty and deprivation
Poverty is still the single most important factor affecting the health of children, both worldwide and within the UK. It is discussed in more detail in the section on inequalities.

The media and commercial world
Aspects of the wider world have a growing impact on children as the reach of the media (including the worldwide web) push forward **globalization** and **consumerism.** **Marketing** (especially of unhealthy food) to children is an increasingly worrying trend. Politics, social policy and the legal world also have an impact on the circumstances in which children live.

Individual lifestyle factors
Lifestyle and health-related behaviour are important determinants of health in older children and parental lifestyles can affect children directly (e.g. smoking in pregnancy and around young children; choices between breast- and formula feeding) and indirectly, by helping to shape habits (e.g. of diet and exercise) which children will carry into later childhood and adulthood. Such 'choices' are significantly affected by socioeconomic and environmental factors (e.g. the 'obesogenic' environment; social class gradients for smoking). Important aspects of lifestyle include:
- **Nutrition,** including breastfeeding and establishing a healthy diet at and after weaning. Many foods which are high in fat, calories, sugar and salt are cheap and readily available. The national School Fruit and Vegetable scheme aims to increase consumption of healthier foods.
- **Physical activity:** 40% of boys and 60% of girls get less than the recommended hour of physical activity a day. Fewer children walk to school, PE provision is poor in schools, many playing fields have been sold off and parents are often reluctant to allow children to play outside because of the lack of safe play areas.
- **Smoking:** Smoking in pregnancy increases the risk of low birth weight, stillbirth and infant death. Smoking in the same household as a young child increases the risk of sudden death and respiratory problems.
- **Risk behaviour** is on the rise among older children and adolescents, e.g. alcohol and drug misuse, sexual behaviour, physical risks and accidents, deliberate self-harm.

Social, family and community networks
- **Relationships between parents and children** affect the child's wellbeing and resilience in responding to stress and adverse events. Particularly important are:
  – **Early care and nurture** and the degree of **attachment** at 1 year of age.
  – **Parenting style,** boundary-setting and support, communication, shared family pursuits and culture.
  – **Abuse and neglect,** which are extreme examples of unhelpful parenting.
- **Family break-up and conflict:** Conflict and domestic violence can have a serious effect on children's health and wellbeing. Around 150 000 children in the UK live through parental divorce every year in the UK, of whom a quarter are under 5 and two-thirds are under 10.
- **Family structure:** 23% of dependent children now live in single-parent households, and more than 10% live in reconstituted families. For children who receive continuous loving care this may be important, but for others living in a non-traditional family may have disadvantages. Other factors include birth order and number of siblings, and the proximity of extended family members.
- **Childcare and working patterns:** The government's plans for 'wraparound childcare' aim to support working parents and mean that more young children will spend more time in daycare. Benefits from extended contact with other children include a decreased risk of asthma and leukaemia, but extended separation at an early age may have less desirable implications for both mother and baby.
- **Maternal age, status and income:** Around 8% of babies are now born to a teenage mother, and 40% outside marriage (although most of these are jointly registered by both parents). Younger mothers tend to be on lower incomes and the health prospects for teenage mothers and their babies are poorer.

Fig. 14.1 The Dahlgren & Whitehead model of determinants of health

Physical environment

Several aspects of the physical environment affect children's health, including:

- **Housing,** e.g. quality (fitness for human habitation criteria), size, amenities. Damp housing increases the risk of childhood asthma; overcrowding increases the risk of infectious diseases, domestic violence and accidents. 58 000 children aged under 2 live in high-rise accommodation, two storeys or more above ground level.
- **Neighbourhood,** e.g. availability of parks and safe play areas; traffic (which causes pollution and road traffic accidents).
- **Poor air quality,** e.g. in inner city areas, can cause exacerbations of respiratory conditions.
- Exposure to **infectious agents,** e.g. food hygiene, handwashing practices, time spent in daycare and nurseries.

Wider social environment

- Qualities of local communities and networks such as **social inclusion** and **social capital** can have a significant impact on health, offering protection against some of the adverse effects of poverty and deprivation.
- Conversely, **social exclusion and stigma** may have a detrimental effect on the health and wellbeing of children from marginalized and minority groups who are less able to access services and participate in community life. These include the very poor, travelling families, asylum seekers, and ethnic and religious minorities, as well as children with disabilities or chronic illnesses.
- The **school environment** is very important for children: the healthy schools movement aims to promote positive ethos, pupil involvement and strong self-esteem, and to tackle bullying and unhealthy environments.
- Respect for **children's rights** is a fundamental responsibility for all. The United Nations Convention on the Rights of the Child is an international treaty which enshrines basic rights for all children, including the right to life, identity, protection and education.

Access to services

Many public services have an impact on children's health, either directly or indirectly. They include:

- **Health services,** including preventive, acute and community services, delivered by a range of health professionals.
- **Education services:** Educational attainment has a significant impact on self-esteem and wellbeing in children, and on later health.
- **Social services,** e.g. child protection and family support for children with disabilities.
- **Leisure services,** e.g. sporting facilities, youth clubs, after-school and holiday activities.
- **Transport services,** e.g. public transport, cycle lanes and safe routes to school.

Fig. 14.1 (*cont'd*)

and the debate continues about the relative contribution of each.

Absolute poverty reflects the resources a family has available to pay for basic necessities such as accommodation, heating and lighting, food, clothing, transport etc. Various formulae (sometimes described as 'consensus' or 'subjective' measures of poverty) have been devised to calculate the minimum weekly or monthly requirement for a family of different sizes, and any whose income falls below this level is deemed to be living in absolute poverty. Absolute poverty can be tackled by boosting the resources of the very poor (e.g. by increasing state benefit levels, which are generally judged to be lower than the minimum needs of an average family), but most experts believe that is not enough to mitigate the health effects of poverty, because relative poverty also plays an important role.

Relative poverty reflects income inequality: how a family's resources compare to those of others. The European Union defines as poor those households whose income is 50% or less of the national average — sometimes known as the 'poverty line'. The number of UK children living below the poverty line increased sharply in the last two decades of the 20th century, and the UK continues to compare poorly with other similar countries. Relative poverty is important at every geographical level. In Scandinavian countries with a more even distribution of wealth, the health status of the whole population is better, not just that of people in lower-income brackets. At a local level, it is better in health terms to be poor in a poor neighbourhood than to be surrounded by better-off households. Relative poverty is believed to exert its effects partly through psychosocial factors such as a sense of marginalization and exclusion, low self-esteem and powerlessness, which can result in physiological changes such as hypertension and lowered immune response.

Poverty affects children's health in several different ways:

- *Effects of absolute poverty*: lack of money to pay for healthy food, suitable housing, clothing, heating, toys and outings.
- *Effects of relative poverty*: psychosocial stresses on parents increase the risk of conflict and domestic violence, depression and poor supervision of children (which may lead to accidents); children themselves can also experience psychosocial effects such as low self-esteem and hopelessness.
- *Effects of living in poor neighbourhoods*: lack of facilities (e.g. outdoor play areas) and services (e.g. poor schools); poor built environment, derelict spaces etc.; crime and violence.
- *Effects of social, cultural and environmental norms and constraints*: unhealthy lifestyle choices (e.g.

143

smoking, binge drinking) may be encouraged by the limited alternative opportunities for pleasure or escape.

Stigma and social exclusion

Social exclusion is described as follows by the UK government's Social Exclusion Unit:

Social exclusion happens when people or places suffer from a series of problems such as unemployment, discrimination, poor skills, low incomes, poor housing, high crime, ill health and family breakdown. When such problems combine they can create a vicious cycle. Social exclusion can happen as a result of problems that face one person in their life. But it can also start from birth.

www.socialexclusionunit.gov.uk

Social exclusion is often closely related to poverty, but other factors affect an individual's, a family's or indeed a whole group's ability to benefit from the opportunities offered by their community and society. The sociological term 'stigma' refers to the negative interpretation placed by society on outward differences, including:

- Bodily characteristics (e.g. disability, obesity, significant birth marks)
- Skin colour
- Religious observance
- Language
- Clothes or other cultural appurtenances
- Illness (especially mental illness)
- Family and social background (e.g. children looked after by the local authority, asylum seekers and refugees)
- Age
- Gender
- Behaviour or lifestyle (e.g. travellers)
- Sexual orientation
- Evident poverty
- Poor hygiene
- Any other factors that set individuals apart.

Children have the capacity to be very accepting of others, but are also quick to pick up prevailing disapproval or mockery and, in circumstances that allow such behaviour, can rapidly learn that falling in with the disparaging of others reinforces their own position as part of the crowd. Thus children (as well as their parents and families) can feel the breath of intolerance directly and suffer the handicapping effects of social exclusion. These may include bullying, low self-esteem, anxiety and depression, a sense of worthlessness and lack of opportunities, difficulties in accessing services (including education and health services) and, in extreme cases, self-harm or physical violence at the hands of others. It is especially tragic when health and

social inequalities are perpetuated through generations as a direct result of intolerance and inhumanity.

Vulnerable and at-risk children

Some children are at particular risk of poor health and/or social exclusion and may need help from one or more public agencies (health, social services, education etc.) to maintain their physical, mental and social wellbeing. These vulnerable children include those:
- With disabilities
- With emotional and behavioural problems
- With a history of abuse or who are at risk of abuse
- Whose families are homeless
- Who are looked after by the local authority ('in care')
- Who have a history of truancy or crime
- Who care for others (e.g. parents with health problems)
- Who have chronic illnesses, especially mental health problems
- Who misuse drugs or alcohol
- Who are teenage parents
- Who are children of asylum seekers, or have arrived in this country as unaccompanied minors.

Some of these children are considered to be in need of more formal public support, and constitute a subgroup of vulnerable children deemed 'at-risk' and includes those:
- In need of protection
- In need of family support
- In public care.

Measuring poverty and social deprivation

Absolute and relative measures of poverty have been described above. Social deprivation is harder to measure than family income and outgoings, but various instruments have been developed to assess deprivation in a broader sense in local areas. The Townsend Index and Jarman Index have both been much used, and are often cited in studies that examine the correlation between deprivation and mortality, morbidity or hospital admission rates for certain conditions (e.g. childhood asthma or accidents), or which plot 'hot spots' of deprivation across a town or Primary Care Trust area. These indices use four and eight items respectively, such as the percentage of the local population that is unemployed or does not own their home.

More recently, the UK government has developed more comprehensive indices that draw on a wide range of routinely collected local data, can be regularly updated and are available for the whole of England at

Table 14.2 Patterns of inequalities in childhood injuries*

Category	Examples
Age	• 40% of the 1071 child deaths from unintentional injury in England and Wales in 1997–99 were in children aged 0–4 • Around two-thirds of deaths from injuries at home (e.g. from suffocation or fire) were in this age group • However, 99% of cyclist deaths and 78% of pedestrian deaths were in children aged 5–14 • A steep gradient, with older children predominating, is also seen for non–fatal injuries to cyclists
Gender	• 66% of the 1071 child deaths from unintentional injury in England and Wales in 1997–99 were in boys • This includes 74% of cyclist deaths, 81% of drowning deaths, 71% of falls and 61% of poisoning deaths • Boys also have higher rates of both major and minor non-fatal accidents than girls
Socioeconomic group	• The death rate from injury for children in social class V was 3.5 times higher than for social class I in 1979–83, and 5 times higher in 1989–92 (both England and Wales) • This increased ratio was due to differential declines in injury death rates (i.e. to a greater fall in social class I) • Death rates in social classes I and V respectively fell over this decade by 30% and 1% for motor vehicle accidents, and by 28% and 5% for fires • The ratio of child death rates for social class V to social class I in 1989–92 was 5:1 for pedestrian injuries and 16:1 for fires • A study in Nottingham found a 'dose–response' relationship between local area deprivation scores and child pedestrian accidents in different wards
Ethnicity	• National routine data sources do not record ethnic group of injured children, so evidence is limited and the effect of ethnicity and culture is hard to tease out from socioeconomic factors (e.g. poverty and deprivation) • Some studies suggest increased risk for children from minority ethnic groups, especially for pedestrian injuries, but others do not
Geography	• Child accident death rates vary by region: in 1989–91, the average rates were 7.2 per 100 000 in England and 8.1 per 100 000 in Wales, but regional rates ranged from 5.4 in the South-West to 9.8 in the North-West • Child pedestrian casualty rates in big cities were twice the UK average, and the rate in inner London was twice that for outer London

* Adapted from: Health Development Agency 2005 Injuries in children aged 0–14 years and inequalities.

a small area level in a consistent form. The Index of Multiple Deprivation 2004 (IMD 2004) is available online (see below) and has a supplementary index on income deprivation affecting children. The IMD 2004 includes seven 'domains':

1. *Income deprivation* (e.g. number of households receiving benefits such as income support, working families' tax credit or asylum seekers' support)
2. *Employment deprivation* (e.g. number of claimants for unemployment or incapacity benefit)
3. *Health deprivation and disability* (e.g. comparative illness and disability ratio, emergency admissions to hospital)
4. *Education, skills and training deprivation* (e.g. children's average scores at Key Stages 2, 3 and 4; proportion leaving school at 16; secondary school absence rate)
5. *Barriers to housing and services* (e.g. overcrowding and homelessness; distance to nearest GP, supermarket, primary school and post office)
6. *Living environment deprivation* (indoors, e.g. housing in poor condition or without central heating; outdoors, e.g. air quality, road traffic accidents with injury to pedestrians or cyclists)
7. *Crime* (e.g. recorded burglary, theft, criminal damage and violence).

Local scores are available for every 'Super Output Area' (SOA) in England — of which there are almost 32 500, with an average population of around 2000 — for each domain separately, together with an overall (weighted) score and rank. Summary scores are also available at district and county level. In the most deprived quintile (20%) of SOAs:

• A fifth of adults are 'employment-deprived'
• Almost half of children live in families which are 'income-deprived' (usually meaning on benefits)

Geographical inequality can be clearly illustrated by looking at the distribution of these most-deprived SOAs; most are in the North-East and North-West regions.

 www.odpm.gov.uk

Preliminary report on Index of Multiple Deprivation 2004

The impact of health inequalities: childhood injuries

Childhood injuries offer a useful case study for examining the impact of health inequalities. A recent report from the Health Development Agency (*www.nice.org.uk*) reviews differences in the pattern of injuries to children for most of the categories of inequality listed above. Some of its key findings are shown in Table 14.2.

The explanations for these differences are complex and incompletely understood, but some relevant factors

Table 14.3 Reasons for inequalities in childhood injuries*

Category	Examples of relevant factors
Age	• Physical development and motor coordination affect ability to avoid (or tendency to encounter) risk: e.g. ability to manage climbing frame/swings • Perceptual and intellectual development affect e.g. ability to judge traffic, awareness of danger • Changing attitudes, behaviour and nature of play/leisure activity with increasing age affect exposure to risk: e.g. deliberate risk-taking in adolescence, hazardous sport • Levels of supervision/independence affect degree of safeguards: e.g. cycling/walking alone to school or shops
Gender	• Differences in rates of development: motor, spatial, cognitive, intellectual • Differences in behaviour: gender-specific norms such as 'macho' risk-taking, nature of peer pressure and attitude to safety (e.g. cycle helmets) • Different choices of sport/leisure activity: e.g. contact sports such as football and rugby; greater overall physical activity levels in boys • Differences in levels of supervision/independence: perhaps greater tendency for parents to protect girls
Socioeconomic group	• Cost of safety equipment: e.g. stair gates, car seats, cycle helmets, reflective clothing, safety harnesses, cordless kettles, smoke alarms • Different levels of exposure to hazards, inside and outside: e.g. cigarette smoking (can lead to fires), unsafe electrical wiring, overcrowded housing, lack of garden/safe play areas, living on main road • Differences in parents'/carers' ability to supervise: e.g. single-parent families, very young mothers, stress/illness (especially mental health problems), parents' working patterns and childcare arrangements • Parents' attitudes to and awareness of risks, and access to information and services to help manage risk
Ethnicity	• Differences in environment and exposure to risk: e.g. different activities and patterns of behaviour, supervision/childcare arrangements • Access to information and services to help manage risk: e.g. language barriers, awareness of services (e.g. lower attendance at child health clinics where health promotion and safety advice is offered) • Especially for first-generation immigrants, lack of familiarity with hazards (e.g. road environment) and differences in expectation (e.g. children 'falling in with' peers)
Geography	• Factors relating to physical environment: e.g. safety of roads (including on-street parking, traffic volume, cycle lanes, pavements, underpasses) • Factors relating to social environment: e.g. community safety, level of collective responsibility for children, familiarity of neighbours

* Adapted from: Health Development Agency 2005 Injuries in children aged 0–14 years and inequalities.

are listed in Table 14.3. It is helpful to bear in mind the different levels at which factors influencing injury risk can operate:

- The event itself and immediate circumstances surrounding the child's exposure to the hazard
- Intermediate factors affecting the child's exposure to risk
- Wider social, economic, cultural and environmental factors that shape the child's experience.

Approaches to preventing injuries in children are discussed in Chapter 17; you may like to consider whether targeted approaches might be needed for some of the different groups considered here.

Other examples of socioeconomic inequalities in child health include:

- *Infant mortality rate (age 0–1 year)*. Social class V has double the mortality rate of social class I, and the gap is still rising.
- *Child mortality rate (age 1–15 years)*. Social classes IV and V have almost double the rate of social classes I and II.
- *Mental health problems*. Prevalence in social class V is three times higher than in social class I.

Ethnicity and health

There is a dearth of child health data to illustrate differences in health outcome between ethnic groups, but infant mortality provides a good 'summary measure' that is routinely available and shows significant variation. For example, in 2003 the infant mortality rate (in England and Wales) for babies whose mothers were born in Pakistan was 10.5 per 1000 live births — more than double the national average — and for babies whose mothers were born in the Caribbean the rate was 8.5 per 1000.

Several factors may affect the health and wellbeing of children from black and minority ethnic groups, including:

- *Socioeconomic factors*. Children from minority ethnic groups are on average more likely to live in poverty, and to suffer the effects of deprivation such as unsuitable, overcrowded accommodation.
- *Stigma and social exclusion*. Children from minority ethnic groups are more likely to suffer the effects of bullying and exclusion; lack of recognition of foreign qualifications may bar entry to employment for parents.

- *Cultural factors.* Differences in child-rearing and lifestyle may affect children's health. For example, family composition and relationship with the extended family affect the home environment; late weaning practices in Asian families can increase the risk of anaemia; lack of availability of culturally familiar food may lead to the adoption of the least healthy aspects of British diet; peer pressure and cultural norms (especially in adolescence) may act in very different ways for children from different groups.
- *Barriers to access.* Language difficulties (and lack of interpreting services) and cultural barriers (e.g. women needing a chaperone to visit the doctor, lack of familiarity with GP registration/appointments system, lack of awareness of entitlements) may impede access to health services (including antenatal and preventive child health services), social services, education and others (including transport, leisure, benefits).
- *Recent history.* Recent immigrants may be separated from extended family and friends and feel very isolated; poor healthcare (e.g. immunization programmes) and/or prevalence of infectious diseases (e.g. HIV, tuberculosis) in their home country may affect health directly; in addition, asylum seekers and refugees have often suffered traumatic experiences before and during their flight, may have lost relatives and friends to war or torture, and may have suffered the effects of infrastructure breakdown (including the loss of possessions or profession).
- *Genetic factors.* Some inherited conditions are more common in certain ethnic groups, e.g. sickle cell disease and thalassaemia; consanguineous marriage increases the risk of a range of rare congenital conditions.

It is clear that the picture is complicated, and that the experience of children from different backgrounds may be dramatically different — which is why simply comparing 'white' and 'non-white' children is over-simplistic and generally unhelpful in elucidating health inequalities and exploring their causes.

The different factors that might affect the health of children in ethnic minority groups are illustrated on the MasterCourse website. Look at these and consider the differences between them.

What can health professionals do to help?

- Adequate interpreting services are very important. They should always be provided by professionals, not members of the family, to avoid problems of incomplete communication or disclosure.
- Patience, persistence and sensitivity to cultural and other barriers are needed to ensure full and equitable access to services for children from all backgrounds. Failure to attend appointments is frustrating, but should not be accepted as a reason for giving up on a child.
- The school environment is crucially important to children's wellbeing, and much can be done at whole-school level to improve the experience of all pupils — and staff.
- Advocacy, partnership working and information sharing with other agencies are essential to ensure a coordinated and effective approach to addressing the needs of individual children and young people (e.g. ensuring that vulnerable children do not miss out on education — including Foundation Stage (nursery and reception year)).
- It is very important that all professionals working with children are sensitive to cultural issues but do not allow them to cloud their judgment about a child's wellbeing, as the Victoria Climbié case tragically illustrated.

Tackling health inequalities: policy, targets and progress

Official recognition of the problem of health inequalities in the UK was marked by the publication of the Black Report in 1980, although action was slow to follow from its findings. The Acheson 'Independent Inquiry into Inequalities in Health' (1998) has also been highly influential; although wide-ranging in its approach, it included a focus on ethnic and gender inequalities, and identified families, mothers and children as a priority group. It set out policy approaches to tackling the determinants of health that sit behind health inequalities, including poverty, tax and benefits; education and employment; environment and housing; transport and pollution; and diet and nutrition. Important developments in recent years include:

- The establishment by the government in 1997 of the Social Exclusion Unit, managed by the Office of the Deputy Prime Minister and including children and young people as a key area (*www.socialexclusionunit.gov.uk*)
- The establishment by the Economic and Social Research Council in 1996 of the Health Variations Programme, which focuses on the causes of health inequality (*www.esrc.ac.uk*)
- The development of the Health Poverty Index, a web-based tool for visualizing the 'health poverty' of different geographical, social, cultural or

Infant mortality

- 'Starting with children under one year, by 2010
to reduce by at least 10 per cent the gap in
mortality between routine and manual groups*
and the population as a whole' — part of a
national public service agreement (PSA) target
set in 2001

Child poverty

- A commitment to reducing by half the number
of children in low-income households (below the
'poverty line') between 1998–99 and 2010, and
eradicating child poverty by 2020

* 'Manual groups' means social classes IIIM, IV and V; classes
I, II and IIIN are defined as 'non-manual'.

economic groups, drawing on a range of indicators
including health status, health behaviours,
prevention and service access (*www.hpi.org.uk*).

The UK government has subsequently included a
commitment to reduce inequalities in a number of
national public health targets, including two focused
specifically on children (Box 14.3). Addressing health
inequalities is also a key theme of the Children's
National Service Framework.

The government's 2003 Programme for Action sets
out wide-ranging plans for tackling health inequalities
by improving the health of the worst-off in society,
providing financial support for families (e.g. tax credits
and benefits) and introducing public service changes
to improve children's life chances. Some examples of
action are set out in Box 14.4.

Progress against national targets

Infant mortality

The latest Office for National Statistics (ONS) figures
for infant mortality (quoted in a 2005 Department of
Health update on the inequalities targets) show that
the gap between manual groups and the population
as a whole has *widened* since the target was set; infant
mortality in manual groups was 19% higher than the
total population in 2001–03, compared with 13%
higher in the baseline period of 1997–99.

Child poverty

The government's preliminary target was to reduce
child poverty by a quarter by 2004–05. Early indications are that this target may be met: the number of
children in low-income households in the UK fell by
around half a million between 1998–99 and 2002–03,

- Helping to ensure a decent income for all
families, through work or benefits
- Improving housing conditions, educational
attainment and access to services, especially
high-quality antenatal care
- More support for preschool children and their
families, building on the lessons learned in Sure
Start pilot areas
- Addressing risk factors for sudden unexplained
death in infancy (SUDI, Ch. 17)
- Promoting breastfeeding (only 59% of mothers
from social class V chose to breastfeed in 2000,
compared to 91% of mothers from social class I)
- Promoting immunization (lower coverage rates
are seen in practices serving socially deprived
areas)
- Reducing smoking and improving nutrition in
pregnancy and early childhood
- Reducing teenage pregnancy and providing more
support to teenage parents (halving the number
of teenage births would make a significant
contribution to the infant mortality target)
- Developing one-stop centres, such as extended
schools and Children's Trusts
- Ensuring health services are better orientated
towards the needs of children and young people,
e.g. more outreach services

* Adapted from: Department of Health 2003, Tackling health
inequalities: a programme for action, and Department
of Health Health Inequalities Unit 2005, Tackling health
inequalities: what works.

and the proportion of households with children below
the poverty line fell from 23% to 20.9% between
1996–97 and 2000–01 after rising steadily for some
time before this. The longer-term targets remain challenging, however.

Key causes of morbidity and mortality in children

The health of children in the UK has improved significantly over the last century, and at the same time
the pattern of morbidity and mortality has changed
dramatically. Immunization and antibiotics have helped
reduce the impact of infectious diseases, and 'high-tech'
interventions have improved the chances of survival
of premature babies and of children with conditions
such as cancer or congenital heart disease. Social and

BOX 14.5 Some key child health problems in the 21st century

Childhood obesity

Prevalence has risen by 0.8% per year over the last decade, due to changes in both caloric intake (diet) and output (physical activity). The government has set a high-profile target to halt this trend. If it is not successful, life expectancy for current and future generations of children may be significantly reduced.

Emotional and behavioural/mental health problems

These are on the increase in children and young people. There are knock-on effects on the individual (jeopardizing educational achievement, employment prospects, success in establishing relationships), the family (increasing stress on parents and siblings; increasing the risk of violent behaviour towards future partners and children), teachers (who find it harder and harder to teach, and may be physically threatened by pupils) and society (increasing truancy and youth crime).

Teenage pregnancy and sexually transmitted infections

The UK has the highest rates in Europe. The impact on the health and wellbeing of teenage mothers and their children is substantial.

Accidents and injuries

These remain a significant cause of morbidity and mortality. The UK has the highest rates in Europe for injuries to child pedestrians.

Child abuse and neglect

These include fatal cases, estimated by the National Society for the Prevention of Cruelty to Children to number at least 100 per year.

Poor vaccine uptake

This is due to media scares and mistrust of official sources, leading to a significant risk of outbreaks of measles and increasing the exposure of pregnant women to rubella.

Increase in disabilities and chronic illness

Many disabilities are due to the improved survival of premature babies.

Substance misuse

This includes alcohol (binge drinking is an especially worrying trend), tobacco (smoking rates continue to rise, especially among teenage girls), drugs and glue-sniffing.

Suicide and self-harm

These are also on the rise; suicide now accounts for a third of deaths in 15–24-year-olds.

Social and health inequalities

These continue to increase as society becomes generally richer and healthier. The UK has the worst record in Europe on child poverty.

environmental factors have played an even larger role, including the beneficial effects of increasing wealth, improved sanitation and housing quality, family planning and safer environments. Society faces new problems today — consumerism, the over-availability of processed and unhealthy food, the prominence of sedentary lifestyles, disaffection and the decline in traditional family structures, a growing gap between the income and health of the richest and poorest — and the pattern of child health reflects them all (Box 14.5).

The leading causes of death among children in the UK (Box 14.6) also reflect our society, and pose a stark contrast to those for children in developing countries.

Causes of child deaths in the UK vary by age and sex (Figs 14.2 and 14.3). There is an excess of male deaths, particularly in the later years. Approximately 50% of adolescent deaths result from road traffic accidents (RTAs).

The pyramid of care (Fig. 14.4)

By no means all children who become ill are cared for in hospital or even see a healthcare professional. Informal care by parents or others in the home is the norm, and advice may be sought from a variety of sources before a doctor is consulted: friends and relatives, the Internet or family health reference books, the community pharmacist and increasingly NHS Direct. Around 80% of sick children are cared for entirely in the community, 17% in primary care (which may include nurses, health visitors and others as well as the GP) and only 3% at

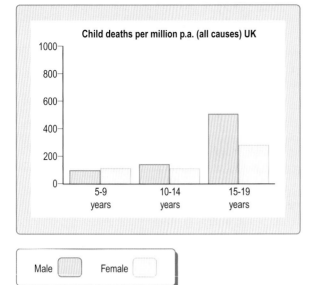

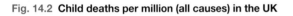

Fig. 14.2 **Child deaths per million (all causes) in the UK**

Fig. 14.3 **Causes of child death in the UK by age and sex.**
(Source: National Statistics booklet *Child Health Statistics*, 2000.)

BOX 14.6 Main causes of death among children under 5

UK

Death rates for under-5s are more than ten times lower in the UK than the worldwide average, amounting to a total of around 5000 deaths per year. The leading causes (excluding neonatal deaths — those occurring in the first 28 days), with approximate percentages, are:

- Congenital anomalies (18%)
- Sudden unexplained death in infancy (14% — but 20% of infant deaths)
- Prematurity, low birth weight and other conditions of perinatal origin (13%)
- Injury and poisoning (11%)
- Cerebral palsy and other diseases of the nervous system (9%)
- Respiratory disease (9%)
- Infections (9%)
- Childhood cancer (5%).

Worldwide

A total of 70% of the 10.6 million child deaths every year in children under 5 are due to six causes:

- Pneumonia (19%)
- Diarrhoea (18%)
- Neonatal infection (10%)
- Preterm delivery (10%)
- Malaria (8%)
- Birth asphyxia (8%).

Many of these are potentially preventable through simple interventions, such as providing clean water supplies, immunization and basic healthcare (especially antenatal and intrapartum care). Overall, 54% of child deaths are due to infections, and many occur as a direct or indirect result of absolute poverty.

Sources: National Statistics booklet 2000 *Child Health Statistics*; Bryce et al 2005 Lancet.

---

the hospital — of which an even smaller percentage will be admitted.

Surveillance of health in the population

Many aspects of child health are monitored routinely. Child health surveillance is important for many reasons, for example:

- To find out about the child population in order to plan services (e.g. birth rate, mortality

rate, proportion from minority ethnic groups, number with disabilities or particular diseases)
- To find out about usage of health services (e.g. children's admission rates to hospital)
- To pick up changes and trends that may require action (e.g. falling immunization coverage rates, which may leave the population susceptible to outbreaks of infectious disease)
- To assess progress against a target (e.g. prevalence of childhood obesity, infant mortality rates)

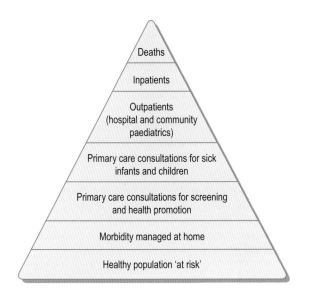

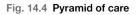

Fig. 14.4 Pyramid of care

- To evaluate the success of public health programmes (e.g. the School Fruit and Vegetable scheme)
- To compare the health status of different groups and assess health inequalities (e.g. low birth weight or infant mortality in babies of mothers from different socioeconomic, ethnic or age groups, or childhood admissions to hospital in different areas of the country).

Some of these require the examination or assessment of every child in a particular age group or population; others rely on statistically valid sampling methods to draw conclusions about the population as a whole after studying a relatively small number of children. In general, public health surveillance does not require identifiable data about individual children, although it may need some demographic information about them to help interpret the results.

Collecting and interpreting health information relies on understanding a few basic measures:

- *Incidence* is the number of new events or cases in a population in a given period (e.g. number of babies born with congenital anomalies each year in the UK).
- *Prevalence* is the overall number (or proportion) of cases in a population at a particular moment in time (e.g. number of children with asthma in a Primary Care Trust (PCT) population).
- *Numerators* are the numbers of children, events or cases measured; they do not usually mean much without knowing how big the population is (e.g. 500 cases per year in a national population of 13 million children is a very rare condition; 500 cases a year in a PCT population of 30 000 children is a fairly common condition).

- *Denominators* provide the population size. They may include all children in a geographic area, a selected population group (e.g. children under 5, children looked after by the local authority) or another measure (e.g. infant mortality is expressed as a proportion of live births).
- *Rates* measure the frequency with which particular events occur in a defined population, taking the average population during a specified period (e.g. a year) as the denominator.

Health needs assessment

Health needs assessment is a key tool for public health practice. Although public health focuses on populations rather than individuals, the first step in most public health projects is still to make a 'diagnosis' and identify the problems to be addressed. Health needs assessment is also an important way of ensuring that the health service uses its resources in the most efficient and effective way to improve the health of the population.

Health needs

But what are 'health needs'? Clearly, this is partly a matter of opinion and perspective, so it is important to be clear about what kind of need is being considered:

- *Felt needs* involve a subjective perception of poor health — or of a risk to health — by an individual (e.g. abdominal pain) or a community (e.g. concern about a dangerous road).
- *Expressed needs* are felt needs that have been articulated, usually to gain the attention of those who might help address them (e.g. a doctor or the local council).
- *Normative needs* are needs defined — usually by a professional — in relation to an objective norm or standard, and may be perceived as requiring or justifying intervention (e.g. acute appendicitis, or a traffic 'black spot' where there has been a consistent pattern of fatal accidents).
- *Comparative needs* are identified by weighing up the health needs of one individual or community against another.

Public health may be concerned with all of these: with uncovering felt needs that have not been articulated; with balancing the expressed needs of communities and normative needs perceived by 'experts'; with comparing the health status and health needs of different communities to ensure that healthcare commissioning and service provision across a given area adequately reflect differences in need. Needs assessment also encompasses:

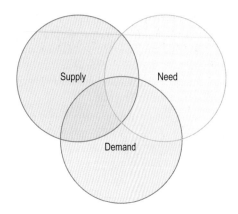

Fig. 14.5 **Triad of need, supply and demand**

- *Health needs* — literally a 'need for health' — which include anything that affects children's (or communities') wellbeing, whether or not they can be 'treated' by health services. Some health needs require action outside the health sector to tackle determinants of health such as poverty, nutrition, housing, pollution, transport policy or employment opportunities.
- *Healthcare needs,* which are those for which effective healthcare interventions are available (e.g. infectious diseases, diabetes, congenital heart disease).

Healthcare needs can be considered in more detail by looking at the triad of need, supply and demand (Fig. 14.5), which compares healthcare needs (usually normative needs), demand for healthcare (similar to expressed needs) and the supply of healthcare services for a particular condition.

The ideal is for need, supply and demand to coincide as far as possible, but where they do not, some action may be indicated. If healthcare is needed and demanded but not supplied (e.g. a local allergy clinic, or school-based sexual health advice for adolescents), then local commissioners may want to consider introducing it. If it is demanded and supplied but not strictly needed (e.g. many instances of tonsillectomy, or antibiotic treatment for acute otitis media that will probably resolve spontaneously), then discontinuing or reducing provision may be appropriate. However, services that are needed and supplied but not demanded (e.g. child protection, some kinds of immunization) may be important.

Approaches to needs assessment

Health needs assessment can focus on a *condition* (e.g. childhood asthma), a *service* (e.g. the paediatric emergency department) or a *population group* (e.g. hearing-impaired children). Stevens and Raftery have identified three main approaches to needs assessment:

BOX 14.7 What information do we need to conduct an epidemiological needs assessment for childhood diabetes?

- *Population*. How many children with diabetes live in the area and what projections there are for the future?
- *Effectiveness*. What evidence is there about effective ways of managing children with diabetes (e.g. community-based versus hospital-based care)?
- *Availability*. What services are currently provided locally?

The needs assessment might result in recommendations for change in service provision to meet the needs of young diabetics better.

Epidemiological needs assessment: what data do we have?

- Essentially sets out to identify gaps in services for which there is both a need and an effective intervention.
- Brings together data from many sources to look at the characteristics and health status of the *population*, the *effectiveness* of interventions for the problem(s) under scrutiny, and the current *availability* of services locally.
- Offers a 'scientific' approach to health needs assessment, which considers the issues logically, and largely from the perspective of health professionals and policy makers.

A simple epidemiological needs assessment for childhood diabetes is outlined in Box 14.7.

Comparative needs assessment: what do other areas do?

- Compares services available locally with those provided for similar populations in other areas. For example, might look at models of care for children with diabetes in neighbouring districts to see whether any of them have services that seem more effective, more efficient or better suited to the needs of the local population.
- May seem an overly simple approach, but allows those commissioning healthcare to 'benchmark' their own local services against others, and looking at examples of good practice elsewhere is often very helpful.

Corporate needs assessment: what do stakeholders think?

- Involves a wide range of people and organizations who have views about health and healthcare, including children, parents, healthcare workers, support groups, policy makers, teachers and social workers.

- Brings together their different perspectives and experience to identify problems and make recommendations to address them.
- Major advantages are in allowing the views of professionals, parents, children and everyone who works with them to be considered together and in avoiding an overly technical or professional focus — vital if services are to be child-centred and to properly reflect the wishes and needs of children and families.

These three approaches are complementary, and are often used in conjunction to build up a full picture of health needs. The balance between the three depends largely on the focus of the needs assessment. The example in Box 14.7 concerns a medical condition, but sometimes needs assessment is more exploratory, starting without any particular agenda or focus and aiming to find out about the problems and health needs of a particular community (e.g. children on a large deprived estate). In this case, the corporate element is likely to be the most important.

Specific techniques have been developed for conducting this type of needs assessment:

- *Participatory needs assessment* aims to involve members of the community fully, with 'experts' facilitating rather than leading the process.
- *Rapid appraisal needs assessment* allows a picture of health needs and problems to be built up very swiftly by gathering and sifting through a wide range of evidence and information from different sources.

Outcomes of needs assessment

The action taken as a result of needs assessment can be very varied and is certainly not limited to changes in health service provision. The outcomes depend very much on the problem and population studied. Before looking at the examples in Box 14.8, see how many different kinds of action, intervention or change you can list that might result from a health needs assessment for a particular condition or population group: for example, a sexual health needs assessment for young people in a local authority area with high rates of teenage pregnancy and sexually transmitted diseases.

Data sources

Child health surveillance and needs assessment both rely on information about the health of individuals and

> **BOX 14.8 Examples of action taken as a result of needs assessment**
>
> - Health promotion programmes (e.g. school-based projects to tackle smoking or provide sexual health advice to young people)
> - Changes to healthcare commissioning to reflect changed perception of priorities: developing new services (e.g. interpreting services for asylum seeker and refugee families) or reconfiguring others (increasing or decreasing availability, or changing the way they are delivered) to ensure that service provision reflects local need
> - Changes to other services (e.g. transport, leisure, community safety)
> - Community development projects (e.g. helping a community to start a new nursery or youth group)
> - Advocacy (e.g. championing children from traveller families or those caring for relatives, to help ensure their needs are met)
> - Developing new policies or strategies to tackle complex or long-term problems (e.g. promoting breastfeeding, reducing emotional and behavioural problems in a community)

populations, but where does this come from? Much (though not all) is collected, directly or indirectly, by doctors and other health professionals. It is helpful to have some idea about what happens to information within the NHS and how it is used — and to be aware of the wide range of information from other sources that can be useful in assessing or monitoring the health of the population.

Different kinds of health information

Figure 14.6 illustrates some kinds of information which it is useful to collect; these are explored further below.

Different sources of health information

Box 14.9 illustrates the wide variety of sources of information about health.

Demographic data

Birth

Information recorded on birth certificates includes birth weight, the marital status of the mother, and whether the birth is registered jointly (i.e. by both parents) or singly. It also includes parents' occupations and places of birth. Hospitals pass basic information on each birth to the local Registrar of Births and Deaths, and parents are required to register the birth

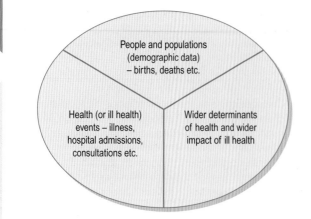

Fig. 14.6 **Different kinds of health information**

(and provide more information, including the child's name) within 6 weeks of delivery. Birth information is collected and analysed nationally, but is also accessible to local public health information specialists. Birth registration is linked to the allocation of an NHS number, which entitles the child to use health services (e.g. register with a GP).

Death

Information recorded on death certificates includes the place and cause of death. The Public Health Mortality File allows information specialists in PCTs and other organizations to access data for their area. Unexpected or unexplained deaths are referred to the Coroner (or Procurator Fiscal in Scotland), whose records will contain more information, e.g. whether an inquest was held or a post-mortem conducted. Information on deaths in children can be used to generate neonatal, infant and child mortality rates, to examine causes of death (see above), and to compare rates in different areas, ethnic groups and sexes.

Census data

Censuses of the population have been conducted in England and Wales every 10 years since 1841 — most recently in 2001. They provide detailed information about the population, including age distribution, ethnic origin, occupation and long-standing illness and disability.

Health data

Information on morbidity and contacts with the NHS is less comprehensive than demographic information, but data is collected about all NHS hospital attendances and admissions and some GP consultation data is available too.

Morbidity

Information on illness is collected through various sources, including routine surveys, doctor-diagnosed illness (e.g. GP data) and screening programmes (e.g. the neonatal blood spot programme). Incidence and prevalence can be calculated if the denominator population is known.

The Health Survey for England is based on a sample of households and currently collects data on 4000 children (as well as adults) each year. It includes information on lifestyle (e.g. smoking, fruit and vegetable consumption), certain key conditions and long-standing illnesses, and nurse-measured height and weight. It is used to provide estimates about health status and trends in the population as a whole.

Contacts with NHS services

Hospital Episode Statistics (HES) include a range of information about patients attending outpatients or admitted to hospital, including discharge information recorded by junior doctors. They contain:

- Details about the hospital and consultant (e.g. specialty)
- Demographic information about the patient (e.g. NHS number, sex, birth date, postcode of usual address)
- Admission information (e.g. referring GP, admission/discharge dates, method/source of admission)

BOX 14.9 Sources of health information		
National or	**Local** or	**International**
(e.g. UK childhood diabetes register)	(e.g. child health information system — surveillance and immunization data)	(e.g. WHO Health Behaviour of School Children survey)
By the NHS or	**Other agencies**	
(e.g. Hospital Episode Statistics)	(e.g. police data on traffic accidents, social services child protection register, education data on school attendance and attainment)	
Routinely or	**Ad hoc**	
(e.g. communicable disease surveillance cross-systems, health visitors' records)	(e.g. research projects collecting specific data — may be longitudinal, sectional or experimental)	

- Clinical information: diagnoses and procedures, coded using ICD–10 (International Classification of Diseases) and OPCS (Office of Population Censuses and Surveys) coding systems to allow analysis by type of disease and operation.

GP consultation data from the Royal College of General Practitioners are based on selected ('sentinel') practices. READ codes are used to classify health problems presenting in general practice.

Preventive health care

Local child health information systems provide a computerized database of all children living in the area. They are used to manage — and to record data about — preventive care services (e.g. immunization and routine health checks), and may also contain data on disability.

Chronic diseases

Information about the incidence and prevalence of some diseases — including congenital malformations, cancer, cerebral palsy, cystic fibrosis and diabetes — is recorded in disease registers.

General Household Survey

This is an interview-based survey administered to a sample of around 12 000 households. There are questions about acute and chronic illness, healthcare contacts and health-related lifestyle. It also covers wider determinants of health such as housing, employment, pensions, leisure activities, education and the family.

Wider aspects of health

Wider determinants of health

In addition to the Health Survey for England and the General Household Survey, which collect data on health-related lifestyles and risk factors for ill health, there have been specific surveys recently to assess the prevalence of disability and mental illness among children in the UK. At a more local level, the Schools Health Education Unit in Exeter conducts surveys of health and lifestyles within schools, and at an international level, the WHO's survey of Health Behaviour of School Children allows comparisons to be made between the UK and other countries.

Wider impact of health issues

Information from many other sources also adds to what we know about children's health in the broader sense and about the impact of ill health on children's lives: for example, school attendance and educational achievement (both can be affected by health — and in turn have repercussions for later health); data from social services on children looked after by the local authority or on the child protection register; and police data on traffic accidents and incidents of domestic violence.

Structure of health and other related services

The NHS was set up on 5 July 1948 to provide health-care for all citizens, based on need, not the ability to pay. The NHS is funded by the taxpayer and managed by the Department of Health, which sets overall policy on health issues. It is the responsibility of the Department of Health to provide health services to the general public through the NHS.

It was launched as a single organization based around 14 regional hospital boards. This new NHS was originally split into three parts:
- Hospital services
- Family doctors, dentists, opticians and pharmacists
- Local authority health services, including community nursing and health visiting.

Since 1948 there have been huge changes to both the organizational structure of the NHS and the way that patient services are provided (Boxes 14.10 and 14.11).

The foundation of the new service was the family doctor or GP. Then, as now, the family doctor acted as gatekeeper to the rest of the NHS, referring patients where appropriate to hospitals or specialist treatment and prescribing medicines and drugs.

Who's who in services for children in the UK?

Parents

Parenting is arguably the most important factor contributing to the health and wellbeing of children, yet it is assumed that it comes naturally and does not need to be taught. The breakdown of the extended family compounds the situation, as parents are often isolated in bringing up children and responsibilities go unshared. Where parenting is good, children in quite adverse circumstances develop resilience to adversity. Where parenting is poor, particularly where it is neglectful or abusive, difficulties are passed from generation to generation.

It is now being recognized that parenting should be taught to young people while at school. The curriculum

BOX 14.10 NHS milestones, 1952–90

- Prescription charges of 1 shilling (5p) were introduced in 1952
- In the 1962 Porritt Report, the medical profession criticized the separation of the NHS into three parts — hospitals, general practice and local health authorities — and called for unification
- Enoch Powell's Hospital Plan, published in 1962, approved the development of district general hospitals for population areas of about 125 000, and in doing so, laid out a pattern for the future
- The Salmon Report of 1967 detailed recommendations for developing the senior nursing staff structure and the status of the profession in hospital management. Then, also in 1967, the first report on the organization of doctors in hospitals (known as the Cogwheel Report) proposed speciality groupings that would arrange clinical and administrative medical work more logically
- NHS management tried to improve efficiency and there were attempts to set priorities in 1979, to restructure the NHS again in 1982 and to introduce a tier of general management between 1983 and 1985. Resource management formulae were developed to share NHS resources out fairly
- The 1990 GP contract rewarded GPs for preventive care, including immunization and child health surveillance

BOX 14.11 NHS milestones: 1990s to the present day

- NHS Direct, the nurse-led 24-hour telephone health advice service was launched in March 1998. Thought to be the largest single e-health service in the world, it handles over half a million calls each month, plus half a million online enquiries through its Web-based service, NHS Direct Online. A number of other alternatives to traditional GP services were developed, including NHS Walk-in Centres, which offer patients treatment and advice for a range of injuries and illnesses without the need to make an appointment or to register permanently
- In April 2001 'Shifting the Balance of Power' was launched to give greater authority and decision-making power to patients and frontline staff
- In 2002 locally based Primary Care Trusts (PCTs) were created — organizations that control 80% of the NHS budget and have the role of running the local NHS and improving the health of people in their areas. At the same time, 28 new Strategic Health Authorities replaced the former Health Authorities and took on a strategic role in improving local health services, while also making sure local NHS organizations are performing well
- In October 2003 consultants in England voted in favour of a new contract aimed at rewarding them more fairly so that more NHS patients benefit from their skills, while also encouraging them to embrace new ways of working in, for instance, multidisciplinary teams
- In April 2004 new contracts were also introduced for GPs and local family practices, accompanied by new, extra funding for local health services. The new contracts meant that, for the first time, all practices were significantly rewarded for the quality of care given and not just the numbers of patients treated
- The National Service Framework for Maternity, Children and Young People was launched in 2003–05

should address emotional wellbeing and discipline as much as the practicalities of caring for babies and young children. A further opportunity to impart good principles and practice comes at antenatal classes. Parenting groups too are helpful and are now becoming popular.

Childcare providers

Increasingly, mothers are working outside the home and have to find alternative care for their young children. Options include a nanny or minder in the home, or childcare outside the home. Child-minders who take other children into their own home have to be legally approved and registered with the Department of Social Services.

Alternative care includes:
- *Day nurseries* staffed by nursery nurses. These may be run by social service departments, privately or by voluntary organizations. Unfortunately, they are in limited supply and are often expensive. In disadvantaged areas, family centres may be available, which not only provide childcare but also offer support to parents in improving parenting skills.

- *Mother and toddler groups and playgroups* are available in most areas. The former are for children accompanied by a carer. Playgroups are run by trained and registered leaders.
- *'Sure Start'* programmes are a new initiative in disadvantaged areas that provide a variety of facilities and programmes for young families.

Education professionals

In Britain compulsory education begins at the age of 5 years:

- *Nursery school* (limited availability, with places from the age of 3 years)
- *Primary school* (5–11 years)
- *Secondary school, sixth form, sixth form college or college of further education* (optional at 16 years).

Educational provision for children with special needs is discussed on page 198.

Professionals involved in child health promotion and screening

Health visitors

Health visitors are nurses who are specially trained in childcare and development. They work either in the framework of a baby clinic or with GPs, and carry out the bulk of the child health surveillance and health promotion programme for preschool children. This includes running child health clinics, visiting at home and providing support, particularly for those children and families identified as being in need or at risk.

School nurses

School nurses are specially trained nurses who work in a group of local schools. They are responsible for identifying children with medical needs, facilitating their care at school, providing liaison between professionals and supplying medical information to school staff. As school doctors are no longer required to see every child at school entry, the school nurse is now responsible for reviewing all children and selecting those who need to be seen by the community paediatrician.

General practitioners

In recent years, GPs have taken over responsibility for some of the routine aspects of the preschool and school child health surveillance programme, which is mostly delivered by health visitors and school nurses. A small number of community paediatricians may still run baby clinics in disadvantaged areas. Approximately 60% of GPs have had a formal training in paediatrics. In many countries in Europe and the USA, preventive and curative care is provided by primary care paediatricians. Paediatricians are secondary care specialists in the UK, accepting referrals from GPs and other primary care staff.

Practice nurses

These nurses are attached to GP practices and provide immunization and other healthcare services to children, e.g. asthma review clinics.

Parents

Parents have a central role in enhancing the health of their children and they should be seen as partners in child health promotion.

Secondary care

Paediatricians

Paediatricians work in both hospital and community settings. Hospitalists tend to specialize in providing acute care which requires inpatient facilities, and also run outpatient clinics, taking referrals from GPs and others. More specialist paediatrics (e.g. respiratory, cardiac) are based in tertiary care children's hospitals.

Paediatricians who specialize in working in the community are sometimes known as consultant paediatricians with a special interest in community child health. Community paediatric teams provide specialized services in the areas of social paediatrics and child protection, behavioural paediatrics, neurodisability services and child public health. In recent years there has been increasing recognition of the importance of fully integrated and seamless services across primary, secondary and tertiary care and of involving the local authority education and social services more fully.

The case studies shown in Table 14.4 illustrate the range of professionals who might be involved in the care of different children.

The Children's National Service Framework

The Children's National Service Framework (NSF) standards are divided into three parts. Part One contains Standards 1–5, which apply to services for all children and young people, while Standards 6–10 in Part Two set standards in services for particular groups of children and young people. Part Three contains Standard 11, which is about maternity services. In this NSF, children and young people are defined as under 19 years. However, the age ranges for service provision vary according to the statutory obligations of the different agencies.

The Children's NSF standards are described in detail on the MasterCourse website.

'Every Child Matters'

The implementation of the Children's NSF will be a major part of the 'Change for Children' programme, driving up standards and leading to improved outcomes for children. The publication 'Every Child Matters' sets out a vision of the outcomes to be achieved, as part of a commitment to support all children to:
- Be healthy
- Stay safe
- Enjoy and achieve
- Make a positive contribution
- Achieve economic wellbeing.

Table 14.4 Individuals involved in the care of children

Child	Health	Education	Social	Voluntary
14-year-old female known drug misuser who is pregnant	School nurse Adolescent worker (teenage pregnancy coordinator) Child and adolescent mental health care team Drug and alcohol team	Welfare assistant Class teacher	Educational social worker Police	Church youth workers
3-year-old with cerebral palsy	Health visitor GP Paediatrician Audiology department Speech and language therapist Psychologist Physiotherapist Occupational therapist	Early years nursery staff Educational psychologist Portage Special educational needs coordinator (SENCO)	Social worker for disability team Benefits advice service	Parent support groups Sure Start
12-month-old with fever and rash	NHS Direct Pharmacy GP Walk-in urgent treatment centre Public health department (communicable disease) Accident and emergency staff Paediatrician Ward nurse	School nurse (of older siblings)		Playgroup

The NHS will have a key role to play in helping to achieve all of these outcomes.

The evidence-based standards in the Children's NSF will feed into the new integrated inspection framework, and the Children's NSF delivery strategy will be closely aligned to the wider 'Change for Children — Every Child Matters' implementation programme. The government is also promoting the development of Children's Trusts, which will have a key role to play in coordinating and integrating the planning, commission and delivery of health, social care and education services. Other key components of the agenda to improve delivery of services are the development of information-sharing arrangements, a Common Assessment Framework, lead professionals and a common core of training across agencies and disciplines.

Improving access to services is a priority for achieving good outcomes for children. More co-located, multidisciplinary services will be put in place, providing personalized support throughout childhood and into adolescence. There are an increasing number of Healthy Schools, which will help lead the way to improving children and young people's health. In addition, schools are being encouraged to develop into 'extended schools', providing health, social care and other services for children and young people, their families and the wider community. Starting in the most disadvantaged areas, the government is also establishing Children's Centres, offering integrated early years education, family and parenting support, and health support.

Implementation

Full implementation of the standards will take up to 10 years. There is already good practice in services in many areas of the country; however, delivering all aspects of the standards in all areas requires a long-term programme of change. The pace of change and immediate local priorities will vary. Nevertheless, the NHS and local authorities will increasingly be assessed on the quality of their services and on whether they are making progress towards meeting the standards.

www.dh.gov.uk/PolicyAndGuidance/
HealthAndSocialCareTopics/ChildrenServices/
ChildrenServicesInformation/fs/en

Reference

Acheson 1986. From Public Health in England: the report of the Committee of Inquiry into the Future Development of the Public Health Function (Cm 289) London: HMSO, 1988
Bryce J, Boschi-Pint C, Shibuya K, Black RE; WHO Child Health Epidemiology Reference Group 2005 WHO estimates of the causes of death in children. Lancet 365:1147–1152

Rachel Crowther   CHAPTER

Screening   15

LEARNING OUTCOMES

By the end of this chapter you should:

● Understand the place of screening in preventive healthcare and why it is an important element of child health services
● Understand the theoretical background to screening and the parameters used to assess screening tests (sensitivity, specificity, positive and negative predictive value)
● Be familiar with the criteria used to evaluate new and existing screening programmes
● Appreciate the difference between screening and surveillance
● Appreciate the potential benefits and disadvantages of screening and the ethical issues involved for parents and professionals
● Understand the role of the National Screening Committee in overseeing screening programmes and the policy context for child health screening in the UK
● Be familiar with current antenatal, neonatal and childhood screening programmes in the UK, and those under development or consideration
● Appreciate the difficulties involved in ensuring universal coverage in screening programmes.

MODULE THREE

Introduction

Screening is an example of secondary prevention (Ch. 17), and which aims to prevent or mitigate the effects of a condition by identifying it early (usually before it is clinically apparent) so that treatment is more effective. Much attention has been focused on screening in early life, when there is considerable scope for identifying potentially serious conditions and reducing — or even eliminating — their impact. Consequently many of the

UK's routine screening programmes operate before birth and in childhood. Together they offer considerable benefits and form an important element of child health services.

In recent years, however, appreciation of the potential drawbacks of screening has grown. It is essential to have an appropriate means of testing before introducing a new screening programme, but that is not enough: careful thought must go into evaluating and designing screening programmes in order to maximize the balance of

159

Table 15.1 Screening and diagnostic tests

Condition	Screening test	Diagnostic test
Down's syndrome	Serum markers (e.g. β-human chorionic gonadotrophin, β-hCG) and/or nuchal translucency	Amniocentesis or chorionic villus sampling (CVS)
Newborn hearing	Oto-acoustic emissions (OAE)	Auditory brainstem responses (ABR)

Table 15.2 False positives and false negatives

	Affected individuals (those with the condition — 'cases')	Unaffected individuals (those without the condition — 'non-cases')
Positive screening test	True positive	False positive
Negative screening test	False negative	True negative

benefit and harm (p. 162). The impact of screening, in economic, social and personal terms, needs to be considered alongside any beneficial health effects. It is also vital that the public understands that screening is not infallible, and that screening tests are offered with as clear an explanation as possible of what the results actually mean (p. 164). This chapter introduces the theory and practice of screening, considering the nature of screening tests, the policy context and the ethical and practical issues involved in delivering a screening programme.

Theoretical background: screening tests

A *screening test* is the first building block in a screening programme. Sometimes the screening test is a 'one-stop shop' that identifies affected or susceptible individuals immediately; examples include serological tests for rubella or HIV antibodies, or certain elements of the neonatal physical examination (e.g. checking for simple abnormalities such as extra digits). Often, however, the initial screening test merely identifies individuals who have a higher chance of having a particular condition, and a positive result leads to a second stage of testing involving a *diagnostic* test. Two examples are given in Table 15.1. Note that for Down's syndrome the diagnostic test is invasive and carries a small but significant risk of abortion, while for newborn hearing screening the diagnostic test is simply a more accurate audiological test.

False positives and false negatives

Most screening tests are not 100% accurate either in detecting individuals who have the condition being tested for or in identifying those who do not. There are almost always 'false positives' and 'false negatives' (Table 15.2).

Individuals with both false positive and false negative are done a disservice by the screening test results. Although

false positives can usually be reassured after further testing (the diagnostic test), they (and/or their parents and families) may suffer considerable anxiety in the meantime, and there may be a more serious impact, such as lost time at work or school, or social stigma. In addition, the diagnostic test, which would have been unnecessary if the screening test had been more accurate or had not been offered at all, may be unpleasant or carry some health risk.

False negatives, on the other hand, are given false reassurance, which may have serious consequences later on: the birth of a child with a congenital condition the parents believed to have been excluded, for example, or the risk that individuals may ignore early symptoms of a condition they believe they do not have.

Sensitivity and specificity

It is clearly important to keep the number of false negative and false positive results from any screening test to a minimum. In technical terms, any test needs to be as *sensitive* and as *specific* as possible. Since the development of a test usually involves reaching agreement about where to set the cutoff for positive/negative results (e.g. at a particular level of a serum marker), there is generally a trade-off between sensitivity and specificity; set the cutoff too high and sensitivity will decline, although specificity will rise, and vice versa.

Sensitivity

- Is related to the number of false negatives: a test is less sensitive if it produces large numbers of false negatives (missed cases)
- Describes the proportion of affected individuals who are picked up by the test (i.e. who have positive test results)
- Is calculated by dividing the number of affected individuals with a positive test by the total number of affected individuals, i.e. (referring to Table 15.2)

A new serum marker for Down's syndrome has recently been piloted. The results are shown below. Calculate the sensitivity and specificity if this marker were to be used on its own as a screening test for Down's syndrome.

- *Trial population*: 1000
- *Positive screening test results*: 82, of which all proceeded to amniocentesis or CVS and 17 were found to be carrying fetuses with Down's syndrome
- *Missed cases*: 2 women with negative screening tests had an amniocentesis for other reasons, which detected Down's fetuses, and another woman subsequently delivered a baby with Down's syndrome

	Affected fetuses	Unaffected fetuses
Positive test	17 (true positives)	65 (false positives)
Negative test	3 (false negatives)	915 (true negatives)

Sensitivity = 17 ÷ (17 + 3) = 85%
Specificity = 915 ÷ (915 + 65) = 93.4%

In the second stage of the pilot, the cutoff for the new marker was lowered in an attempt to increase sensitivity. The results for this stage are shown below. Has the screening test improved? Which do you think is more important in this case: sensitivity or specificity? (Think about the implications of false negative and false positive test results.)

- *Trial population*: 2000
- *Positive screening test results*: 296, of which all proceeded to amniocentesis or CVS and 36 were found to be carrying fetuses with Down's syndrome
- *Missed cases*: 4

	Affected fetuses	Unaffected fetuses
Positive test	36 (true positives)	260 (false positives)
Negative test	4 (false negatives)	1700 (true negatives)

Sensitivity = 36 ÷ (36 + 4) = 90%
Specificity = 1700 ÷ (1700 + 260) = 86.7%

by dividing true positives by (true positives + false negatives).

Specificity

- Is related to the number of false positives: a test is less specific if it produces large numbers of false positives
- Describes the proportion of unaffected individuals who are cleared by the test (i.e. who have negative test results)
- Is calculated by dividing the number of unaffected individuals with a negative test by the total number of unaffected individuals, i.e. (referring to Table 15.2) by dividing true negatives by (true negatives + false positives).

Both sensitivity and specificity are usually expressed as a percentage (Box 15.1).

Positive and negative predictive value

Other terms used to describe how well a screening test performs are *positive and negative predictive value*.

Positive predictive value (PPV)

- Asks the question: how helpful is a positive result in predicting whether an individual is affected by the condition being tested for?
- Describes the proportion of individuals with a positive test who actually have the condition
- Is calculated by dividing the number of affected individuals with a positive test by the total number of positive test results, i.e. (referring to Table 15.2) by dividing true positives by (true positives + false positives).

Negative predictive value (NPV)

- Asks the question: how helpful is a negative result in predicting whether an individual is unaffected by the condition being tested for?
- Describes the proportion of individuals with a negative test who are free of the condition
- Is calculated by dividing the number of unaffected individuals with a negative test by the total number of negative test results, i.e. (referring to Table 15.2) by dividing true negatives by (true negatives + false negatives).

Like specificity, PPV is lower when there are more false positives; and like sensitivity, NPV is lower when there are more false negatives. However, there is an important difference between the two sets of terms. Sensitivity and specificity are intrinsic properties of the screening test that remain the same whatever the characteristics of the population being tested. PPV and NPV, however, vary according to the prevalence of the condition in a particular population. Generally, where prevalence is low, PPV is lower too, but NPV is higher.

 A case study which illustrates this point is available on the MasterCourse website.

The development of new screening tests may raise important issues such as the acceptability of the test for families, the cost to the NHS of the test and also the cost of care for a case *not* detected. It is clear that a framework for assessing a potential screening programme is required. Such a framework is shown in Box 15.2 facing.

Policy and practice: screening programmes

Screening programmes and the National Screening Committee

Responsibility for managing screening programmes and shaping screening policy in the UK rests with the National Screening Committee (NSC), which advises government ministers in England, Wales, Scotland and Northern Ireland on screening issues, and states its purpose as follows:

Screening programmes are public health services that need to be managed at the level of a large population to monitor quality effectively. In the UK, this is carried out by the National Screening Committee (NSC). The first task of the NSC is to use research evidence to identify programmes that do more good than harm; the second is to make policy recommendations about those programmes that will do more good than harm at a reasonable cost. In policy-making, the evidence for screening is often limited, because of the rarity of the conditions being screened for.

http://libraries.nelh.nhs.uk/screening

It is clear from the previous section that evaluating any proposed screening programme involves considering many complex issues.

Although the general public has become more cautious in accepting medical opinion wholesale (witness falling immunization rates for the measles/mumps/rubella (MMR) vaccine following the 'autism scare'), faith in clinical tests tends to be high and lay people may find it hard

to understand that a screening test may not necessarily give them the 'right answer'. The NSC recognizes the dangers of this situation and is committed to presenting and explaining screening programmes so that the balance of benefit and harm is understood. Screening should be seen as a way of reducing the risk of suffering the ill-effects of a condition, rather than an infallible means of distinguishing those with and without it, and individuals should always be given fully informed choice about screening tests.

In order to fulfil its role, the NSC draws information from a wide range of sources, and makes it available through the National Electronic Library for Health.

http://libraries.nelh.nhs.uk/screening

In addition, the 'Health for all Children' (4th edition) report set out carefully considered recommendations for screening and health promotion throughout childhood.

Other recent government documents that shape the policy context for screening are listed on the MasterCourse website.

Criteria for screening programmes

In order to ensure that screening does more good than harm, and that all the relevant issues, difficulties and drawbacks are considered, the NSC has developed a set of criteria for appraising the viability, effectiveness and appropriateness of existing and potential screening programmes (Box 15.2). These build on the criteria first established by Wilson and Jungner, but set screening in the context of planned service provision for each condition, of meticulous quality control, and of informed choice for the public.

Benefit and harm: ethical issues in screening

Some ethical implications of screening programmes have been alluded to earlier (e.g. drawbacks for those with false positive and false negative results on screening tests). As well as ensuring that screening does more good than harm at population level, it is important to bear in mind the experience of individuals and to strive to maximize the balance of good over harm for each.

Screening in pregnancy and childhood is different from screening in adulthood. It requires parents to make decisions about and on behalf of their children, often before birth or very early in life. These are often emotionally charged times, and such decisions may be the first experience of the responsibilities of parenthood. Antenatal screening is usually directed at

The condition

- The condition should be an important health problem
- The epidemiology and natural history of the condition, including development from latent to declared disease, should be adequately understood and there should be a detectable risk factor, disease marker, latent period or early symptomatic stage
- All the cost-effective primary prevention interventions should have been implemented as far as practicable
- If the carriers of a mutation are identified as a result of screening, the natural history of people with this status should be understood, including the psychological implications

The test

- There should be a simple, safe, precise and validated screening test
- The distribution of the test values in the target population should be known and a suitable cutoff level defined and agreed
- The test should be acceptable to the population
- There should be an agreed policy on the further diagnostic investigation of individuals with a positive test result and on the choices available to those individuals
- If the test is for mutations, the criteria used to select the subset of mutations to be covered by screening, if all possible mutations are not being tested, should be clearly set out

The treatment

- There should be an effective treatment or intervention for patients identified through early detection, with evidence of early treatment leading to better outcomes than late treatment
- There should be agreed evidence-based policies covering which individuals should be offered treatment and the appropriate treatment to be offered
- Clinical management of the condition and patient outcomes should be optimized by all healthcare providers prior to participation in a screening programme

The screening programme

- There should be evidence from high-quality RCTs that the screening programme is effective in reducing mortality or morbidity
- Where screening is aimed solely at providing information to allow the person being screened to make an 'informed choice' (e.g. Down's syndrome, cystic fibrosis carrier screening), there must be evidence from high-quality trials that the test accurately measures risk. The information that is provided about the test and its outcome must be of value and readily understood by the individual being screened
- There should be evidence that the complete screening programme (test, diagnostic procedures, treatment/intervention) is clinically, socially and ethically acceptable to health professionals and the public
- The benefit from the screening programme should outweigh the physical and psychological harm (caused by the test, diagnostic procedures and treatment)
- The opportunity cost of the screening programme (including testing, diagnosis and treatment, administration, training and quality assurance) should be economically balanced in relation to expenditure on medical care as a whole (i.e. value for money)
- There should be a plan for managing and monitoring the screening programme and an agreed set of quality assurance standards
- Adequate staffing and facilities for testing, diagnosis, treatment and programme management should be available prior to the commencement of the screening programme
- All other options for managing the condition should have been considered (e.g. improving treatment, providing other services), to ensure that no more cost-effective intervention could be introduced or current interventions increased within the resources available
- Evidence-based information, explaining the consequences of testing, investigation and treatment, should be made available to potential participants to assist them in making an informed choice
- Public pressure for widening the eligibility criteria for reducing the screening interval, and for increasing the sensitivity of the testing process, should be anticipated. Decisions about these parameters should be scientifically justifiable to the public
- If screening is for a mutation, the programme should be acceptable to people identified as carriers and to other family members

Source: National Screening Committee 2003: http://libraries.nelh.nhs.uk/screening

offering parents the choice of terminating an affected pregnancy, a life-or-death decision about a child who may be very much wanted, and neonatal screening involves facing up to the possibility that an apparently perfect baby may have something seriously wrong with him or her before the parents have even got used to this new presence in their lives. Cultural, religious and social factors may strongly influence parents' thinking, and the views and interests of others, including older children and perhaps the extended family, may need to be taken into account. Sometimes screening may be offered for a condition (e.g. sickle cell disease) that already affects one child in the family, and may therefore involve implicit judgments about the value of that child's life and stimulate reflection about what the parents might have done, had they known in advance that the first child was affected.

It is important not to underestimate the gravity of the burden these decisions place on parents. However, where testing will be, for the majority, no more than a brief incident soon forgotten, there is a balance to be struck between the obligation to provide full information and the risk of causing undue alarm by insisting that every single parent is briefed on the full range of consequences of every single test. Doctors and others involved in delivering screening programmes are often advised to test the water by asking parents whether they would like to know everything about every test in advance, or whether they would prefer the healthcare team to 'do what is usually done' and leave detailed discussion until there is an indication that something might be wrong. Does this seem a good approach to you? If you were a parent, how would you answer this question?

Two case studies are presented on the MasterCourse website to encourage you to think further about the ethics of screening in antenatal and child health, and about the personal, social and cultural context in which it takes place. Read these scenarios and reflect on the questions.

Some of the advantages and disadvantages of screening programmes are summarized in Box 15.3.

Screening and surveillance

It is important to be clear about the distinction between screening and surveillance: both useful public health activities, but with different purposes. Surveillance is concerned with the collection of data on health and disease from a variety of possible sources, with analysing and interpreting it, and with feedback to 'those who need to know' (e.g. those planning and delivering health services or responsible for healthcare policy).

BOX 15.3 Advantages and disadvantages of screening

Advantages

- Better outcome for true positives if picked up early: may include lower morbidity and/or mortality, avoiding more unpleasant and severe treatment for later disease etc.
- Opportunity for parents to decide whether or not to proceed with affected pregnancy, and/or to prepare for birth of baby with health problems
- Reassurance for true negatives that they do not have the condition or are at very low risk
- Public health benefits: may include lower prevalence of condition, lower mortality, lower overall expenditure on the condition

Disadvantages

- Anxiety, further intervention and other possible risks for false positives
- False reassurance and possibly worse outcome for false negatives
- Cost of screening test for individuals: time, worry, discomfort or risk associated with procedure
- Those with positive screening test may face difficult decisions about how to proceed
- Cost of screening programme for NHS: N.B. opportunity cost (what else could this money be spent on?)
- Unless benefit of early intervention is absolutely clear, early diagnosis may mean longer period of 'illness' and/or unnecessary or excessive treatment

---

Surveillance is an epidemiological rather than a clinical tool, and does not generally involve patient-identifiable data (although sometimes individuals' records are identified in order to facilitate further investigation and follow-up).

The term 'surveillance' is sometimes used more loosely in paediatrics, to cover the broader elements of child health services that involve regular contact between health visitors, GPs and others and the children and families they look after, and which aim to spot problems early, to offer reassurance and advice, and to 'keep an eye' on the child: a group of functions closer to the lay definition of surveillance as 'close observation'. This use of the term is potentially unhelpful, however, for a variety of reasons, unless it involves collecting and collating data (rather than simply recording it in the parent-held record), it is *not* surveillance, and it may involve activities that are in effect screening but which do not meet the NSC's criteria (often because there is insufficient evidence for the validity of the 'screening test' or the benefits of early intervention).

A topical example is childhood obesity. Although weighing and measuring all children in certain years of primary school is a useful public health surveillance exercise, until there is a remedy of proven effectiveness for those found to be obese (and everything possible has been done to prevent obesity in children), the NSC could not support the introduction of a screening programme for childhood obesity in which results are fed back to individual children and parents. It is better to divide child health 'surveillance' into screening and health promotion activities and to be clear about their precise purpose and justification.

Current antenatal, neonatal and child health screening programmes in the UK

A summary of NSC policy (current in July 2005) on antenatal, neonatal and childhood screening in the UK is set out in Boxes 15.4–15.7.

 http://libraries.nelh.nhs.uk/screening

Contains more information on any screening programme or condition

Antenatal screening

Antenatal screening (Box 15.4) is included here because it inevitably involves the fetus as well as the mother. It falls into one of several categories, including programmes that aim to:

- Ensure optimal general health for mother and fetus, and identify complications of pregnancy and threats to the fetus early so that they can be mitigated through optimal antenatal care (e.g. screening for anaemia, atypical red cell antibodies and risk factors for pre-eclampsia)
- Identify specific conditions for which planned changes in management can benefit mother and fetus (e.g. screening for HIV and hepatitis B)
- Identify fetal abnormalities early so parents can be offered counselling and options for management, including termination of pregnancy (e.g. screening for Down's syndrome, neural tube defects and other fetal anomalies).

Down's syndrome (p. 93)

The NSC surveyed the availability and quality of existing piecemeal Down's screening services across the country and established the basis for a coordinated national service with clear standards and infrastructure.

The national Down's syndrome screening programme aims to ensure that all pregnant women are offered

---

BOX 15.4 NSC policy on antenatal screening

Conditions for which all pregnant women should be offered screening (in most cases as part of routine antenatal care)

- Anaemia
- Bacteriuria
- Blood group, rhesus D status and atypical red cell alloantibodies
- Down's syndrome
- Fetal anomalies
- Hepatitis B
- HIV
- Neural tube defects
- Risk factors for pre-eclampsia
- Rubella immunity
- Syphilis

Conditions for which screening should be offered in some cases

- Placenta praevia (given relevant history)
- Psychiatric illness (given relevant history)
- Sickle cell and thalassaemia (in high-prevalence areas — see below)
- Tay–Sachs disease (in at-risk populations)

Conditions for which screening should not be offered

- Bacterial vaginosis
- *Chlamydia*
- Cystic fibrosis (for review in 2005)
- Cytomegalovirus
- Diabetes (for review in 2005)
- Domestic violence (for review in 2005)
- Familial dysautonomia (review commissioned)
- Fetomaternal alloimmune thrombocytopenia
- Fragile X syndrome
- Hepatitis C
- Herpes (for review in 2005)
- Human T-cell lymphotrophic virus (HTLV) 1
- Postnatal depression
- Predictors of preterm labour (review commissioned)
- Streptococcus B
- Thrombophilia (Health Technology Assessment report due 2005)
- Toxoplasmosis

Source: http://libraries.nelh.nhs.uk/screening

---

screening that conforms to NSC guidance, in order to give parents informed choices about pregnancy outcome and reduce the number of babies born with *undiagnosed* Down's syndrome.

Down's syndrome tests

A variety of testing combinations have evolved, including up to four serum markers (various proteins and hormones assayed in a blood sample taken between 10 and 20 weeks' gestation) and ultrasound scanning for nuchal translucency (NT; the fluid area at the back of the fetal neck, the size of which is related to the risk of Down's syndrome).

A combination of ultrasound and serum methods is ideal, but where NT measurement is not yet available, serum testing alone is acceptable. Markers used for second-trimester screening include alpha-fetoprotein (AFP), free β-human chorionic gonadotrophin (β-hCG), unconjugated oestriol (UE3) and inhibin A. First-trimester (10–14 weeks) screening generally uses β-hCG and placenta-associated plasma protein-A (PAPP-A).

Estimating the risk of Down's syndrome from the results of any testing combination requires the use of specialist software that calculates the risk of an affected baby given the mother's age. (The background risk increases sharply with age, from 1:1500 at age 20 to 1:270 at age 35 and 1:100 at 40.) Women with an adjusted risk over 1:250 (about 5% of those tested) should be offered diagnostic cytogenetic testing, involving amniocentesis between 15 and 20 weeks, or chorionic villus sampling (CVS) between 11 and 13 weeks, together with appropriate counselling. Both carry a risk of miscarriage: around 2% for CVS and 1% for amniocentesis. Currently, around 90% of women choose to terminate confirmed Down's syndrome fetuses. Testing should ideally take place early in pregnancy to avoid late decisions about termination.

As for any screening programme, maximizing sensitivity and specificity is important. The targets for the Down's syndrome programme are:

- Detection rate of 60% or more and false positive rate of 5% or less by April 2005, progressing to
- Detection rate over 75% and false positive rate less than 3% by April 2007.

www.screening.nhs.uk/downs/home.htm

Fetal anomalies

A recent Health Technology Assessment (HTA) review found that ultrasound screening before 24 weeks offered some benefits. In many hospitals all women are already offered a fetal anomaly scan at 18–20 weeks of pregnancy, and a national programme is now planned with working standards that aim to ensure a high-quality universal service. Anomaly scans cannot detect all abnormalities, but aim to identify those that:

- Are incompatible with life
- Are likely to be associated with high morbidity and long-term disability

- Might benefit from intrauterine therapy
- Will need investigation or treatment after birth.

HIV (Ch. 44)

Antenatal serological screening for HIV was introduced in 2000, following a period of anonymous testing in pregnancy for surveillance purposes. Most children in the UK infected with HIV acquire the infection from their mothers during pregnancy, birth or lactation ('vertical transmission'). If maternal infection is diagnosed during pregnancy, interventions are available that can reduce the risk of vertical transmission from 25% to around 2% (including antiretroviral drugs, delivery by caesarean section and advising against breastfeeding). Women found to be HIV-positive are also referred for specialist HIV treatment and advice, and virological follow-up is arranged for the baby.

Sickle cell disease and thalassaemia (Ch. 43)

Sickle cell and thalassaemia screening is now part of a national linked antenatal and neonatal screening programme that has three elements:

- Antenatal screening for thalassaemia
- Antenatal screening for sickle cell disease
- Neonatal screening for sickle cell disease.

Antenatal screening for sickle cell disease and thalassaemia aims to identify couples at risk of carrying an affected fetus early in pregnancy and to offer them the choice of prenatal diagnosis, potentially followed by termination. Screening is being introduced on a phased basis. It should be offered in high-prevalence areas (where the estimated fetal prevalence of sickle cell disorder is 1.5 per 10 000 or more) from April 2005 and will ultimately be offered to all women as a routine part of antenatal care. In the interim, testing for relevant haemoglobin variants (e.g. HbS, HbC) should be offered to some women in low-prevalence areas on the basis of a question about ethnic origin (targeting high-risk groups, including those originating from Africa, the Caribbean, the Middle East, Asia and the Mediterranean).

Neonatal screening for sickle cell disease has been found to reduce morbidity and mortality in infancy. Identifying affected infants before the disease presents clinically (often with severe infections and splenic sequestration crises) enables babies to be given penicillin and vaccine prophylaxis and parents to be trained to recognize complications early and seek help. It is being introduced as part of the universal newborn blood spot programme, to complement antenatal screening.

www.kcl-phs.org.uk/haemscreening

Neonatal blood spot screening

The neonatal blood spot test is offered to all babies at 5–8 days of age. It is usually delivered by midwives as part of the routine postnatal home visiting programme and involves the collection of capillary blood from a heel prick on to a card. Since 1969 all babies in the UK have been tested for phenylketonuria (PKU), and congenital hypothyroidism (CHT) was added in 1981. These are both rare conditions for which early intervention is highly effective, preventing irreversible neurological damage and consequent disability. Cystic fibrosis and sickle cell disease (both disorders for which testing is already established in some parts of the UK) are being added to the national programme, using the same blood sample as for PKU and CHT screening. For sickle cell disease, implementation began in 2003 and coverage was estimated at 87% by April 2005. For cystic fibrosis the aim is to screen all babies born in England by April 2007, and in other areas in the UK by 2008.

The neonatal blood spot programme is one of the largest and most successful screening programmes in the UK; over 600 000 babies are screened each year, with uptake levels of over 99%, and about 250 babies with PKU or CHT are identified each year. As for most screening programmes, a positive screening result means that further diagnostic tests are indicated to confirm whether or not the child is affected. The UK Newborn Screening Programme Centre has been set up to monitor newborn blood spot screening (Box 15.5).

The HTA programme has recently reviewed neonatal screening for other inborn errors of metabolism, stimulated by the development of tandem mass spectrometry. Rapid developments in biochemistry and genetics mean that screening for other conditions will continue to be regularly reviewed.

www.newbornscreening-bloodspot.org.uk

Medium-chain acyl-CoA dehydrogenase deficiency (MCADD, Ch. 34)

An evaluative study has been commissioned by the NSC to examine the effectiveness of MCADD screening. Six laboratories are taking part in the study, which is due to report in 2008. Screening for MCADD should not currently be offered outside the study.

Duchenne muscular dystrophy (Ch. 28)

The condition was assessed against the NSC's criteria in 2004 and newborn screening was not recommended. However, screening was introduced on a pilot basis in Wales and has not been discontinued.

BOX 15.5 NSC policy on neonatal blood spot screening

Conditions included in the neonatal bloodspot programme
- Congenital hypothyroidism
- Phenylketonuria
- Cystic fibrosis (soon to be added)
- Sickle cell disease (soon to be added)

Conditions for which screening is under review
- Medium chain acyl CoA dehydrogenase deficiency (MCADD)

Conditions for which screening should not be offered
- Biotinidase deficiency
- Cannavan's disease (review against NSC criteria commissioned)
- Congenital adrenal hyperplasia
- Duchenne muscular dystrophy
- Galactosaemia
- Gaucher's disease
- Organic acid metabolism disorder

Source: http://libraries.nelh.nhs.uk/screening

BOX 15.6 NSC policy on other neonatal screening

Conditions for which screening forms part of the routine physical examination of newborn babies
- Congenital cataract
- Congenital heart disease
- Congenital malformations
- Cryptorchidism
- Developmental dislocation of the hip

Conditions for which screening should also be offered
- Hearing

Conditions for which screening should not be offered
- Biliary atresia
- Neonatal alloimmune thrombocytopenia
- Neuroblastoma

Source: http://libraries.nelh.nhs.uk/screening

Other neonatal screening

All newborn babies should be offered a routine physical examination that aims to detect a range of congenital conditions (Box 15.6). Universal newborn hearing screening is also in place in most areas now.

Conditions for which screening is currently recommended*

- Growth
- Hearing
- Hyperlipidaemia
- Vision defects

Conditions for which screening is being reviewed

- Dental disease

Conditions for which screening should not be offered

- Autism
- Developmental and behavioural problems
- Hypertension
- Hypertrophic cardiomyopathy
- Iron deficiency anaemia
- Lead poisoning
- Obesity
- Scoliosis
- Speech and language delay

* See below for qualifications.

Universal newborn hearing screening

Approximately 900 babies with permanent hearing loss are born every year in the UK. Universal newborn hearing screening (UNHS) was first introduced in 2001 as a more accurate — and earlier — alternative to the infant distraction test (IDT). It offers benefits for:

- *Parents.* Parents would generally rather know earlier if their child has a hearing problem and can be helped to come to terms with and manage their child's condition.
- *Children.* There is increasing evidence of the benefits of appropriate intervention before 6 months of age in terms of language skills, speech, social and emotional development.
- *The NHS.* UNHS is cheaper per child than the IDT and far more cost-effective, given its superior sensitivity and specificity.

The UNHS is discussed in detail in Chapter 32.

www.nhsp.info/index.php

Screening in later childhood (Box 15.7)

Growth

Children should have their height and weight measured around the time of school entry and the 0.4th centile cutoff for height should be used to initiate referral.

Hearing

Screening for hearing loss in school-age children should continue while further research is undertaken.

Hyperlipidaemia

Screening should only be offered as part of a project on cascade screening of the relatives of patients with confirmed familial hypercholesterolaemia, which is not a screening pilot but an initiative under the 2003 Genetics White Paper.

Vision defects

In line with the recommendation in the 4th edition of 'Health for All Children', screening for visual impairment in 7-year-old children should be discontinued, and screening should instead be offered between 4 and 5 years of age.

Obesity

A Department of Health expert advisory group has been set up to consider surveillance of childhood obesity, and how to monitor the national target for this condition. The NSC does not support screening for obesity.

Coverage in screening programmes

National screening programmes aim to offer testing to all individuals within the target population on the basis of informed consent. Among the parameters for quality control of screening programmes is the coverage rate achieved in practice (what percentage of eligible individuals have actually been offered screening, and/or have taken it up?). Several factors may affect coverage:

- Local difficulties within the programme — shortage of staff, problems with the call–recall system, laboratory issues etc. — which require the attention of the programme coordinator.
- Problems with access, which may — as for other aspects of healthcare — affect different groups differently, and often mean that deprived groups are less likely to benefit from services. It is important that screening programmes take account of 'hard to reach' groups (including, for example, women who book very late, or not at all, for antenatal care) and ensure that they promote equity and reduce health inequality, rather than increasing it by allowing those with the greatest health needs to miss out on screening.

- Individuals may make informed choices not to accept screening or not to proceed to diagnostic testing: for example, those who would not accept termination of an affected fetus.

The objective is to ensure that universal programmes offer universal access, and provide individuals with full information on which to base their decisions.

Reference

Hall DMB, Elliman D 2003 Health for all children, 4th edn. Oxford University Press, Oxford

MODULE THREE

Kathleen Skinner

Immunization

LEARNING OUTCOMES

By the end of this chapter you should:
- Understand passive and active immunity
- Understand the principles and rationale behind the national immunization policy for children in the UK
- Understand the indications and contraindications of routine childhood immunizations, and know them
- Understand the reasons why some parents are resistant to immunization
- Understand the principles of disease outbreak control.

Introduction

Immunization is the process of protecting individuals from infection through passive or active immunity. Passive immunity is provided by administering antibodies, whilst active immunity is achieved through stimulating the individual's immune system by an inactive vaccine (toxoid such as tetanus, inactivated organism such as hepatitis A vaccine, or subunit vaccines such as acellular pertussis vaccine) or a modified, attenuated live organism such as measles/mumps/rubella (MMR).

Historical impact

After clean water, vaccination is the most effective public health measure for saving lives and promoting good health. Vaccination now refers to all procedures for immunization but first originated 200 years ago from the procedure to protect people from smallpox using the first vaccine derived from a cow infected with the vaccinia virus.

Diseases such as smallpox and polio used to cause widespread illness, disability and death but, because of vaccination, smallpox has been eradicated and polio is present in only a few countries in the world, with strong efforts ongoing to eradicate this as well. Most people in the UK will never have seen a child crippled by polio.

In the late 1990s, meningitis C was a major killer of children under 5 but since the introduction of the vaccine in 1999, the incidence rates and subsequent complications have plummeted.

Because immunization is so successful it may be easy to think that outbreaks cannot occur today; however, most childhood diseases have not disappeared. In Ireland, the Netherlands and Italy there have been outbreaks of measles in the last 5 years. Immunization is the safest way to protect children and the new diphtheria, tetanus, pertussis, polio and Hib (DTaP/IPV/Hib) immunization provides protection from five diseases in one vaccine.

Rationale

Infectious disease is different from other disease in many respects, including its non-linear nature. Herd immunity refers to the immunity of a group or community. The resistance to infection is the product of the number susceptible and the probability that those susceptible will come into contact with an infected person. The proportion of the population required to be immune varies with the agent, its transmission dynamics, the geographical distribution of susceptibles and immunes, and other environmental factors.

The herd immunity threshold is the proportion of immunes in a population above which the incidence of infection decreases. Therefore immunizing a greater proportion than this will ensure that infection will always decline and herd immunity is achieved.

For measles vaccination, coverage of 90% is required to prevent ongoing transmission, whilst for mumps this threshold is much lower.

The age at which vaccination is carried out is crucial; vaccination after the average age of infection cannot interrupt transmission.

Note that herd immunity is based on the following assumptions:

- Natural immunity is solid and lifelong.
- Vaccine immunity is solid and lifelong.
- Dynamic effects of antigenic diversity are negligible.

Since none of these is strictly true, eradication becomes more difficult.

Routine UK schedule of vaccination

The current routine schedule in the UK is outlined in Table 16.1. There have been several recent changes to the routine schedule.

Inactivated polio vaccine (IPV)

IPV is used instead of the live oral polio vaccine (OPV) because the present risk of imported polio infection in the UK is low now that polio has been eliminated from large parts of the world through the global vaccination programme. OPV provided more effective community-wide protection but carried a small risk (about 1 case in more than 1.5 million doses used) of causing vaccine-associated paralytic polio (VAPP). IPV

Table 16.1 Routine UK vaccination schedule

When to immunize	What is given
2, 3 and 4 months old	Diphtheria, tetanus, pertussis (whooping cough), polio and Hib (DTaP/IPV/Hib) *and* meningitis C (MenC)
Around 13 months old	Measles, mumps and rubella (MMR)
3 years and 4 months to 5 years old	Diphtheria, tetanus, pertussis and polio (dTaP/IPV or DTaP/IPV) *and* MMR
13 to 18 years old	Diphtheria, tetanus, polio (Td/IPV)

provides effective individual protection but carries no risk of VAPP.

Diphtheria, tetanus and acellular pertussis (DTaP)

A change has been made from using whole-cell pertussis vaccine to using acellular pertussis, which has been shown to be just as effective at protecting babies from whooping cough. The acellular vaccine causes fewer minor reactions of the type that was previously associated with the whole-cell vaccine.

Thiomersal

Thiomersal is a mercury-based preservative that has been used in some vaccines to prevent microbial contamination, or in the process of producing inactivated vaccines. Recently concern has been raised over the safety of thiomersal in vaccines, particularly regarding organo-mercury compounds linked to neurotoxicity.

All vaccines in the childhood immunization programme are now thiomersal-free in order to meet with World Health Organization (WHO) and internationally agreed aims of reducing the exposure of children to mercury where it can be avoided and where a safe effective alternative can be provided.

Additional non-routine vaccines available for children

Tuberculosis (TB, Ch. 44)

The schools programme offering BCG (bacille Calmette-Guérin) to school leavers is now being phased out. A new programme targeting neonatal and other at-risk children will be implemented.

Those now recommended to receive BCG are:
- All infants living in areas where the incidence of TB is greater than 40/100 000 or greater
- All infants whose grandparents or parents were born in a country with a TB incidence of 40/100 000 or greater

- Previously unvaccinated recent immigrants from high-prevalence countries
- Children who would otherwise have been offered BCG through the school programme, who will now be screened for TB risk factors and tested and vaccinated if appropriate.

The contact recommendations remain unchanged. The Mantoux test will be the standard method of tuberculin skin testing.

Pneumococcal vaccine

Pneumococcal vaccine is also recommended for children who are at increased risk of contracting pneumococcal disease because of one of the following conditions:

- Serious breathing problems, such as chronic bronchitis or emphysema
- Serious heart conditions
- Severe kidney disease
- Long-term liver disease
- Diabetes that needs medication
- Immunosuppression due to disease or treatment.

There are two types of pneumococcal vaccine: pneumococcal conjugate vaccine and pneumococcal polysaccharide vaccine.

Pneumococcal conjugate vaccine (PCV)

This contains polysaccharide from seven common capsular types, which are then conjugated to protein using similar technology to that for Hib and MenC vaccines. The seven capsular types cause about 66% of all pneumococcal disease and 82% of pneumococcal disease in children less than 5 years. The pneumococcal conjugate vaccine is recommended for at-risk children aged between 2 months and 5 years of age. These children should also receive PPV from age 2 years to protect them against a wider range of serotypes.

Pneumococcal polysaccharide vaccine (PPV)

This can be used for adults and children over the age of 2 years. The antibodies it produces help protect against 23 types of pneumococcal bacteria, which cause about 96% of pneumococcal disease in the UK.

Hepatitis B

Hep B vaccine (HBV) is recommended for all babies whose mothers or close family have been infected with hepatitis B. The vaccine is very effective in babies and children, although it is not known how long immunity lasts. The evidence so far suggests that people who develop immunity after vaccination stay immune for life.

The first dose is given within 2 days of birth; a second dose is given at 1 month old; and a third dose given at 2 months old. A booster dose is given at 12 months of age and blood titres are checked.

www.immunisation.org.uk
www.dh.gov.uk/PolicyAndGuidance/
HealthAndSocialCareTopics/GreenBook/
GreenBookGeneralInformation/
GreenBookGeneralArticle/fs/en?CONTENT_
ID=4097254&chk=isTfGX

Immunisation Against Infectious Disease 1996 — 'The Green Book' with updated chapters

www.advisorybodies.doh.gov.uk/jcvi/foi_
classesofinformation.htm

Joint Committee on Vaccination and Immunisation

www.hpa.org.uk/infections/topics_az/
vaccination/vacc_menu.htm

Health Protection Agency guidelines on immunization

Maintaining coverage in the face of complacency

Today it is clear that fear of the vaccine-preventable diseases has declined. Many UK parents will never see a case of measles. Whilst fear of the diseases themselves has diminished, fear of the potential side-effects has increased, especially since it requires parents taking a proactive step to give their child vaccinations. In the 1970s, many parents were concerned about a possible link between pertussis immunization and 'brain damage', with major consequences for the uptake and consequent protection of the child population from pertussis disease (Fig. 16.1).

Overwhelming evidence shows the benefits and safety of childhood vaccination, and whilst it may seem that parental concern is misplaced, these are genuine anxieties that should be treated seriously and sympathetically whilst being countered with evidence from robust scientific trials.

MMR: the facts

Parents have been refusing MMR vaccine based on a belief that it is associated with autism. No vaccine has ever been studied in as much detail as MMR, and making a decision on whether to immunize with MMR should be easy for both doctors and parents, but it is the most frequently questioned and contested of all vaccines by parents from all walks of life.

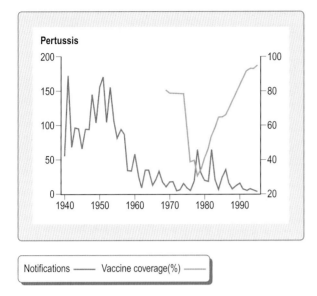

Fig. 16.1 **Graph showing relationship between coverage and notifications of pertussis disease**

The Wakefield et al study published in the Lancet in 1998 actually said, 'We did not prove an association between MMR vaccine and the syndrome described' and none of the studies since has found a link.

A review of the case histories of all autistic children born in the North Thames region between 1979 and 1994 (the time before and after the introduction of MMR in the UK in 1988) found:

- No increase in autism associated with the introduction of MMR in 1998
- No difference in age of diagnosis of autism between children who had been immunized with MMR and unimmunized children
- No difference in the MMR immunization rates between those children with autism and the general population in North Thames
- No link between the timing of MMR and the onset of autism.

It concluded there was no causal link between the MMR vaccine and autism.

Parents should be informed of all the ongoing trials and given the opportunity to study the evidence by themselves. They may worry that they cannot trust 'the government' but it should be remembered that vaccines are recommended for children on the advice of independent expert groups:

- The Royal College of Paediatrics and Child Health, the Health Protection Agency and the WHO all have a responsibility and mission to protect health and each recommends the MMR.
- MMR is the vaccine of choice in 90 countries.
- Single vaccines leave children vulnerable to diseases for longer periods of time.

- Past experience shows that uptake of single vaccines will be much lower.
- It is unfair and unkind to give children six injections when they can be better protected by just two.

www.mmrthefacts.nhs.uk/

Some frequent parental concerns

- *Vaccines cause long-term side-effects.* On the contrary, there is strong evidence to support the fact that allowing children to develop infections that were once considered part of growing up is much more dangerous.
- *Vaccines cause disease.* Vaccines have been linked to autism, bowel disease, brain damage, diabetes, multiple sclerosis and rheumatoid arthritis. No robust trials have ever proved this link. Many robust trials have indeed failed to find any link.
- *Vaccines do not work.* Evidence from notifiable disease statistics testifies to the dramatic drop in measles, mumps and rubella incidence, the almost complete eradication of Hib meningitis in the UK and the plummeting incidence of group C meningitis.
- *Clean water and healthy living are better than vaccines.* Undoubtedly these contribute to the decrease in spread of diseases but living standards increased in the 1960s and 1970s and whooping cough came back when vaccination coverage fell.
- *Multiple vaccines 'overload' the child's immune system.* From birth the immune system copes with many challenges every day. Highly purified, safety-tested vaccine is introduced into muscle tissue at the lowest effective dose, causing a natural immune response.

The bottom line is that having a vaccine is safer than having the disease.

Indications and contraindications

Withholding immunization may have consequences for both the individual concerned and the general public; therefore serious consideration should be given to all risks and benefits before taking this step. No opportunity for immunizing children should be missed, and so when in any doubt, advice should be sought from a consultant paediatrician, a consultant in communicable disease control or the immunization coordinator based in the local Health Protection Agency. Hospitals may provide specialist immunization clinics for those

Table 16.2 Contraindications to immunization

General contraindications	What to do
Acute illness with fever or systemic upset	Immunization should be postponed until recovery has occurred in order to ensure symptoms are not wrongly attributed to an adverse vaccine reaction. Minor illness is not a reason to postpone immunization
Hypersensitivity or previous anaphylactic reaction to egg	Previous anaphylactic reaction to egg contraindicates influenza and yellow fever vaccines. MMR vaccine can be given safely

children thought to be at high risk from severe adverse reactions. Contraindications to immunizations are shown in Table 16.2.

Siblings and close contacts of immunosuppressed children should be immunized against measles, mumps and rubella.

Conditions that are *not* contraindications

- Personal history of seizure not associated with fever (with no evidence of neurological deterioration)
- Personal history of seizure associated with fever with no evidence of neurological deterioration (but advice to be given on management of fever)
- Family history of seizures or any adverse reaction post-immunization
- Previous history of natural pertussis, measles, rubella or mumps infection
- Contact with an infectious disease
- Asthma or hay fever
- Personal or family history of autistic spectrum disorders or inflammatory bowel disease
- Treatment with antibiotics or topical or inhaled steroids
- Breastfed child
- Pregnancy of child's mother
- History of neonatal jaundice
- Being under a certain weight
- Surgery (neither is recent immunization a contraindication to surgery or anaesthesia).

There are a number of 'special risk' groups where further consideration of the risks of the disease or vaccination need to be considered (Table 16.3). Figure 16.2 shows an algorithm for children with neurological disease.

www.rcpch.ac.uk/publications/recent_
publications/Immunocomp.pdf

RCPCH February 2002 Immunisation of the immunocompromised child: best practice statement

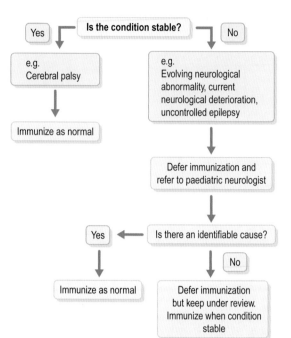

Fig. 16.2 Neurological conditions prior to immunization

Live vaccines — special risk groups

Certain individuals cannot mount a normal immune response to live vaccines and could suffer from severe complications, such as disseminated BCG infection or paralytic poliomyelitis. Do not offer live vaccines to the following:

- All patients treated currently or within last 6 months with chemotherapy or radiotherapy for malignant disease
- All post-operative organ transplant patients currently on immunosuppressant drugs
- All patients receiving a bone marrow transplant within the last 6 months
- Children receiving prednisolone at a daily dose of 2 mg/kg for at least 1 week or 1 mg/kg/day for 1 month
- Patients with evidence of impaired cell-mediated immunity: for example, HIV-positive patients with current symptoms, those with severe combined immunodeficiency syndrome, those with DiGeorge syndrome.

Individuals from this list, who are exposed to measles or chickenpox and are susceptible on the grounds of history or antibody titres, should be given the appropriate immunoglobulin as soon as possible.

HIV-positive children

Whether or not they have symptoms, these children should receive the following:

Table 16.3 Special risk groups

Special risk groups	What to do
Certain conditions increase the risk of complications from infectious diseases, e.g. Asthma Chronic lung disease Congenital heart disease Down's syndrome HIV (not all routine vaccines — p. 174) Small-for-dates babies Premature babies — the schedule should start from 2 months after their birth *not* from their expected due date	Immunize as a matter of priority following routine UK schedule
Unimmunized children	Assume they are unimmunized and begin a full course of immunization following the standard UK schedule with some modifications for those 10 years and over
Uncertain immunization histories	Assume they are unimmunized and begin a full course of immunization following the standard UK schedule with some modification for those 10 years and over
Incomplete but known immunization history: for example, from coming to the UK part way through	Start on the UK schedule according to the child's age at presentation
Asplenia or functional hyposplenia increase the risk of bacterial infections, most commonly due to encapsulated organisms, particularly in the first 2 years after splenectomy	Follow the routine schedule and *also* give pneumococcal vaccine, Hib vaccine, influenza, meningococcal A and C
Haemodialysis increases the risk of hepatitis B and C	Screen patients for serological evidence of hepatitis B immunity; antibody-negative patients should receive three doses of hepatitis B vaccine
Renal transplant recipients and those with chronic renal disease	Consider annual influenza immunization, Hib and pneumococcal immunization

- *Live vaccines*: MMR
- *Inactivated vaccines*: inactivated polio vaccine, pertussis; diphtheria; tetanus; polio; typhoid; cholera; hepatitis B and Hib
- *Contraindicated*: BCG vaccination
- *May also receive*: pneumococcal, rabies, hepatitis A and meningococcal A and C vaccines.

Safety of the yellow fever vaccine is not established; therefore it is contraindicated.

Consider measles, chickenpox or zoster normal immunoglobulin after exposure.

Principles of outbreak control

It is not uncommon for the paediatric team to be asked for advice about control of an outbreak of an infectious disease in either a home, a nursery or a school setting. Meningococcal disease (Ch. 44) is a good example.

The peak ages for meningococcal disease are in children under 5 (especially infants) and in the late teens (15–19 years, including first-year college students). MenC vaccine is now given as part of the routine UK schedule to infants and is available to young people if they are under 24 years of age and unimmunized. During the first winter after its introduction in 1999

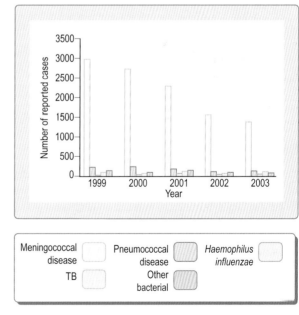

Fig. 16.3 Reported cases of meningococcal disease and other bacterial meningitis, England and Wales, 1999–2003

there was a 75% reduction in incidence of group C disease in children under 1 and in young people between 15 and 17 years (Fig. 16.3). The previous year had seen 1500 cases of group C disease, with 150 deaths.

Meningococcal disease is communicable and close, i.e. household or mouth-kissing, contacts are at increased risk; however, the risk of a secondary case is only about 1 in 200.

Between 5 and 10% of adults carry meningococcus in the nasopharynx, whilst 25% of young adults, especially those living in close proximity in boarding schools or residential establishments, may be carriers. Smoking and concurrent upper respiratory tract infections (URTIs) increase the risk of invasive disease.

Public health responsibilities

Below are given some of the steps you need to consider.

Step 1

Decide whether the case is confirmed, probable or possible:

- *Confirmed case*: invasive disease (meningitis, septicaemia, or infection of otherwise normally sterile tissue) in which *Neisseria meningitidis* has been isolated or identified
- *Probable case*: clinical diagnosis in which the Health Protection Team, in consultation with the clinician managing the case, considers that meningococcal disease is the likeliest diagnosis
- *Possible case*: as for probable, but it is considered that diagnoses other than meningococcal disease are at least as likely (including cases treated with antibiotics whose probable diagnosis is viral meningitis).

Public health action is required for confirmed and probable cases only.

Step 2

Ensure specimens are taken to maximize the possibility of identification of the organism; throat swab, blood culture and polymerase chain reaction (PCR) on EDTA blood, and acute serum should always be carried out. Consider a cerebrospinal fluid/rash aspirate.

Step 3

Identify the group of close contacts and ensure they receive appropriate prophylaxis within 24 hours when possible:

- Rifampicin, ciprofloxacin and ceftriaxone are all recommended for use in preventing secondary cases of meningococcal disease, but rifampicin is the only antibacterial licensed for this purpose. Rifampicin is recommended for all age groups. Ciprofloxacin is recommended as an alternative

agent to rifampicin in adults and children aged 5 years and above.
- Close contacts of confirmed cases due to vaccine-preventable strains of *N. meningitidis* (A, C, W135 and Y) should be offered vaccination up to 4 weeks after onset of symptoms in the index case.
- MenC vaccine should be offered to all unimmunized index cases under 25 years, irrespective of serogroup found.

Chemoprophylaxis acts in two ways: by eradicating carriage in established carriers who pose a risk of infection to others, and by eradicating carriage in those who have newly acquired the invasive strain and who may themselves be at risk. There is a small risk of meningitis developing in contacts, even if they are given prophylaxis; therefore, close contacts should be made aware of key meningitis symptoms and advised to seek urgent medical treatment if they occur.

Chemoprophylaxis is rarely required for cases now that first-line treatment is with ceftriaxone, which efficiently eradicates carriage.

Step 4

Give advice and information about the risks of secondary cases.

Risks of second cases within 4 weeks are as follows:
- *Background risk*: 2–6 in 100 000
- *Household members*: 1 in 300 if prophylaxis not given
- *Pre-school group*: 1 in 1500
- *Primary school child*: 1 in 18 000
- *Secondary school student*: 1 in 33 000.

Step 5

Investigate whether there are linked cases. If there is a second related case, e.g. in the same school, this constitutes an outbreak and would require a multidisciplinary Outbreak Control Team to manage it.

Step 6

Liaise with and inform GPs, employers and head teachers, where appropriate.

Step 7

Be available to reassure the public when the case reaches the media.

Step 8

Decide who else needs to be informed.

Health promotion and disease prevention

LEARNING OUTCOMES

By the end of this chapter you should:

- Understand the terms health promotion, disease prevention and health protection, and how these relate to different definitions of health
- Understand the importance of thinking 'upstream' about the determinants of health — 'prevention is better than cure'
- Understand why improving the health of the population is everyone's concern and the importance of partnership working to improve health
- Know about different approaches to improving health
- Appreciate the different levels at which health promotion and disease prevention can operate
- Be able to suggest examples of health promotion and disease prevention at various levels for different conditions
- Understand the difference between universal and targeted approaches to health promotion and disease prevention and the 'population paradox'
- Be aware of opportunities for health promotion in everyday practice, and the skills required to be a health-promoting doctor.

MODULE THREE

Health and health improvement

Definitions and meanings are important in the area of health promotion and preventive health care because they help to identify what we are trying to achieve. Before reading further, think for a moment about what you understand by the following terms, which will be explored in this chapter. How easy is it to come up with succinct definitions?

- Health
- Health improvement
- Health promotion
- Health protection
- Disease prevention.

- The absence of disease (medical or deficit model)
- A state of complete physical, mental and social wellbeing and not merely the absence of disease or infirmity (WHO)
- A function of individual lifestyle, the environment, human biology and healthcare provision (Lalonde)
- The ability to realize aspirations, satisfy needs and change or learn to cope with the environment
- A resource for living, not the object of living … a positive concept emphasizing social and personal resources as well as physical capabilities (Ottawa Charter for Health Promotion 1986)

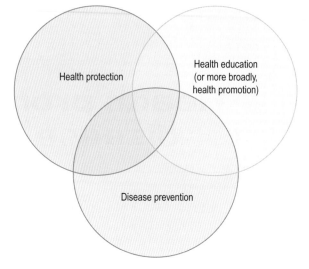

Fig. 17.1 **Summary of different means of improving health**

What is health?

Although it may seem a straightforward concept, the question of what health is, and how to define it, has generated considerable debate. Doctors have tended to see it simply as an absence of disease — sometimes called the 'deficit model', since it does not recognize the positive aspects of good health. The World Health Organization (WHO) has addressed this shortcoming in its much-used (though arguably rather idealistic) definition, which conceives of health as a state of complete wellbeing. Others have seen it in terms of its determinants — what affects health — or in terms of function: not what health is, but what it enables us to do.

Some commonly used definitions of health are listed in Box 17.1. The most appropriate choice depends partly on the circumstances, but in the field of health promotion, when we are seeking to foster optimum health across a population, a wider interpretation is needed that embraces the notion of wellbeing and includes different dimensions of health.

Health improvement

'Health improvement' is often used in a very general way to encompass all activities that aim to enhance health — including both preventive and curative medical services, and other functions undertaken by a wide range of organizations and individuals. Health improvement plans have been used, for example, as a means of setting out clearly the means by which the NHS, local authorities and other partners aim to maximize the health of their local population.

In this chapter, health improvement is defined more narrowly, as a broad term for 'upstream' interventions that tackle the determinants of health, as opposed to 'downstream' therapeutic interventions. Acting upstream to prevent ill health and to promote health in its broadest sense is one of the key features of public health and, as will become clear in this chapter, improving health is an important responsibility for everyone involved in healthcare, as well as many other fields of public and private life. Different means of improving health have been summarized by Tannahill (Fig. 17.1).

Health protection involves specialist activities that aim to protect the population from hazards, including infectious diseases and environmental threats. This is now overseen by the Health Protection Agency, formed through the integration of a variety of agencies and functions. The term has also been used to describe other measures such as seatbelt legislation, usually introduced (and often enforced) by the government or government agencies.

Whose responsibility is health improvement?

Improving health is very much part of the NHS agenda; indeed, if the health of the population is not improved by the combined activities of the NHS, then it might be seen to have failed in its main purpose. The government has recently laid increasing emphasis on transforming the NHS from a 'National Sickness Service' to a true National *Health* Service, and on making health improvement the responsibility of all its staff. Health professionals' commitment to improving health as well as tackling disease is vital. This is especially so in the case of children: all professionals share a responsibility to protect and care for children and to promote their best interests, and this includes ensuring the best possible health for them, now and in the future.

It is also very important to recognize that improving health is not just the business of the health sector. A very wide variety of factors affect health, many of which are beyond the scope of health professionals; consider, for example, poverty, traffic, pollution, parenting and school attendance, to name just a few key influences on child health. Partnership working is therefore crucial, and our achievements would be severely limited if we were to ignore the potential contribution of others.

Some of those with important roles to play in tackling the wider determinants of health and improving the health of children are listed on the MasterCourse website.

Evidence-based health improvement

The value of evidence-based medicine is well established in medical practice and education. It is just as important in public health practice as in clinical practice to ensure that what we do is effective and makes the best use of scarce resources, but it is less easy to establish an evidence base for health improvement than it is for many therapeutic interventions. Evidence-based medicine relevant to this course is discussed in Chapter 13.

Disease prevention

Disease prevention can be seen as the 'medical' end of the health improvement spectrum, related to the deficit model (health as absence of disease) rather than the positive WHO model. It tends to focus on the prevention of specific diseases or conditions, but quite often involves reducing risk factors that have a more general benefit for health; for example, tackling obesity to prevent type 2 diabetes in children confers many other advantages too. Three different levels of prevention are usually described.

Primary prevention

This involves stopping a disease, condition or insult from occurring in the first place.

Examples include the prevention of:
- Infectious diseases, by immunization
- Sudden unexplained death in infancy (SUDI, SIDS), through the 'Back to Sleep' campaign
- Child abuse, through interventions to support vulnerable children and families

- Teenage pregnancy through the provision of appropriate contraceptive advice
- Neural tube defects, by encouraging folic acid consumption before conception and in early pregnancy.

Secondary prevention

This involves preventing or mitigating the *effects* of a disease, condition or insult, often by identifying it early so treatment is more effective. Examples include child health screening programmes.

N.B. Sometimes 'secondary prevention' is used in a different way, to mean preventing recurrence after a first episode: for example, of child abuse.

Tertiary prevention

This involves slowing the progress and/or managing the consequences of an established disease, condition or insult.

Examples include:
- Optimum management of children with chronic diseases, such as diabetes mellitus, asthma or cystic fibrosis, to maximize their health (now and in the longer term) and minimize the impact of the disease on the child's everyday life
- Appropriate education, therapy (physiotherapy, occupational therapy, speech and language therapy), medical treatment and family support for a child with complex disabilities (p. 199).

Example: dental caries

The prevention of dental caries offers a good illustration of preventive action at all three levels.

Primary prevention

- Fluoridation of the water supply
- Regular tooth-brushing and good oral hygiene (involves providing advice to parents and children through a range of channels — dental health promotion)
- Avoiding sweets and fizzy drinks, or limiting them to specific times after meals (involves providing advice — link to nutrition and healthy eating, and the prevention of obesity)
- Fissure sealants (preventive dental care).

Secondary prevention

- Regular dental checkups to ensure decay is spotted and treated early (involves ensuring that

all children in the local area have access to NHS dentistry)
- Identifying gingivitis and advising on treatment
- Removal of plaque by hygienist.

Tertiary prevention

- Filling of cavities — or in extreme cases, removal of teeth.

Example: childhood injuries

Key facts

- Childhood injury prevention has been very successful; the number of deaths in the UK has dropped significantly in recent years.
- However, injuries and accidents remain very common; 1 in 5 children attend the accident and emergency department each year, having sustained an injury. 'Injury and poisoning' is a leading cause of death in children (p. 149) and also causes significant morbidity.
- There is a strong social class gradient in childhood injuries, with those in lower socioeconomic groups being most at risk.
- Non-accidental injury is an important cause that must always be borne in mind.
- Childhood injuries occur in many different settings — at home, on the roads, in other public places — as the clinical histories below illustrate.
  Head injuries, and other types of injury, can occur at any age, but the patterns vary at different ages. Common types of injury include:
  - *Toddlers*: falls, scalds, poisoning, drowning
  - *Older children*: road traffic accidents (usually as pedestrian or cyclist), and injuries sustained while playing sport
  - *Adolescents*: often related to risk behaviour— joy riding, extreme sports, experimenting with substance use etc.

Problem-orientated topic:

head injury

Three children have been admitted to the local hospital via the accident and emergency department in the last fortnight with moderate to severe head injuries.

Hassam is 18 months old and was brought to hospital by ambulance after falling at home. His mother was out at the time, running an errand for her mother-in-law, and Hassam was being looked after by his 6-year-old brother and an uncle with learning difficulties. The history is confused but the brother reports that Hassam wanted to come downstairs, and when they tried to stop him the toddler screamed and struggled and eventually fell down the stairs, landing on the uncarpeted floor in the hall.

Cara is $2^1/_2$ years old and sustained her injury in the local supermarket while out shopping with her mother. She had refused to be strapped into the trolley and insisted on climbing to and fro between the main part of the trolley and the seat at the back, helping herself to chocolate biscuits, while her mother made her way round the shop. A member of the public was worried by her behaviour and tried to intervene, whereupon Cara became angry and frightened and lost her balance, falling head-first on to the tiled floor. She was unconscious on arrival.

Sam is 10 and was out with friends riding his bike around their housing estate at dusk. When a car came round the corner he tried to swerve to the side of the road but lost control of the bike, colliding with the car's bumper, and was thrown across the road and on to the pavement. He was not wearing a cycle helmet or any reflective clothing. The other children reported that the car was going 'very fast', but it may not have been travelling over the 30 mile an hour speed limit. The council has recently put up signs on the roads in the estate warning motorists of children playing nearby, and has been deliberating about imposing a 20 mile an hour limit and installing speed bumps and other traffic calming measures to help enforce it. Sam had multiple injuries including a skull fracture.

Q1. What could be done to prevent these injuries?

Q2. Can you give examples of primary, secondary and tertiary preventive measures?

Q1. What could be done to prevent these injuries?

It can be helpful to think about the kinds of action that can be taken at different organizational levels — individual, community/environment and policy (p. 182) — and by different agencies. For example:

Individual level
- Advice to parents and children from health visitors, GPs, school nurses and others
- Providing access to safety equipment for those who cannot afford it.

Community/environmental level
- Action by supermarkets to encourage the use of safety straps in trolleys
- Action by local authorities to improve road safety (traffic calming, safe areas for playing, cycle lanes)
- Installing soft flooring in community playgrounds and other improvements to the environment to protect or separate children from hazards.

National/policy level
- Legislation on seat belts
- Reduction of speed limits in built-up areas.

Q2. Can you give examples of primary, secondary and tertiary preventive measures?

Primary prevention — preventing accidents from occurring
Examples include:
- Promoting the use of safety equipment such as stair gates, safety harnesses and fluorescent clothing for cyclists. Approaches include individual advice to parents from health visitors, GPs and others; health education in schools; programmes linked to hospital accident and emergency departments (e.g. injury minimization and prevention — IMPS) and media campaigns to raise awareness of hazards.
- Promoting road safety to reduce the likelihood of road traffic accidents. Approaches include cycle proficiency training, traffic calming and the provision of cycle lanes and safe areas to play and cycle (e.g. parks with cycle tracks).

Secondary prevention — mitigating the impact of accidents and reducing the likelihood of them resulting in serious injury
Examples include:
- Promoting the use of seatbelts in cars, cycle helmets etc. Approaches may be similar to those

---

BOX 17.2 Exercise

Can you apply the same approach to identify examples of primary, secondary and tertiary prevention for congenital malformations and meningococcal disease?

Prevention of congenital malformations: some examples
- *Primary*: folic acid before conception and in early pregnancy; advice on eating and other activities in pregnancy to avoid listeria and toxoplasmosis
- *Secondary*: antenatal screening to pick up malformations early and offer information/ termination
- *Tertiary*: information/support/discussion of treatment options after delivery

Prevention of meningococcal disease: some examples
- *Primary*: immunization (especially group C)
- *Secondary*: prophylaxis for contacts after a single case
- *Tertiary*: rehabilitation for children damaged by meningitis, e.g. providing hearing aids for those with deafness resulting from the disease

---

listed above, but also include legislation (e.g. for seatbelts, motorcycle helmets).

Secondary prevention — preventing a second episode
Examples include:
- Offering support to families where children are at risk of injury through poverty, poor supervision or neglect (in extreme cases) through the child protection system.

Tertiary prevention — managing the consequences of injury
Examples include:
- Provision of effective emergency services, neurosurgical units and rehabilitation facilities to optimize the long-term outcome for children with head injuries.

More examples are given in Box 17.2.

Health promotion

Health promotion is a broader endeavour than disease prevention. The definitions in Box 17.3 capture the key features of health promotion.

The aims of health promotion

Health promotion seeks to benefit both individuals and whole populations. At the individual level, it is most

Health promotion is:

- 'The process of enabling people to increase control over the determinants of health and thereby improve their health' (Nutbeam 1985)
- 'Any activity or program designed to improve social and environmental living conditions such that people's experience of well-being is increased' (Labonte & Little 1992)
- 'A combination of health education and related organizational, political and economic programs designed to support changes in behavior and in the environment that will improve health' (US Department of Health, Education and Welfare 1979)

simply seen as aiming to improve physical, mental and social wellbeing. At population level, the WHO (Health for All in Europe) sets out the aspirations of health promotion as follows:

- *To ensure equity in health* by reducing gaps in health status between and within countries
- *To add life to years* by ensuring the full development and use of people's physical and mental capacity to derive full benefit from life
- *To add health to life* by reducing disease and disability
- *To add years to life* by reducing premature deaths and thereby increasing life expectancy.

Different types of health promotion activity

The Ottawa Charter for Health Promotion (1986) defined five aspects of health promotion, which provide a useful overview of activities in this field:

1. **Building healthy public policy,** e.g.:
   - Taking account of the health impact of all policy decisions — such as the design of new buildings and roads
   - Legislation — including laws on seatbelts, drink-driving, and restrictions on the sale of tobacco, solvents and alcohol
   - Fiscal policy — including taxes on fuel, cigarettes and alcohol
2. **Creating supportive environments,** e.g.:
   - Local and national policies on transport and smoking
   - Encouraging active transport — walking and cycling
   - Increasing the availability and accessibility of healthy food
   - Making healthy choices easier in every aspect of life — the focus of the 2004 Public Health White Paper, 'Choosing Health'

3. **Strengthening communities,** e.g.:
   - Encouraging genuine participation and involvement in local democracy
   - Promoting ownership and control by communities, and enabling them to make decisions about issues affecting their health and to set priorities for action
4. **Reorienting health services,** e.g.:
   - Improving access and reducing inequalities in health service provision
   - Focusing on the health needs of the individual as a whole person rather than on the illness, and sharing power in decision-making
5. **Developing personal knowledge and skills,** e.g.:
   - Providing information and health education
   - Promoting problem-solving and coping skills to help individuals increase control over their health.

Health promotion can thus operate in many different ways and at many different levels. A simpler framework considers action at:

- *Individual level* (e.g. health education and empowerment)
- *Community level* (e.g. social action and community development)
- *Policy level* (e.g. lobbying and advocacy directed at healthy public policy).

It is always more effective to combine action at two or three different levels than to focus only on one, and to involve as wide a range of stakeholders as possible. Health promotion is very much about partnership: with individuals and communities, with other statutory and voluntary agencies, and with the worlds of commerce and the media.

Health promotion at individual level

In the past, there was a tendency to perceive individual-level health promotion as a matter of simply instructing people as to how to live and act in order to be healthy, and seeing it as their own responsibility to make the necessary changes (giving up smoking, losing weight, taking more exercise etc.) to achieve better health. Although individual responsibility and control is an important concept, there is much greater understanding now of the impact of societal and environmental constraints on choices and behaviour; hence the emphasis on structural and social changes to make healthy choices easier (e.g. walking or cycling to school rather than driving children there; eating five pieces of fresh fruit and vegetables a day). This is particularly the case for children. Box 17.4 below summarizes some of the key influences on 'lifestyle choices' for children of different ages.

Infancy and early childhood

- Choices are largely made by parents or other adults, e.g. breast- vs formula feeding; weaning and later diet; second-hand smoking; sleeping position; leisure pursuits (television, playing outside); parenting style, affection and control
- Parental choices are heavily constrained by factors such as cost, convenience, knowledge and perceptions, habit and cultural norms

Later childhood

- Children have increasing scope to make decisions for themselves (e.g. meals at school, physical activity, experimenting with tobacco, alcohol and other substances) and also have an influence over their parents and carers through 'pester power'
- Children's habits and decisions are strongly shaped by parental and family norms, by peer pressure, by media campaigns aimed at children, and, as for adults, by cost and convenience

Health education

There is still, nevertheless, an important role for health education, which was defined by Ewles and Simnett as 'planned interventions or programmes for people to learn about health, and to undertake voluntary changes in their behaviour'. In terms of the Ottawa Charter categories set out above, this involves developing personal knowledge and skills.

Health education is often delivered to individuals in groups (e.g. children in schools) and includes not simply providing information, but also building skills and self-esteem. The key outcome is often seen as improved *health literacy*, defined by Nutbeam as 'cognitive and social skills which determine the motivation and ability of individuals to gain access to, and understand and use information in ways that promote health'. Health education is an active, rather than a passive, activity, recognizing that interventions to change behaviour and lifestyle can only succeed through individuals' conscious participation.

Empowerment

Another important concept in the field of individual health promotion is that of empowerment, defined as the process of helping people to develop a sense of:

- *Agency* (the ability to have an influence on the world)
- *Self-efficacy* (belief in the capacity to have an influence)
- *Personal autonomy* (the ability to speak and act independently of others).

Together, these enable individuals to take charge of their own destinies and their health.

Health promotion at community level

Community level health promotion is important for a number of reasons:

- The physical and social environment has a powerful influence on health, both directly (e.g. pollution, bullying) and indirectly, by affecting individual behaviour (e.g. choices about food), and the local environment is best tackled through a local approach.
- There are important group effects when programmes operate at the level of settings (e.g. schools, young offenders' institutions), involving all members of these communities and seeking to improve policies, ethos and culture (p. 188).
- The participation of users in the planning and running of services makes them more appropriate to the local population.
- Communities have untapped resources that may be directed towards promoting health concerns.
- People have the right, and responsibility, to be involved in improving their collective life.

In terms of the Ottawa Charter categories set out above, action at this level includes creating supportive environments and strengthening communities.

Community development

Community development involves working with a community (which may be a village, a housing estate, a school, or an interest group such as a parents' collective) to identify areas of concern and to improve health and wellbeing. It is 'done with' the community rather than 'done to' them and indeed, in an ideal world, involves only minimal support and advice from 'experts' to encourage and enable local action.

Healthy Schools

The National Healthy Schools Programme defines a Healthy School as one that 'promotes the health and wellbeing of its pupils and staff through a well-planned, taught curriculum in a physical and emotional environment that promotes learning and healthy lifestyle choices'.

 www.wiredforhealth.gov.uk

The programme focuses on a whole-school approach to the five national outcomes for children set out in 'Every Child Matters':

- Being healthy
- Staying safe
- Enjoying and achieving
- Making a positive contribution
- Achieving economic wellbeing.

There are four core themes for healthy schools:

- *Personal, social and health education*, including sex and relationship education and drug education (alcohol, tobacco and volatile substance abuse)
- *Healthy eating*
- *Physical activity*
- *Emotional health and wellbeing* (including bullying).

The government aims to involve every school in the UK in the programme by 2009. The aims include supporting children and young people in developing healthy behaviours, helping to reduce health inequalities and promoting social inclusion. The intended benefits for schools as a whole include:

- Improving behaviour and attendance (schools with Healthy School status have less fear of bullying)
- Improving educational achievement (schools with Healthy School status have better results for government assessments at Key Stages 1 and 2)
- Reducing and halting the increase in childhood obesity
- Promoting positive sexual health and reducing teenage pregnancy
- Reducing young people's drug, alcohol and tobacco use (schools with Healthy School status have less use of illegal drugs).

The programme emphasizes pupil involvement as well as the commitment of staff, parents, governors and others associated with the school. Examples of projects that might contribute to a school achieving National Healthy Schools status include:

- Introducing a breakfast club or break-time stalls selling healthy drinks and snacks
- Introducing a school council with pupil representation to feed into policy decisions and ensure pupils' voices are heard
- Introducing a peer listening and counselling service run by pupils, for pupils
- Improving playground facilities or introducing lunch-time activity clubs.

Health promotion at policy level

The third level for health promotion involves policy: often at national level, though international (and more local) policy is important too. In terms of the Ottawa Charter categories set out above, action at this level includes building healthy public policy and reorienting health services (although the latter can also be seen as operating at local and individual level). Healthy public policy includes areas outside health, e.g. transport, education, and social and fiscal policy.

Clearly, 'high-level' decisions can have a significant impact on individuals' health — affecting, for example, their disposable income (including benefits), the cost and availability of goods, public sector service provision, their exposure to advertising and other media influences, the safety of their environment, and opportunities for employment and training. Although such decisions are largely the responsibility of local and national government, individuals can influence them not merely by participating in elections, but through advocacy and lobbying. *Advocacy* means speaking out publicly in support of an individual, group or cause, and *lobbying* means putting pressure on government: for example, to encourage healthy public policy.

Examples of health promotion and disease prevention in key areas of child health

Childhood obesity (Box 17.5 and p. 255)

The importance of the childhood obesity 'epidemic' has been recognized by the UK government in setting a national target to 'halt the year-on-year rise in obesity in children aged 2–10 years by 2010, in the context of a broader strategy to tackle obesity in the population as a whole' (Public Service Agreement 2004).

The impact of childhood obesity is far-reaching, and obese children are more likely to suffer from:

- Early signs of risk factors for heart disease (e.g. high blood pressure or arterial intimal changes)
- Type 2 diabetes, traditionally 'maturity onset', which is being seen increasingly in obese children and has been dubbed 'diabesity'
- Other medical problems, including sleep apnoea, orthopaedic problems and benign intracranial hypertension
- Social isolation and bullying, poor self-esteem and depression
- Reduced mobility and lower levels of participation in sport and physical activity, which in turn perpetuate obesity
- Lower levels of educational achievement

BOX 17.5 Childhood obesity: facts and figures

- Childhood obesity is rising fast: the UK is outstripping other European countries and is not far behind the United States. Obesity in children rose by an average of 0.8% per year between 1995 and 2002
- Obesity rates have doubled in 6-year-olds (to 8.5%) and trebled in 15-year-olds (to 15%) in the last 10 years
- Rates are higher for girls than boys: up to 30% of girls aged 2–15 are overweight or obese in some areas of England
- Asian children are four times more likely to be obese than their white counterparts
- If the increase continues, parents' life expectancy may exceed their children's, with obesity becoming the chief cause of premature death
- Both energy input (diet) and output (physical activity) play a part
- Children in England eat on average double the necessary amounts of saturated fat, salt and sugar per day
- 40% of boys and 60% of girls get less than the recommended hour of physical activity a day

- A higher risk of becoming obese adults (up to 25%), with all the associated long-term health risks. The risks are even higher if both parents are overweight or obesity persists into adolescence.

Action to tackle obesity

Childhood obesity is a key public health problem that needs a collaborative, multisectoral approach. Since treatment is difficult and of limited effectiveness, the emphasis must be on prevention. Concerted action is needed, which tackles both the input and output sides of the equation, operates at different levels and involves a wide range of stakeholders and agencies.

Examples of action at different levels might include:
- Physical activity:
  - *At individual level*: exercise prescriptions, cycle proficiency training
  - *At community level*: better and more equitable access to local leisure facilities and sports clubs
  - *At policy level*: transport policy designed to promote walking and cycling and reduce traffic danger to child pedestrians and cyclists
- Food:
  - *At individual level*: classroom activities to teach children about healthy eating and food preparation
  - *At community level*: farmers' markets and local food cooperatives to increase availability of cheap, fresh, local produce

- *At policy level*: agreement on labelling to help consumers choose healthy food.

Examples of action by different agencies might include:
- Schools (e.g. as part of the National Healthy Schools Programme):
  - 'Safe Routes to School' schemes and 'walking buses' (organized and supervised walking routes for groups of children)
  - Changing to healthy vending machines (e.g. selling fruit and other healthy snacks)
- Local authorities:
  - Allotment schemes to encourage growing fruit and vegetables
  - Improving street safety and outdoor play spaces
- Media and commercial worlds:
  - Schemes to market sport and exercise as 'cool' by celebrities
- Food manufacturers:
  - Reducing sugar, salt and fat content of food
- Supermarkets:
  - Offering ranges of fruit and vegetables to appeal to children
  - Promoting the '5 a Day' message
- Agriculture:
  - Research into production of lower-fat foods
- National government:
  - Food pricing policies to shift balance away from junk foods
  - Setting nutritional standards for school catering.

The Health Development Agency's evidence briefing, 'Management of obesity and overweight' (Oct 2003), summarizes evidence of effectiveness of strategies to tackle obesity, including those that aim to:
- Prevent obesity and overweight in children (e.g. multifaceted school-based interventions)
- Treat obesity and overweight in children (e.g. interventions that involve parents, including exercise and behaviour modification programmes).

The 2004 White Paper, 'Choosing Health: Making Healthy Choices Easier', and its delivery plan set out details of the government's plans to prevent and treat obesity in children.

Parenting

For most children, parents and families make up the closest 'layer' of their environment and constitute the most immediate influence on their health and wellbeing. Particular aspects of family life that affect children's health (apart from lifestyle factors such as eating and smoking habits, and economic factors such as employment and family income) include:
- Family size and composition, including the extended family

- Attachment is measured by the baby's response to temporary separation from the mother at around 1 year of age
- Poor attachment leads to lower self-confidence, higher anxiety, aggression and stress, and less success in forming relationships in later childhood and adulthood
- Secure attachment leads to greater resilience to stress and adversity and seems to mitigate some of the detrimental health effects of poverty and deprivation

BOX 17.7 Parenting in later childhood

- Different styles of parenting may be 'helpful' or 'unhelpful' in nurturing the child's emotional health and self-esteem, and his or her later predisposition to conduct disorder and antisocial behaviour
- The parents' approach to discipline is particularly important; a balance is needed between clear, consistent and appropriate boundary-setting, and warmth, empathy and encouragement
- Less helpful parenting styles may be cold and punitive, overly permissive or neglectful of the child and his or her needs

- Family relationships, culture and communication
- Early relationships and attachment
- Parenting skills and style
- Domestic violence, conflict and family breakup.

Parenting is an important determinant of mental health in children, and is an often-undervalued skill. Parenting is important both in very early life (e.g. establishing secure attachment to the mother in the first year) and throughout childhood (Boxes 17.6 and 17.7).

Abuse and neglect (Chs 21 and 37)

Child abuse is the most extreme example of unhelpful parenting and can have a serious and long-lasting effect on children's physical and mental health. Abuse may be physical, emotional or sexual, and severe neglect is also recognized as a form of abuse. Around 100 child deaths from abuse are identified every year in the UK, and many more may go undetected. Children who have been abused are more likely to abuse their own children and partners when they grow up, perpetuating a vicious cycle. Identifying and tackling child abuse is the responsibility of all who work with children.

Action to tackle unhelpful parenting

Individual level

- Several programmes have been shown to help promote attachment, especially for 'high-risk' mother–baby relationships (e.g. teenage mothers, mothers with mental health problems or families living in poverty).
- Interventions can also help parents of older children to alter their parenting style and improve the health and wellbeing of their children — and often themselves.
- Family support (often involving several agencies) can help prevent abuse in families where a risk has been identified.

Community level

- Some parenting programmes are offered to parents through schools, and may have a component delivered to children in the classroom too.
- Linking to a Healthy Schools project can be helpful in achieving a consistent change throughout the child's environment.

Policy level

- Recent legislation on physical punishment of children by parents aims to reduce violence against children, which is an inappropriate element of parenting.
- Criminal Records Bureau checks on all staff working with children can help prevent known abusers from coming into contact with children.
- In the case of abuse or an identified risk of abuse, all agencies working with children should have identified child protection procedures, overseen by local Safeguarding Children Boards (replacing Area Child Protection Committees).

Sudden unexplained death in infancy (SUDI, SIDS, Ch. 50)

Risk factors for SUDI include:
- Sleeping prone
- Parental smoking
- Co-sleeping (bed-sharing) with parents, especially on a sofa or when parents have taken alcohol or drugs
- Premature and low-birth weight babies
- Children of very young mothers
- Poverty and deprivation
- Postnatal depression
- Male gender (male babies being at slightly increased risk).

Inappropriate medical advice that babies should sleep on their fronts has been blamed for a rise in

SUDI deaths in the 1960s and 1970s. The rate of SUDI remained around 2 per 1000 live births in the 1970s and 1980s. Following clear evidence that prone sleeping increased the risk of SUDI, the 'Back to Sleep' (or 'Reduce the Risk') campaign was introduced in 1991, since when the rate of SUDI in the UK has fallen by 75%. This is a powerful example of a successful prevention campaign and also illustrates the importance of ensuring that the health promotion messages conveyed to parents and the population at large are the right ones.

Action to tackle SUDI

The most important aspect of prevention is consistent and appropriate advice to parents, delivered through as many routes as possible and including action at individual level (e.g. contact with health professionals), at community level (e.g. communication through antenatal and postnatal groups) and at policy level (e.g. clear policies and guidance for health professionals, supported by leaflets, media campaigns etc.).

Advice should include:

- Putting babies to sleep on their backs, with the head uncovered and feet placed to the foot of the cot to prevent wriggling down under the covers — ideally in a cot in the parents' room for the first 6 months
- Preventing the baby getting too hot
- Stopping (or reducing) smoking in pregnancy — mothers and partners
- Keeping babies away from cigarette smoke
- Avoiding co-sleeping on a sofa or armchair, or if either parent smokes, has been drinking or taking drugs, or is very tired.

Smoking

Cigarette smoking affects children's health in a variety of different ways. Smoking by parents and other adults is an important starting point, since it significantly affects a child's intrauterine and early postnatal environment and subsequent health:

- *Smoking in pregnancy* increases the risk of stillbirth, preterm delivery and low birth weight.
- *Smoking by parents or others in the household during a child's early life* increases the risk of asthma and other respiratory problems, pneumonia, meningitis, glue ear and SUDI.
- *Exposure to smoke during childhood and modelling of smoking behaviour by parents and others* increase the chances of the child taking up smoking, which confers a long and familiar list of long-term risks.

Smoking is more common in low-income families, so that children in lower social classes are more likely

---

BOX 17.8   Antenatal smoking

- The national target ('Smoking Kills') is to reduce smoking in pregnancy from 23% in 1998 to 18% by 2005 and 15% by 2010
- Rates are falling (from 23% to 20% between 1998 and 2000) but significant differences between social classes remain. Rates are 4%, 8%, 21% and 26% respectively in social classes I, II, IV and V (Infant Feeding Survey 2000)
- Many complex factors affect 'choosing' to smoke

BOX 17.9 Smoking in children and young people

- The national target ('Smoking Kills') is to reduce smoking in children from 13% in 1998 to 11% by 2005 and 9% by 2010
- 10% of 11–15-year-olds smoked regularly in 2002; rates are higher in 16–19-year-olds and are falling more slowly
- More children from manual social classes smoke
- Girls are a particular worry: 29% of 15-year-old girls are regular smokers
- Rates are lower in young people from several ethnic minority groups: Indian, Pakistani, Bangladeshi and Chinese

Source: Office for National Statistics 2004 The health of children and young people

---

to be exposed to all these risks. Although young people from all social classes experiment with smoking in their teens, those from higher social classes are more likely to quit as they enter adulthood. Marketing campaigns aimed at adolescents (e.g. giving away cigarettes in clubs), peer pressure and low self-esteem (e.g. related to lack of educational attainment and poor opportunities for employment) also encourage unhealthy choices in young people (Boxes 17.8 and 17.9).

Action to tackle smoking

Action can be taken at different levels:

- *Individual level*: e.g. offering information, advice, access to expert help. The availability of specialist smoking cessation services is important.
- *Community level*: e.g. interventions in schools and with community groups, enforcing ban on under-age cigarette sales.
- *Policy level*: no smoking in public places, taxation — but raising taxes on cigarettes deters rich smokers more than poor.

The Health Development Agency's evidence briefing, 'Smoking and Public Health' (April 2004), summarizes evidence of effectiveness of smoking cessation strategies, including:

- Deterring young people from starting smoking (e.g. school- and community-level interventions, media campaigns, interventions with tobacco retailers)
- Helping all smokers stop (e.g. role of health professionals, counselling, pricing of cigarettes, media campaigns)
- Helping pregnant women stop (e.g. giving stop smoking leaflets during routine antenatal care)
- Tackling inequalities (little evidence available).

The 2004 White Paper, 'Choosing Health: Making Healthy Choices Easier', and its delivery plan set out details of the government's plans to tackle smoking in both children and adults.

Problem-orientated topic:

health promotion

You are charged with planning a health promotion programme to promote sexual health in teenage girls.

Q1. What would you aim to achieve?

Q2. Can you come up with examples of action at individual, community and policy level to illustrate how you might approach the problem?

Q1. What would you aim to achieve?

The major aim would be to reduce sexually transmitted diseases and prevent teenage pregnancy by:
- Improving access to contraceptive advice
- Improving knowledge of sex and sexual health
- Empowering young women to take charge of their bodies and control their sexual activity
- Building self-esteem (the best way to reduce under-age conceptions).

Q2. Can you come up with examples of action at individual, community and policy level to illustrate how you might approach the problem?

- *Individual level*: peer-led sessions to discuss sexual health issues and build confidence and self-esteem; Teenage Health Freak website
- *Community level*: 'BodyZone' project in schools to offer confidential accessible information, advice and contraceptive services

BOX 17.10 Advantages of a universal approach

- Often everyone stands to benefit: e.g. from adding fluoride to drinking water to prevent caries
- No stigma attached: e.g. difference between health visiting and social services involvement
- Often hard to define who is 'at risk'; therefore treat all
- May have 'knock-on' benefits for others: e.g. herd immunity, altered attitude or behaviour in peer group
- May be easier and/or cheaper to deliver to all than to select out target group: e.g. School Fruit and Vegetable Programme

BOX 17.11 Advantages of targeted approach

- May be a better use of limited resources
- Those who perceive themselves as low-risk may ignore advice or opt out of programme, thus wasting resources
- Sometimes very clear who is at risk and who is not: e.g. by family history, sex, ethnic group
- Even if everyone would benefit a little, may be better to focus on those who could benefit a lot
- More effective for reducing inequalities (direct resources at worst off or those with poorest health, to reduce gap)

- *Policy level*: improve facilities for teenage mothers to continue their education, to try to break the cycle of deprivation and recurrence.

Universal and targeted approaches

Sometimes there is a choice between a universal approach to health promotion or disease prevention, which encompasses a whole population or community, and a targeted approach, which focuses on an identified high-risk group (e.g. defined by age, race, gender, occupation or geography) (Boxes 17.10 and 17.11).

Think about the following examples while you consider the advantages and disadvantages of each approach:
- Immunization
- Screening for thalassaemia
- Screening for Down's syndrome.

Clearly much depends on the particular condition, intervention and situation. Factors to consider when choosing between universal and targeted approaches include:

- How common is the condition?
- How well defined are the risk factors (and the cutoff for the at-risk group)?
- How will the programme be delivered (e.g. water fluoridation vs individual screening)?
- How will the intervention be perceived?
- How expensive is the intervention (and how expensive to select out an at-risk group)?
- Is there likely to be a 'group effect'?

The population paradox

The population paradox was described by the famous epidemiologist, Geoffrey Rose, and provides a powerful argument for the universal approach to health promotion and disease prevention. Rose noted that even when a risk factor can be clearly linked to a disease, most cases may occur in low-risk groups simply because these contain far more people. To take a simple numerical illustration, a 1 in 10 risk applied to 10 000 people will lead to 1000 cases — ten times fewer than the number of cases produced by a 1 in 100 risk applied to a million people. The classic example in adult health is serum cholesterol or blood pressure and the risk of myocardial infarction; in child health an obvious example is Down's syndrome and maternal age.

The paradox can be represented as in Figure 17.2, where a universal approach would seek to shift the entire risk distribution to the left, while a targeted approach would aim to 'cut off the tail' at the top end of the distribution. It is clear which would have a more significant effect at the population level. However, the 'number needed to treat for benefit' is much higher for the universal approach, so much still depends on the cost of the intervention.

Improving health in everyday practice

The government is committed to improving health across the population and to making health improvement the responsibility of all its staff. But what can individuals do in their everyday clinical practice to promote health and prevent disease? What is the role of doctors, in a field that relies on partnership working across such a wide range of individuals and agencies? What opportunities are there and what skills are required?

The most important answer is to be aware of the importance of this aspect of practice, and to ask yourself regularly, 'How could I, as a doctor working with other professionals and agencies, make a difference to the way this patient, condition or service is managed?' The list

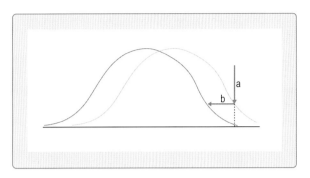

Fig. 17.2 Is it better to 'cut off the tail' (a) through a targeted approach, or to shift the whole population's risk profile downwards (b) through a universal approach?

below is not exhaustive, but contains some examples of action that individual doctors can take to promote child health:

- Advising parents about avoiding risks:
    - Sleeping position and SUDI
    - Safety in the home (cordless kettles, stair gates, smoke alarms)
    - Cycle helmets and cycle proficiency training
    - Child car seats and restraints
    - Pets, smoking and asthma
- Being alert to the presence of conditions or risks that might threaten health and offering appropriate advice and/or referral:
    - Obesity and overweight
    - Smoking (children or adults)
    - Short stature, failure to thrive etc.
- Knowing about and offering advice on preventive and health promotion services:
    - Immunization
    - Smoking cessation
    - Parenting classes and support for vulnerable families
    - Dental healthcare
- Recognizing and acting on signs of abuse and neglect
- Knowing about services provided by other agencies and liaising effectively with them:
    - *Social services*: asylum seekers; children at risk of abuse or neglect; children with disabilities
    - *Education*: children with complex health needs; using school nursing services to best effect
    - *'Connexions'* careers and employment services
    - *Drug action teams* and facilities
    - In some cases, the *police* and *probation services*
- Advocacy and lobbying:
    - *Individual level*: e.g. supporting request for rehousing for child with severe asthma
    - *Community level*: e.g. supporting campaign for a new NHS dental centre in the middle of a local housing estate

Policy level: e.g. lobbying for more resources for children within the NHS.

Two case studies are included on the Master-Course website, which set health promotion in the context of clinical practice and illustrate the ways in which the general principles introduced in this chapter relate to individual patients. We suggest that you work through these examples.

References

Labonte & Little 1992. From Rootman I et al (eds) 2001. Evaluation in health promotion. Principles and perspectives. WHO Regional Publications, European Series, N° 92, p. 10. WHO Office for Europe, Copenhagen

Nutbeam 1985. From Rootman I et al (eds) 2001. Evaluation in health promotion. Principles and perspectives. WHO Regional Publications, European Series, N° 92, p. 10. WHO Office for Europe, Copenhagen

Ottawa Charter for Health Promotion Downloadable from http://www.who.int/hpr/NPH/docs/ottawa_charter_hp.pdf

US Department of Health, Education and Welfare 1979. From Rootman I et al (eds) 2001. Evaluation in health promotion. Principles and perspectives. WHO Regional Publications, European Series, N° 92, p. 10. WHO Office for Europe, Copenhagen

Edited by Mary Rudolf, Mitch Blair

Community Child Health

MODULE FOUR

Valerie Harpin   Sue Gentle

CHAPTER

18

Childhood disability

LEARNING OUTCOMES

By the end of this chapter you should:

- Understand concepts of disability and be familiar with the terminology in use
- Be aware of cultural attitudes to disability
- Know the causes of disability in childhood
- Be able to identify abnormal patterns of development
- Know when further assessment and investigation is required
- Understand the need for a multidisciplinary approach to management
- Appreciate the impact that disability has on the family
- Know about the role that various agencies have in providing services for the child with a disability.

MODULE FOUR

Concepts of disability and terminology

Before considering clinical aspects of disability we need to think about what the terminology used in relation to disability means and why this might be important. There are three groups of people who need to be considered: our fellow professionals with whom we need to be able to communicate clearly, and importantly the children or young people and their parents who need to understand the terms we use. We need to avoid terms to which stigma is attached. Sadly many words previously used by professionals may now be terms of abuse in the playground, e.g. 'spastic', 'cretin' or 'retarded'.

Four common terms used in association with children with disability are disorder, impairment, disability and handicap (Box 18.1). In Table 18.1 you will see accepted definitions of these terms based on the World Health Organization (WHO) International Classification of Impairments, Disabilities and Handicaps (ICIDH). How do these definitions compare with yours?

The distinction between disability and handicap is particularly important. One of our aims when looking after children with disabilities should be to minimize the handicap that results from that disability. It is also important to consider how people with disability are perceived by society; some disabled people say that the handicap lies in society, not with them. We can help by helping the child to overcome or compensate for the disability and by advocating for changes in attitudes to disability in society.

Some parents prefer to describe their child as a child with 'special needs' rather than as either disabled or handicapped. This terminology is also widely used by professionals, not only in discussions with families, but

What do you understand by these terms? Spend a few moments trying to define them:

- Disorder
- Impairment
- Disability
- Handicap

Table 18.1 Feedback: defining the terminology

Term	Definition
Disorder	Medically definable condition or disease
Impairment	Loss or abnormality of psychological, physiological or anatomical structure or function
Disability	Any restriction or lack (resulting from an impairment) of ability to perform an activity in the manner or within the range considered normal for a child of that age
Handicap	The impact of the impairment or disability on the person's pursuits or achievement of goals that are desired by him/her or expected of him/her by society

BOX 18.2 Exercise

One way to try to decide whether a definition of a term is a working definition is to try to apply it to some clinical situations. Have a go at identifying the disorder, impairment, disability and handicap in the conditions below:

- Spastic diplegia
- Sensorineural hearing loss
- Epilepsy

also in a more formal context, such as the educational setting when a child may have a 'statement of special educational needs' (see below).

An exercise for you to complete is given in Box 18.2 (see Table 18.1 for definitions and Table 18.2 for feedback after doing the exercise).

In response to a move away from the entirely medical model of disability, the ICIDH has developed the International Classification of Functioning, Disability and Health (ICF). The stated aims are as follows:

- To provide a scientific basis for consequences of health conditions
- To establish a common language to improve communications
- To permit comparison of data across countries, healthcare disciplines, services and time
- To provide a systematic coding scheme for health information systems.

The stress is on functioning rather than disability, so the ICF has sections on:

- Body functions and structures rather than impairments
- Activities rather than disability
- Participation rather than handicap.

www.who.int/icf/icftemplate.cfm

Further details of definitions

Cultural attitudes to disability

Cultural issues should be in the back of your mind all the time. These are some key points relating to disability:

- Attitudes to disability differ in different cultures, e.g. acceptance of disability as the will of God,

Table 18.2 Applying the terminology

Disorder	Impairment	Disability	Handicap
Spastic diplegia	Increased muscle tone most marked in lower limbs, although there may be minor/moderate upper limb involvement	Abnormal gait and delayed gross motor milestones May not walk independently	Inability to join in with all playground games/physical education or walk to school
Profound sensorineural hearing loss	Hearing loss secondary to a lesion in the cochlea and/or neural pathways to auditory cortex	Impaired hearing and delay in speech and language development	Inability to communicate with most strangers Difficulty understanding spoken conversation
Epilepsy	Tendency to recurrent seizures resulting from abnormal and excessive activity of cortical neurons	Recurrent seizures may prevent a child from functioning normally at school	May be prevented from taking part in some physical activities, e.g. swimming unsupervised with friends, riding a bike May cause learning difficulties and poor school performance if fits are very frequent May, of course, cause little handicap if fits are well controlled

Table 18.3 The more common causes of childhood disability

Type of disability	Incidence
Physical and multiple disabilities	
Cerebral palsy	2.5 per 1000
Spina bifida	0.3 per 1000
Muscular dystrophy	0.2 per 1000
Severe learning difficulty	4.0 per 1000
Chromosomal abnormalities	4.0 per 1000
Central nervous system abnormality	1–2 per 1000
Special senses	
Severe visual handicap	0.4 per 1000
Severe hearing loss	1.0 per 1000

hiding disabled people away because they are a sign of wrongdoing, seeing disabled people as being specially 'touched by God'.

- Communication: we use a lot of terms that are hard for people to understand, even more so if English is their second language.
- Consanguineous marriages are common in some ethnic groups, giving rise to an increase in the number of children born with recessive genetic disorders. It is important to offer genetic counselling but you need to take cultural differences into account when doing this.
- Attitudes to abortion as a method of preventing the birth of a disabled child have a strong cultural base.
- Expectations of children's development vary from group to group.
- Within the deaf culture, some people choose to have a deaf child rather than a hearing child.
- There are many other issues relating to cultural background that are relevant in all health settings, such as dietary needs, concerns about the gender of the professional treating an adolescent girl, recognition of fasts and festivals, issues around death, and attitudes to medicines, surgery and blood transfusions.

The epidemiology of disability

Disability in childhood is relatively common. The prevalence of physical and multiple disabilities in children is estimated to be approximately 10–20 per 1000. The more common causes of disability are shown in Table 18.3.

Presentation of disability

Children with disabilities may be identified as a result of parental suspicion or concern on the part of health or other professionals. Their presentation occurs at different times, depending on the problem. A syndrome or central nervous system abnormality may be identified in the antenatal period or at birth. Deafness, motor handicaps and severe learning disabilities often become apparent during the first year. Moderate or even severe learning disabilities, language disorder and autism may not be recognized until the child is 2 or 3 years old, when the family or health visitor questions the child's developmental progress. Finally, children may present after life-threatening events such as head injury or encephalopathy.

Developmental problems and disability in primary care

Problem-orientated topic:

developmental delay

Jane is 3 years old. Her parents have been concerned about her development, and have consulted their health visitor. She asks you to assess her.

You find that she falls over frequently; she shows no interest in toys and does not seem to know what they are for; she can only say a few single words; she has difficult outbursts when she seems in a world of her own; and she has major problems with sleeping and is not yet toilet-trained.

Q1. What are the important aspects to focus on in your history and physical examination?

Q2. When should you become concerned that a child's development is delayed and referral is required?

Q3. What is the role of a child development team?

Q4. What impact does a disabled child have on the family?

Q5. What educational options are there likely to be for Jane?

Q6. When a child is disabled, what agencies need to be involved and what support is available?

Q1. What are the important aspects to focus on in your history and physical examination?

The history is of paramount importance. Children are quite likely to be uncooperative when relating to an unfamiliar person and in unfamiliar surroundings, and a reliable parent's report can provide much information.

The history should include an assessment of the following:

- Current developmental skills
- History of developmental milestones
- Birth history
- Past medical history
- Family history
- Parental anxieties.

Allowances for prematurity must be made during the first 2 years, but beyond that period catch-up in development rarely occurs. Parents often find it difficult to recall their child's developmental milestones, but in the event of delay they are likely to be more accurate. Of particular importance in taking a history is the identification of any regression in skills.

Your physical examination should include the following.

Developmental skills

You should attempt to evaluate Jane's development before carrying out any other part of the physical examination, as undressing her is likely to arouse some antagonism. When you meet a child who may have a neurodisability, you will find it helpful to think through the following areas systematically:

- Gross motor
- Fine motor
- Learning
- Communication
- Hearing
- Vision
- Behaviour
- Chronic illness, e.g. chest or heart problems
- Self-care.

In addition, you must assess factors such as alertness, responsiveness, interest in surroundings, determination and concentration, which all can positively influence a child's attainments.

Jane may well not cooperate with particular tasks, particularly if she is tired, shy or at the stage of stranger anxiety. You can gain a great deal of information from simply observing her at play while taking the history.

General examination

You need to carry out a complete physical examination in order to identify medical problems. Particularly relevant are dysmorphic signs, microcephaly, poor growth and signs of neglect.

Neurological examination

This needs to be thorough, looking for abnormalities in tone, strength and coordination, deep tendon reflexes, clonus, cranial nerves and primitive reflexes.

Q2. When should you become concerned that a child's development is delayed and referral is required?

Normal developmental milestones are covered in Module 1. It is important not only to know the normal range of development but also to appreciate when development is so delayed or disordered that an expert opinion should be obtained. Box 18.3 provides you with some developmental warning signs that can guide you in your decision whether to refer.

Jane's development is severely delayed in all areas, notably gross motor, communication and language as well as social skills. Such global developmental delay at the age of 3 is indicative of severe or at best moderate learning disability and she should be referred to your local Child Development Centre.

BOX 18.3 Developmental warning signs

At any age
- Maternal concern
- Regression in previously acquired skills

At 10 weeks
- Not smiling

At 6 months
- Persistent primitive reflexes
- Persistent squint
- Hand preference
- Little interest in people, toys, noises

At 10–12 months
- No sitting
- No double-syllable babble
- No pincer grasp

At 18 months
- Not walking independently
- Fewer than six words
- Persistent mouthing and drooling

At 2$\frac{1}{2}$ years
- No 2–3-word sentences

At 4 years
- Unintelligible speech

Q3. What is the role of a child development team?

The child development team is a multidisciplinary team of professionals who are involved in assessing and managing children with complex difficulties. The

Table18.4 The child development team

Professional	Role
Developmental paediatrician	Diagnosis of medical problems Advice on medical issues
Physiotherapist	Assessment and management of gross motor difficulties, abnormal tone and prevention of deformities in cerebral palsy Provision of special equipment
Occupational therapist	Assessment and management of fine motor difficulties Advice on toys, play and appliances to aid daily living
Speech and language therapist	Advice on feeding Assessment and management of speech, language and all aspects of communication
Psychologist	Support and counselling of family and team Cognitive assessment
Special needs teacher	Advice on special educational needs
Social worker	Support for the family Advice on social service benefits, respite care etc.
Health visitor	Support for the family Liaison with local health visitor

members of the team (Table 18.4) and the manner in which they work may vary from centre to centre, and their roles may overlap considerably in practice.

Jane's management will go beyond diagnosis, explanation of the problem and providing therapeutic input. It will involve supporting the family while they come to terms with the child's difficulties and learn how to cope. It also involves a great deal of liaison work with other professionals, both medical and non-medical.

The major benefit of the team approach lies in the coordination of care, so ensuring that the various professionals communicate with each other well and that the family does not receive a mixture of contradictory advice. The work of the team involves the following aspects.

Giving a diagnosis

The diagnosis of a disability is usually devastating and the way that the news is initially broken is of long-lasting importance to the family. The session should be conducted in private by a senior doctor in the presence of both parents. There should be plenty of opportunity for questions, and a follow-up session should be arranged shortly after. If a baby is born with congenital anomalies, the session should take place directly after birth, when possible with the baby present.

Medical management

Once the child's difficulties have been fully assessed, appropriate therapeutic input is required. This may be delivered in the child development centre, at home or at nursery. Once the child is in full-time school, the services are delivered there by community therapists, whose task is not only to work with the child but also to advise school staff.

Genetic counselling

When a child has been diagnosed as having a disability, the family will want to know the genetic implications for themselves and their relatives. Many disabilities have a genetic basis, in which case informed advice must be provided. However, even if there is no specific underlying genetic cause, the family will need to discuss the risk of further children being affected.

Q4. What impact does a disabled child have on the family?

Families differ greatly in their reaction to having a child with a disability. However, on first receiving the news, they all tend to pass through similar emotional stages to those experienced in coping with bereavement. The first reaction is one of shock, when often only a small proportion of what is said is taken in. Negative feelings of fear and loss, anger and guilt then follow. Gradually adaptation follows and leads to the final stage of acceptance. Some parents have difficulty in reaching this last stage, in which case supportive counselling by a psychologist may be necessary.

The family needs to adapt again at each stage of the child's development. Independence becomes an issue at each step and an important part of the child's education is to foster this, so it must be addressed as part of his or her special educational needs.

Good liaison is needed with school, and the school needs to be prepared and informed about any anticipated difficulties. If the child needs occupational therapy, physiotherapy or speech and language therapy, the staff will need to work with the therapists in order to implement their recommendations. In some circumstances the school may need to make alterations to accommodate physical disabilities. Special guidance or counselling may be required, and help may be needed to integrate the child into the classroom.

Having a child with a disability places extra pressure and stresses on any family. It is important therefore to determine how much support is available. Informal support in terms of family and friends can be variable, and additional support is often appreciated.

Q5. What educational options are there likely to be for Jane?

There are a number of possible educational options for children with special needs.

Preschool
- *Preschool teachers* are often the first contact from the Education Department. They will usually get to know the family well and provide key support in the preschool years. There may be specialist preschool teachers for deaf and visually impaired children. They usually visit the home to work with the child and advise the parents on the best ways to help the child. This should be in the first year of life if it can be confidently assumed that there will be special needs at school age, e.g. Down's syndrome, severe deafness.
- *Portage workers* have a similar role. Portage is a particular method of helping young children, which follows a specific programme of developmental steps.
- *Mainstream nursery school* with or without support.
- *Day nurseries, family centres and preschool playgroups* with or without support.
- *Special nursery school, unit or other group* for children with disabilities.

School age
- *Mainstream school.* The inclusion of children with special educational needs in mainstream school has been a core principle of Education Acts since 1981. The extent still varies across the country but there is a presumption of inclusive education where that meets the parents' wishes, meets the child's needs and is not incompatible with the efficient education of other children.

  The amount and type of support needed will vary according to the disability and severity. Physical disability may best be helped by structural changes in the school (lifts, ramps etc.); visual impairment by modifications for the child (enlargement of written material, better lighting etc.); severe hearing impairment may need the support of a signing assistant. Classroom support can range from occasional advice to one-to-one help full-time, including help during break times.

Local authorities may have specialist teams of teachers (e.g. sensory impairment, autism, behaviour difficulties), whose expertise can be called upon by schools to advise on management.
- *Special schools.* These are schools where all the children have special needs and the staff has special expertise in those needs. They may cater for a particular special need (e.g. deafness, visual impairment, autism) or be available for children with various or multiple special needs. Class sizes are small and children get a lot of individual attention. With education authorities moving to include more children in mainstream schools, local authority special schools have been reducing in size, changing in character and in some cases closing down. There have been major changes in the needs of children attending special schools, with the children generally having the most specialized needs. Special schools may have links with a mainstream school to provide the children with some opportunity to interact with their mainstream peers and to give them access to a wider range of facilities. Some special schools are run by voluntary organizations. There may be boarding facilities at these schools because of the wide geographical area they cover.
- *Special units in mainstream schools.* These are a compromise between special school and full inclusion. The unit may be for a particular type of disability or for a range of disabilities.

The debate continues around the merits of mainstream and special schools for children with disabilities. It is vital to listen to the child/young person and family and consider their needs flexibly.

Identification of special educational needs (SEN)
There have been many legislative measures around education. All the Education Acts since 1944 have now been consolidated into the 1996 Education Act.

In response to the 1996 Education Act and the SEN and Disability Act 2001, a new Code of Practice came into being in 2002. This document is available from the Department for Education and Skills (DFES) website.

www.dfes.gov.uk/publications

The assessment process
When a school and family first recognize that a child has special educational needs, they first consider what can be done by the school to support the child. This is called 'School Action'. If the school needs help from outside agencies, such as educational psychology, speech and language therapy or paediatrician, this is called

'School Action Plus'. If these measures cannot meet the child's needs, an assessment of special educational needs is initiated and a statement of educational needs may be issued.

The special educational needs coordinator (SENCO) is a teacher with special expertise in this area. The SENCO is usually the person you should contact to discuss a child's special educational needs and with whom you should liaise if an assessment of educational need is initiated.

Medical advice for education

There are different levels and different degrees of formality for giving advice to schools about individual children with special needs. This may involve discussion of the child's difficulties with teachers or writing a letter to the school. The child's and parent's consent should always be sought and it is useful to include this request routinely in your outpatient sessions.

Medical reports for statutory assessment

During an assessment of special educational needs, input is sought from the school or nursery, parents/carers and the health services and social services involved.

www.dfes.gov.uk/publications

'The Role of Health Professionals', with helpful information about the health professional's role and guidance on writing medical advice

Q6. When a child is disabled, what agencies need to be involved and what support is available?

See Box 18.4. These services are described in detail below.

Agencies with a responsibility for childhood disability

Statutory services

Statutory services try to meet the needs of children and young people with disabilities and their families. It is particularly important to see how these services are coordinated. Much is said about multidisciplinary, interdisciplinary, interagency and multi-agency working. Putting it into practice so that an individual family can see it working is not so easy. Indeed we know that parents often feel that it is not working for them. Families' views must be taken into account when services are offered to them and in ongoing service review.

Health services

We will start by looking at health services, since these are the ones with which you are going to be most familiar. Also, these are the services that most young children with disabilities come into contact with first. There are two important health teams with overlapping but distinct functions:
- The primary healthcare team (PHCT)
- The disability team.

The PHCT, particularly the GP and health visitor, have usually been involved from the start and it is important that they remain fully informed in order to give continuing support to the family. Once a child gets into school, the school nurse becomes a key health professional in the PHCT.

The disability team varies from place to place. There is usually a core team of at least a paediatrician, physiotherapist, occupational therapist, speech and language therapist and nurse. They usually work from a central base and are involved in the initial assessment of a child referred with a disability. The amount of involvement in follow-up depends on the condition and the local circumstances.

Communication between all involved professionals is vital. In the UK, Parent-held Child Health Records can help with this, as long as they are used and kept up to date. Special pages have been developed in some areas for use with children with disabilities. The only national one is for Down's syndrome.

Disability services and teams

The Court Report, 'Fit for the Future' (HMSO 1976), recommended that each health district established what was called a district handicap team, with two types of function:
- Clinical:
  - To provide investigation and assessment of children with complex disorders, and to arrange and coordinate management
  - To provide parents, teachers and others with advice and support on management of the child

199

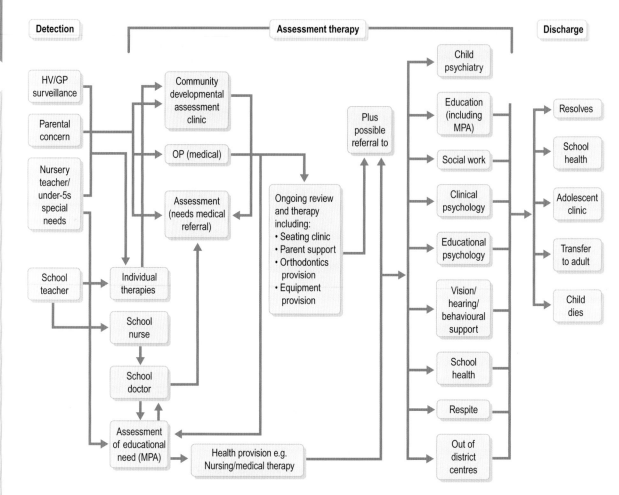

N.B. Links with others, e.g. audiology, orthodontic, general orthopaedic, as needed

Fig. 18.1 Range of services that may be involved for a child with a neurodisability. (OP = outpatients; MPA = multiprofessional assessment.)

– To encourage and assist professional fieldwork staff in management and surveillance
– To provide primary and supporting specialist services to special schools
• Operational:
– To be involved in epidemiological surveys, monitoring effectiveness of services, advising on services and maintaining quality
– To act as a source of information
– To organize training for professional staff.

Over the years these recommendations have been taken up in a variety of ways and to a variable degree. As a result, there is a wide variation in the organization of services across the UK. Hopefully, this reflects the needs of the local population, (e.g. large conurbations, predominantly rural areas, areas of mixed ethnicity etc.). Fundamental principles should remain the same, aiming at high-quality, coordinated, evidence-based and accessible services for all.

Organization of services (pathways of care)

Figure 18.1 reflects possible services involved for a child with a neurodisability. It is complex and may be confusing for both families and professionals! Try to think what a similar diagram may look like for your own area.

One of the key things parents ask for is a 'joined-up service'. This is not only geographical (services on the same site) but also involves professionals who communicate with each other so that the parents do not have to keep repeating the story. Families also highlight their need for general and disorder-specific information.

Social services

Social work input can be invaluable for many families. Input may be diverse, ranging from practical tasks to emotional support, e.g. around the time of diagnosis of severe or complex difficulty. Social services have certain statutory responsibilities:

- To provide services for children in need
- To keep a register of children with disabilities
- To ensure services are coordinated
- To include families in decision-making
- To make provision for respite care
- To safeguard the welfare of children in respite care in health or educational facilities
- To collaborate with the education authority to assess the needs of school-leavers with disabilities.

Social work services may advise on:

- Grants and allowances (although social services do not issue these)
- Respite care facilities
- Leisure activities
- Day care facilities.

Financial help

Caring for a child with a disability is expensive. Consider the following:

- Reduced income:
  - A parent giving up work or not starting work in order to care for the child
  - A parent choosing to turn down a promotion that means moving away
  - Loss of earnings when time is taken off for hospital visits
- Increased expenditure:
  - Transport: for hospital and therapy visits; general increased transport costs, e.g. taxis (imagine taking a child with severe behavioural problems on a bus)
  - Food: parents may want to 'feed the child up'; food wasted through feeding difficulties; less efficient shopping — easier to shop at the corner shop
  - Household goods: telephone needed; washing machine and drier for extra washing; freezer — difficulty getting to the shops frequently
  - Housing: adaptations; moving to a larger house
  - Equipment and special toys
  - Hospital admissions: transport to visit daily; child-minding for other children; new pyjamas; treats for the child.

This is an endless list!

Children with disabilities may be eligible for a number of benefits. Statutory help comes from the Benefits Agency, which is part of Social Security. Anyone involved in caring for the child should be able to advise parents on how to access help and should have a knowledge of what is available.

Disability Living Allowance (DLA)

This is an allowance for any child who has needs 'substantially' higher needs than those of a non-disabled child of the same age. There are two components: care and mobility.

The mobility component of the DLA qualifies you for:

- Help from Motability — a voluntary organization to help people use their higher-rate mobility component of the DLA to buy or hire a car
- The car badge scheme — available for children from 2 years
- No charge or time limit at parking meters
- No-limit street parking
- A maximum of 3 hours' parking where there are parking restrictions indicated by yellow lines
- Exemption from road tax.

Invalid Care Allowance

This is an additional allowance, which is available for the person caring for the child. (DLA is for the children themselves.)

Income Support

This is a means-tested benefit for all low-income families and has a disabled child's premium.

Fares to hospital

These are available for those on income support.

In addition to statutory benefits there are various funds that families can apply to for financial or other help.

The Family Fund Trust

This is an independent organization, registered as a charity. It is funded by the government through the Department of Health. It provides information (such as the benefits checklist) and grants for special requests related to the care of children with disabilities. Provision of grants is means-tested. It is useful for things like laundry equipment, bedding and holidays.

 www.familyfundtrust.org.uk

Contact a Family

Contact a Family also produces guidance for parents on benefits.

www.cafamily.org.uk

An excellent source of information about specific conditions and syndromes, primarily for families but also for professionals. It also provides information about parent support groups

Other possible sources for help for families are:

- Toy libraries
- Equipment loan facilities

- Disabled persons railcard: an accompanying person receives a third off the ticket price
- Local charities
- Local transport schemes
- Holiday organizations (more information from Royal Association for Disability and Rehabilitation, RADAR, tel. 0171 2503222)
- The local Citizens' Advice Bureau.

The voluntary sector

Parents can be helped by local and national support groups with many of the issues so far covered in this chapter. It is a statutory requirement for health professionals to inform parents of any voluntary organizations that might be of help to the family. Most areas will have an umbrella body such as the Council for Voluntary Services, which will have information on what is available locally. There should also be information about the voluntary sector at your child development centre.

Specific conditions causing disabiliity

There are many possible causes of childhood disability. The most common ones are summarized here and are described in more detail in Chapter 29 (Volume 2).

Severe learning disability (Ch. 29)

The incidence of mild/moderate learning disability (IQ 50–70) is 5 per 1000 and that of severe learning disability (IQ < 50) is 3.8 per 1000. In almost all cases of severe learning disability a cause is found. (Around 25% have a chromosome abnormality, and 80% of these have Down's syndrome.) Other important causes include congenital brain malformations, acquired brain injury (e.g. intraventricular haemorrhage in a pre-term infant or encephalitis) and metabolic defects (especially if unexplained illness or seizures occur).

Cerebral palsy (Ch. 29)

Incidence is approximately 1:400 births. Cerebral palsy is the result of a non-progressive disorder in the developing brain. Although the initial brain lesion is non-progressive, the effect on the child changes with time. Cerebral palsy is mostly due to factors before

birth but may also follow infection, difficult or preterm birth or an accident in early life.

Cerebral palsy is usually divided into three main types; spastic, athetoid or ataxic; terms such as hemiplegia, diplegia and quadriplegia denote the body parts affected. Children with this condition frequently have additional difficulties (learning problems, epilepsy, sensory impairment). A multidisciplinary approach to care is essential.

Epilepsy (Chs 24 and 28)

This has been defined as epileptic seizures or attacks, which are transient clinical events resulting from abnormal or excessive activity of a more or less extensive collection of cerebral neurons. Epilepsy is classified as partial (simple or complex) or generalized. Several studies have highlighted the false diagnosis rate in epilepsy, with both under- and over-diagnosis, and this may be as high as 25% of cases. The most important step in making the diagnosis is to take a thorough and accurate history.

Visual and hearing impairment

(Chs 31 and 32)

It is vital to assess vision and hearing in all children with a disability because it may further affect development, often avoidably, and also because vision and hearing problems are more common in this group of children. Sometimes disabled children cannot be accurately assessed by normal testing and specialist referral is required.

Specific learning disabilities (Ch. 29)

Children are defined as having specific learning difficulties if they have more difficulty than expected in an area of learning, which is not accounted for by general learning disability. This is a complex topic covering developmental coordination disorder, attention deficit disorder, dyslexia, dyscalculia, language disorder and social skills difficulties.

Acknowledgments

We would like to thank the contributors to the Sheffield Distance Learning Course in Paediatric Neurodisability, and in particular Dr Helena Davies, Professor David Hall and Dr Connie Pullan.

Aidan MacFarlane

Adolescent health and health problems

LEARNING OUTCOMES

By the end of this chapter you should:

- Understand and be able to apply the concepts of 'confidentiality' and 'informed consent' when dealing with adolescents
- Understand why the needs of adolescents may be different from those of children/adults
- Know broadly what health problems are more specific to adolescents
- Have the skills and sensitivity to deal with the emotional and information needs of young people when they consult you
- Have the skills to diagnose and treat specific disorders relating to adolescence.

What is adolescence?

A definition of adolescence

Adolescence begins with the onset of physiologically normal puberty, and ends when an adult identity and behaviour are accepted. This period of development corresponds roughly to the period between the ages of 10 (from the beginning of the 10th year) and runs till 19 years (the end of the 19th year), which is consistent with the World Health Organization's definition of adolescence.

Note that adolescence contains biological, psychological and social elements (Fig. 19.1).

The key health problems of adolescence include the following, which are not all considered in detail in this chapter, but elsewhere in these books:
- Growth and puberty (Chs 22 and 25)
- Nutrition, exercise and obesity (Chs 4 and 22)
- Sexual and reproductive health

- Common medical conditions of adolescence (including acne, common orthopaedic diseases, functional/psychosomatic disorders, sleep disorders, fatigue and chronic fatigue syndrome)
- Chronic conditions/disabilities (Chs 29 and 33)
- Mental health problems (Ch. 30)
- Eating disorders
- Substance use and misuse, including smoking
- Injuries and violence, including accidents, self-harm, abuse etc. (Chs 37 and 50).

Sex and sexually transmitted infections

Teenagers and sex: some facts

- Average age of first sex is 16 (boys and girls).
- 30% of boys and 26% of girls have sex before 16.

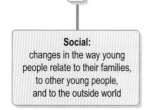

Biological:
changes in body shape, appearance and function (puberty)

Psychological:
changes in the way of thinking about oneself (identity and sexual identity) and the ability to think about the world (thinking pattern)

A

Social:
changes in the way young people relate to their families, to other young people, and to the outside world

Fig. 19.1 **Adolescence (A) contains biological, psychological and social elements**

- The earlier the first sexual encounter, the higher the regret.
- Over 40% of teenagers think the majority of under-16s have had sex.
- 75% of teenage pregnancies are unplanned.
- 46% of under-18 conceptions end in abortion.
- Sexually transmitted infections (STIs) are highest in 16–19-year-old women.
- Rates of infant mortality are 60% higher.
- There is three times the rate of postnatal depression.

Teenage pregnancy: risk factors

Poverty and poor housing are major risk factors associated with teenage pregnancy. Young people who have emotional problems at key ages (7 and 16 years), who have experienced sexual abuse or have been in local authority care are more likely to become pregnant. Teenagers who dislike school, are excluded and/or have low educational attainment are also at risk. Alcohol intake is associated with unprotected sex and higher levels of regret. This is of concern as binge drinking is on the increase; 25% of 15–16-year-olds get drunk at least three times a month.

The evidence base for reducing teenage pregnancy and STIs: the means and motivation

A key aspect in prevention is the availability of accurate information to young people in their own media, and sex education in schools and in out-of-school settings; this should focus on providing knowledge and skills, on delaying first sex, on the risks of unprotected sex,

and on effective contraceptive/condom use. Open discussion with parents and carers has been shown to facilitate healthy sexual practices. Easy access to confidential youth-friendly contraceptive/sexual health services is important. Teenage pregnancy prevention aims at a multifaceted approach, with *all* factors in place and intensive delivery to at-risk groups, combined with additional motivation to delay early pregnancy.

Problem-orientated topic:

vaginal discharge in a sexually active girl

A 15-year-old Muslim girl presents with a vaginal discharge. She has had very little information about sex because her parents refused to allow her to attend sex education classes at her school. She recently began having sex without using any form of contraception, out of fear that she would otherwise lose her boyfriend who is at the same school. She knows this discharge could mean that she has an STI, but she refuses to discuss using contraceptive methods because she now intends to break up with her boyfriend, who she thinks has infected her, and says that she will never have sex again.

Q1. What are the issues here of confidentiality and consent? Do her parents need to know?
Q2. How do you investigate her present discharge?
Q3. How do you ensure that she does get information about sex contraception in the future?

Q1. **What are the issues here of confidentiality and consent? Do her parents need to know?**

Involvement
Article 12 of the United Nations Convention on the Rights of the Child states that:

Parties shall assure to the child who is capable of forming his or her own views, the right to express those views freely in all matters affecting the child, the views of the child being given due weight in accordance with the age and maturity of the child.

Confidentiality
(This is also discussed in detail in Chapter 11.)

The basic philosophy is that 'the professional should not disclose anything learned from a person who has consulted them, or whom he or she has examined or treated — without that person's agreement.' Children and young people are entitled to the same standards of confidentiality as other patients. This means that their rights are not absolute but can only generally be overridden when there is clear justification, such as the risk of significant harm. Where an exceptional reason justifies disclosure without consent, children should be told that their secrets cannot be kept. In the absence of any such reason justifying disclosure, they should be encouraged but not forced to share their health information with their parents.

Consent

Adolescents under 16 years of age can consent to examination and treatment, provided they have sufficient understanding and intelligence to enable them to understand fully what is being proposed. Consent for treatment of a person under 18 can therefore come from any one of the following:

- A competent child
- A person or local authority with parental responsibility
- A court
- A person caring for a child, but only if it is reasonable in the circumstances to safeguard or promote the child's welfare.

Q2. How do you investigate her present discharge?

In 2003, women aged 16–24 accounted for 73% of all *Chlamydia* diagnoses in women, 69% of gonorrhoea, 35% of syphilis and 62% of genital warts diagnosed in genitourinary medicine (GUM) clinics in England, Wales and Northern Ireland.

In 2003, young men aged 16–24 accounted for 55% of all *Chlamydia* diagnoses in men, 41% of gonorrhoea and 44% of genital warts diagnosed in GUM clinics in England, Wales and Northern Ireland.

Reinfection with acute STIs is a particular problem with young people, but the risk decreases with increasing age. STIs generally are on the increase amongst young people (see below and Fig. 19.2).

The common STIs of adolescence

- *Gonorrhoea* has an incubation period of only a few days. Males and females may experience a urethral discharge. Women are at risk of long-term serious complications such as infertility and ectopic pregnancy. It is possible to have long-term infection without obvious symptoms. Treatment is with antibiotics.

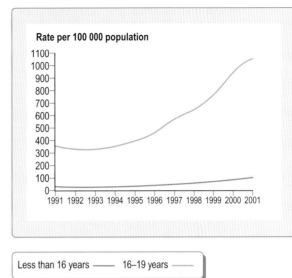

Fig. 19.2 Rates of diagnosis of uncomplicated genital *Chlamydia* infection in females made in GUM clinics by age group, UK.
Teen infection almost doubled during the 1990s.

- *Chlamydia* causes an often symptomless infection but may be associated with vaginal bleeding, discharge, abdominal pain, fever, and inflammation of the cervix in women and watery discharge from the penis in men. Long-term complications may be severe, particularly in women, as it can lead to pelvic inflammatory diseases, ectopic pregnancy and infertility. It is easy to treat with antibiotics.
- *Genital warts* are caused by human papillomavirus (HPV) and are found around the penis, anus and vagina. Certain types of HPV are associated with cervical cancer. Warts often disappear without treatment but can also be removed by freezing, burning and laser treatment.
- *Syphilis* has an incubation period ranging from a few days to 3 months. Symptoms are non-specific, though illness usually begins with painless, highly infectious sores anywhere around the body but usually at the site of infection. Syphilis can cause miscarriage and stillbirth, but can be cured with antibiotics.
- *Genital herpes* is a common infection caused by herpes simplex virus type 2 or type 1. Symptoms include small blisters in the genital area, which break down to give painful ulcers. Herpes may cause pain on urination.
- *HIV infection* — see Table 19.1 and Chapter 44.

Table 19.1 HIV-infected individuals and AIDS cases in the UK by age group at diagnosis and sex (% of total cases)

Age group (years)	Male				Female				Total			
	HIV		AIDS		HIV		AIDS		HIV*		AIDS	
	No	%	No	%	No	%	No	%	No	%	No	%
0–4	471	1	224	1	432	2	223	6	905	1	447	2
5–9	262	1	73	0	157	1	52	1	421	1	125	1
10–14	232	0	49	0	76	0	26	1	309	0	75	0
15–19	949	2	71	0	647	3	34	1	1598	2	105	0

* In some cases sex not given.

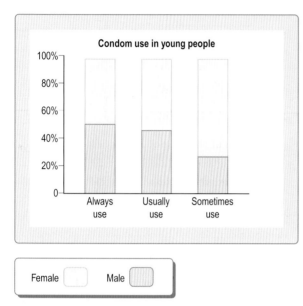

Fig. 19.3 Regular condom use amongst 16–19-year-olds by gender.
The graph shows the clear gender difference for the 'sometimes use' group.

Table 19.2 Psychopathology of eating disorders

	Anorexia nervosa	Bulimia nervosa
Strict dieting	+++	+++
Self-induced vomiting	+	++
Laxative misuse	+	++
Over-exercising	++	+
Bulimic episodes ('binges')	+	+++
Ritualistic eating habits	++	–
Anxiety when eating with others	+++	+++
Over-evaluation of shape and weight	+++	+++
Depressive symptoms	+	+++
Anxiety symptoms	+	++
Obsessional symptoms	++	+
Impaired concentration	+++	+++
Social withdrawal	+++	+
Substance abuse	–	+

Q3. How do you ensure that she does get information about sex contraception in the future?

There has been a sustained increase in condom use and a decline of men and women reporting no contraceptive use at first intercourse (Fig. 19.3). Contraceptive use generally increases with age, and 'the pill' followed by the 'male condom' are by far the most common methods used by adolescents.

Legal issues relating to contraceptive advice to adolescents

A young person can be given contraceptive advice, even under the age of 16, if:
- The young person understands the doctor's advice
- The doctor cannot persuade the young person to inform his or her parents, or to allow the doctor to inform the parents

- The young person is likely to begin or continue having sexual intercourse with or without contraception
- The young person's physical and/or mental health are likely to suffer unless he or she receives contraception
- The young person's best interests require the doctor to give contraceptive advice, treatment or both, without parental consent.

Eating disorders (Table 19.2)

Problem-orientated topic:

eating disorder

A 15-year-old girl comes to the clinic with her mother. Her mother is concerned because her daughter has been losing weight for the past 3 months and the school has reported a falling off in her academic work, despite her previously being a high achiever. The mother says that her daughter has been eating alone

Continued overleaf

in her room and refusing to have dinner with her family. The father is a lawyer and the mother is a retired dancer. The girl started having regular periods at 11, but she has had no menstrual bleeding for the last 2 months. She avoids fat and sweets, never eats breakfast and exercises 5 days a week. Her oldest brother teased her about being fat when she was younger, around the time her periods started. She has few friends. From the school letter, you calculate a body mass index (BMI) of 16, which is under the 5th percentile for age and gender. The girl refuses to be either weighed or examined.

Q1. What initial assessment should you make?
Q2. What tests do you want to arrange?
Q3. Who can you treat yourself and who do you refer?

Q1. What initial assessment should you make?

Recommended screening questions for eating problems
- Do you think you have an eating problem?
- Do you worry excessively about your weight?

Note: early detection normally improves outcome.

Detection of eating disorders: high-risk groups
- Young women who are underweight
- Young women with depressed mood
- Patients with weight concerns who are not overweight
- Children with poor growth
- Menstrual disturbances and infertility
- Gastrointestinal disturbance
- Type 1 diabetes with poor glycaemic control.

Engagement can be difficult but developing a good relationship and getting a clear history are paramount. Over-investigation can lead to delay in diagnosis and such a delay can hold up treatment, resulting in a poorer outcome.

Presentations
- *Anorexia nervosa.* It is often not the patient herself/himself who makes contact, but rather someone else (e.g. parent, school etc.). The presentation features normally include weight loss, undereating and over-exercise, though patients may also present with non-specific physical symptoms. It is also normal for the patients themselves to deny that there is a problem.
- *Bulimia nervosa.* Usually patients consult alone (after a considerable delay), with the complaint that they are unable to control their eating. They may also present with non-specific physical or psychiatric symptoms (e.g. menstrual disturbance, depression).

Q2. What tests do you want to arrange?

Laboratory investigations should be limited to routine blood tests, which can be normal even with extreme weight loss. It is important to monitor electrolytes if there is frequent vomiting or laxative misuse. Consider bone densitometry. Electrocardiography (ECG) at low weight (BMI < 15) can indicate early heart failure. It is important to consider coexisting psychiatric disorders, including depression, anxiety disorders, substance abuse and self-harm, and adverse social circumstances.

Q3. Who can you treat yourself and who do you refer?

The following represents best evidence for the treatment of eating disorders in children and adolescents:
- Weight and BMI alone may be unreliable in children as the sole assessment of eating disorders. Assess growth rates over time.
- Clinicians and teachers should be alert to indicators of abuse (emotional, physical and sexual, Ch. 37). Confidentiality should be respected. Indications for urgent referral of eating disorders include a BMI < 13.5, severe depression and medical complications of severe weight loss.
- In a child with a suspected eating disorder, referral to a paediatrician or child psychiatrist should be made for further assesssment and management.
- Family interventions that directly address the eating disorder should be offered to children and adolescents with anorexia nervosa. This involves individual appointments separate from those with their family members or carers. Carers should be included in any dietary education or meal planning.
- The effects of management on siblings and other family members should be considered and they should be included in therapeutic involvement.
- Admission to hospital is generally avoided unless there is need for urgent weight restoration. Feeding against a child's or adolescent's will must only be done in the context of the Mental Health Act 1983 or the Children Act 1989. An expert in eating

disorders should be involved if there are issues surrounding consent to treatment.

- There is no evidence that drugs have a role in the management of anorexia nervosa in children and adolescents. In older adolescents with bulimia nervosa, antidepressants may be effective.
- Adolescents with bulimia nervosa may respond to cognitive behavioural therapy, including the family as appropriate.
- The aim of treatment is to achieve a weight gain of 0.5 kg per week in an outpatient setting. Regular monitoring of vital signs is essential and follow-up is required for at least a year after sustained weight gain is achieved.

www.nice.org.uk/page.aspx?o=101239

Substance abuse

Problem-orientated topic:

substance abuse

The mother of a 16-year-old boy attends with her son and asks for him to have a urine test for drugs because of a marked change for the worse in his behaviour at home and at school. On questioning, the son says that, although he smokes a packet of cigarettes a day and binge-drinks at weekends, he is not otherwise 'into' taking illegal drugs but would like some information from you about the good and bad aspects of smoking cannabis.

Q1. What advice would you give him about smoking?

Q2. How would you assess the risk of substance abuse in him?

Q3. What is the evidence of the effectiveness of drug intervention programmes?

Q1. What advice would you give him about smoking?

Adolescents who smoke are three times more likely than non-smokers to use alcohol, eight times more likely to use marijuana, and 22 times more likely to use cocaine. Smoking is associated with a host of other risky behaviours, such as fighting and engaging in unprotected sex. The smoking rate in young people rises rapidly between 14 and 16 years of age. By the age of 16, approximately one-third of young people will

---

BOX 19.1 Risk factors for the problem use of substances in adolescence

- Genetic predisposition
- High experience-seeking
- High psychological distress
- Poor life skills
- Conduct disorder, impulsivity
- Mental disorders
- High level of use among friends
- High level of use among family members
- Physical or sexual abuse
- Childhood neglect
- Delinquency
- Poor academic achievement, school disconnectedness
- Unemployment, homelessness
- Separation or divorce of parents during childhood

---

have tried smoking and continue to smoke, one-third have tried smoking and given it up, and one-third have never tried smoking.

Effective methods for the prevention of starting smoking include banning advertising plus banning 'hidden advertising' on TV or in films, as well as increasing the price of cigarettes.

Effective methods for giving up smoking include medical advice if smoking-related problems are present and nicotine patches/gum etc. — although this last has not been proven to work with adolescents.

Q2. How would you assess the risk of substance abuse in him?

When you are taking a history, it is important for you to be aware of factors that are associated with an increased risk of substance abuse (Box 19.1).

General signs of illegal drug use include:

- Physical:
  - Fatigue
  - Repeated health complaints
  - Red and glazed eyes
  - Lasting cough
- Emotional:
  - Personality change
  - Sudden mood changes
  - Irritability
  - Irresponsible behaviour
  - Low self-esteem
  - Poor judgment
  - Depression
  - General lack of interest

- Family:
  - Starting arguments
  - Negative attitude
  - Breaking rules
  - Withdrawing from family
  - Secretiveness
- School:
  - Decreased interest
  - Negative attitude
  - Drop in grades
  - Many absences
  - Truancy
  - Discipline problems
- Social problems:
  - New friends who make poor decisions and are not interested in school or family activities
  - Problems with the law
  - Changes to less conventional styles in dress and music.

Q3. What is the evidence of the effectiveness of drug intervention programmes?

School-based programmes aimed at adolescents can delay the start of substance misuse by non-users for a short time. Universal prevention programmes appear to be more effective for lower socioeconomic adolescents than those at higher risk. Life skills training is one of the only programmes that has been extensively evaluated and for which there is some research evidence of a small but positive impact on drug use.

Acne

The skin produces sebum, an oily substance that helps moisturize and stops hair and skin drying out. Increasing androgen production associated with puberty stimulates sebum production and this can block the pores and result in inflammation of the surrounding skin. The severity of acne increases and, typically, reaches its peak around the ages of 17–19. For most, acne reduces by the mid-20s; however, very sensitive people may continue to have the disorder until they reach their 40s.

The spots are caused by *Propionibacterium acnes*, a common bacterium on the skin that feeds on sebum. This bacterium produces waste products and fatty acids that irritate the sebaceous glands and make them inflamed.

> **Problem-orientated topic:**
>
> **facial spots**
>
> Darren is a 14-year-old boy who consults you and is accompanied by his father. They explain how Darren is being teased because of his many spots and that it has started to affect his mood and confidence. His father is particularly worried about Darren not wishing to continue on the school swimming team because of acne on his torso.
>
> Q1. How would you advise Darren to manage his acne?

Q1. How would you advise Darren to manage his acne?

Factors that exacerbate acne include:
- Working in a damp environment with oil, grease and other chemicals
- Stress or emotional tension
- Squeezing or picking at the pimples
- In adolescent girls, menstrual periods
- Certain medicines and chemicals.

Management includes:
- Washing the face twice a day with a mild cleanser.
- Avoiding hairstyles in which the hair is constantly touching your face and keeping hair clean.
- Not squeezing or picking at the pimples. This makes them worse and may cause scarring.
- Water-based moisturizer. Greasy or oily creams and foundations block the pores and may cause pimples.
- A balanced diet, which is important for skin health generally, although no research has shown that certain foods can cause acne, e.g. chocolate.

Simple skin cleansers and lotion containing benzoyl peroxide can be purchased over the counter and may help, but if there is little improvement after 6 weeks, topical antibiotics or systemic antibiotics, e.g. oxytetracycline, can be used. Isotretinoin can be used in more severe cases.

Melanie Epstein

Emotional and behavioural problems: primary care aspects

LEARNING OUTCOMES

By the end of this module you should:
- Know the common problems presenting in primary care
- Understand the common predisposing and protective factors related to mental health problems
- Know how to manage common problems presenting in preschool and school-age children.
- Have developed an approach to diagnostic formulation
- Be able to approach a consultation with a family presenting with an emotional or behavioural problem.

Take the opportunity where possible of sitting in with an experienced community paediatrician or mental health professional for some observational experience.

Introduction

This chapter covers clinical aspects of child mental health, and how they present and need to be managed in primary care. The RCPCH's 'Child in Mind' project is intended to provide a series of practical courses to teach all paediatricians child mental health as it relates to paediatrics, and a number of the modules are designed for senior house officers in training. This chapter is intended to be complementary to the 'Child in Mind' course.

www.rcpch.ac.uk/education/projects/child_in_mind.html

Children may have mental health needs if their abilities in any one of the following areas are impaired (Spender et al 2001):

- The ability to develop psychologically, emotionally, intellectually and spiritually
- The ability to initiate, develop and sustain mutually satisfying personal relationships
- The ability to become aware of others and to empathize with them
- The ability to use psychological distress as a developmental process, so that it does not hinder or impair further development.

In children, it is vital to consider their developmental stage. Child mental health problems arise when the degree of psychological distress and/or maladaptive behaviour is outside the normal limits for the child's age, developmental stage and context. This may depend on the values, thresholds for concern and culture of the family. Children are therefore presented as having emotional and behavioural problems according to the perceptions of the adults around them. Sometimes the behaviour is appropriate developmentally, but is not understood. Sometimes, a mild problem in some families may be seen as a major difficulty by others. Alternatively, serious problems may be overlooked. It is also important to remember that children may be presented as a symptom of another problem in a parent or the family.

Significant problems can be defined not by symptoms alone, but by interference with a child's functioning. Children present mental health problems in many different ways. Thus a child who is not doing well at school, who stops going to school, who does not make friends and who is very disruptive at home is likely to have mental health needs.

Mental health problems in children are associated with educational failure, family disruption, disability, offending and antisocial behaviour, placing demands on social services, schools and the youth justice system. Untreated mental health problems create distress not only in the children and young people, but also for their families and carers, continuing into adult life and affecting the next generation.

Prevalence of emotional and behavioural problems

Emotional and behavioural problems are relatively common in children and young people. It is likely that, in the UK, between 10 and 25% of 0–18-year-olds are suffering from emotional and behavioural problems. Up to 15% of children and young people have mild emotional and behavioural problems. A further 7–10% have moderate or severe problems requiring specialist psychiatric assessment. Only 2% of children up to 16 years old have mental health disorders that are severe enough to be disabling.

About 2–5% of children seen in the UK in primary care settings are presented by their parents, with emotional and behavioural problems as the main complaint. The rates for particular problems are as follows:

In preschool children (under 5 years of age)

- Waking and crying at night: 15%
- Over-activity: 13%
- Difficulty settling at night: 12%
- Refusing food: 12%.

In middle childhood (age 6–12 years)

- Persistent tearful, unhappy mood: 12%
- Bedtime behavioural rituals: 8%
- Night terrors/other disturbances of sleep: 6%
- Bedwetting: 5%
- Inattentive over-activity: 5%
- Faecal soiling: 1%.

In adolescence (age 13–18)

- Appreciable misery: 45%
- Social sensitivity: 30%
- Evident anxiety: 25%
- Suicidal ideas: 7%.

About 10% of adolescents suffer from more complex depressive moods. This is in addition to those diagnosed as having a psychiatric disorder, such as major depression.

Will the problem go away by itself?

Mild or moderate psychological problems are relatively persistent, particularly when linked with continuing problematic family relationships and attachment difficulties. Two large studies have shown that at least half of 3-year-olds rated as having behaviour problems were still displaying problems several years later.

Factors influencing the development of mental health problems

The presenting features of mental health problems in children can be associated with one or more biological, psychological or social factors. The sorts of factor that can impact on a child's mental health are shown in Box 20.1.

BOX 20.1 Predisposing factors

The child
- Genetics and temperament (the child's inbuilt personality style)
- Acute or chronic illness
- Specific or general learning difficulties
- Language and other developmental disorder
- Sexual, physical or emotional abuse
- Lack of a secure attachment figure in the first few years of life

The family
- Parental discord
- Parental coldness or irritability towards the child
- Parental mental health problems or substance abuse
- Neglect
- Criminality
- Economic circumstances

The environment
- Overcrowding
- Homelessness
- Discrimination
- Refugee status

Life events
- Parental separation
- Acute illness
- Bereavement
- Experiencing or witnessing sudden and extreme trauma

School
- Bullying, victimization
- Inappropriate curriculum

BOX 20.2 Protective factors

The child
- Easy temperament
- At least average intelligence
- The capacity to process experiences in a positive way
- A sense of humour
- A sense of self-mastery

The family
- High warmth/low criticism
- Appropriate boundaries and discipline
- Absence of parental discord
- A secure attachment relationship with at least one parent

The social environment
- Affectionate ties with parent substitutes
- External support system
- Positive school experiences
- Opportunities for meaningful social roles and experiences

Some children who live with adverse circumstances or a combination of risk factors develop fewer or no more long-term problems than others. This is known as resilience.

The overarching factor contributing to resilience is mediated through attachment, and consists of having at least one adult who believes in and cares about the child. Three key groups of factors appear to protect children and adolescents (Spender et al 2001). Factors that are recognized to protect a child from the development of mental health problems are shown in Box 20.2.

Consultation skills

Parents often turn to their doctor for help with their child's emotional and behavioural problems.

If conducted well, the consultation in itself can be therapeutic. To achieve this it is essential that you are skilled at listening and communicating, and convey empathy to the family.

It is useful to start from the premise that all parents want to do the best they can for their children and your role is to build on strengths in order to remove obstacles to a natural state of affairs. In doing this you are modelling the relationship you would like the parents to provide. In prevention, an approach focused on relationship building and treating the mother as the person with responsibility to promote the development of her child has been demonstrated to be more successful than one that is didactic.

Listening

Allow adequate time for the appointment and listen well. Hear a full account of the problem. This in itself can be therapeutic, and can lead the family to find solutions themselves.

Personal skills and attitudes

Know yourself

What are the cultural values, life experiences and personal attributes you bring to the consultation?

Maintain a respectful and non-judgmental attitude

This is best done by drawing on your skills of scientific enquiry and your natural curiosity and empathy. However, being human, we all experience other responses such as feeling critical, hopeless or frustrated, or an identification with the parents at times. It is useful to notice and be aware of the responses that you have. These can all give you more information.

Self-maintenance

Like a well-tuned car, your consultation is more likely to run smoothly if your physical and emotional needs are taken care of. In a busy job, considering work–life balance is sometimes a tall order. However, if you put yourself on hold for too long, your ability to be compassionate and curious is likely to feel harder to access.

Reflections

Sometimes, even with the best of intentions, consultations do not go as planned. If so, ask yourself:

- Does this give me any more information about the presenting problem or the process that is happening with the family?
- Do I need consultation with a colleague or another professional to help make sense of that?
- Does this tell me anything about myself?
- What did I like about how I was with this family?
- Would I do anything differently next time?

The consultation (Box 20.3)

You need to obtain as full a picture as possible of the problem, the child, the family and the environment, and it is important that the focus does not rest on the child alone. You need to understand the broader picture and see the difficulties in the context of the family and the child's environment. It is important to obtain the perceptions of each parent, where possible, as well as those of the child. It is helpful to bear in mind the predisposing and protective factors outlined in Boxes 20.1 and 20.2, and to think how these may be an influence on the child's behaviour.

As in any paediatric consultation, you need to take a structured approach. The following is the relevant background information you should obtain:

- History of the pregnancy and birth. It is usual when dealing with children to ask about the medical aspects of these. Remember also that pregnancy involves psychological preparation

> **BOX 20.3 Key points: approach to the child with emotional and behavioural problems**
>
> - Allow adequate time to make a full assessment
> - Obtain as full a picture as possible of the problem, the child, the family and the environment. Involve the child in a developmentally appropriate way
> - Think about behaviour as a form of communication. Use observation of the family and child, as well as history-taking
> - Address family and school issues, as well as the child's problems. Where relevant, confer with others involved, such as grandparents, teachers or child-minders
> - Support parents in providing developmentally appropriate and consistent boundaries with love and affection. Focus on strengths and encourage parents to praise and reward good behaviour, rather than focusing on negatives
> - Do not wait for a child to grow out of a problem. Problems tend to persist or re-emerge at the next developmental stage
> - Medication has a very limited role and should only be prescribed by specialists

for a child, as well for the mother's changing identity.

- Prematurity and admission to a neonatal unit.
- Developmental milestones.
- Any medical problems.
- Establishment of routines around feeding and sleeping.
- History suggestive of maternal depression.
- Any history of separations.
- Any major losses, e.g. loss of parent, death of family member, moving house.
- The child's temperament and personality.
- Who else looks after the child and, if the child attends playgroup or nursery, how he or she has integrated.
- Sources of support to mother. It is usual to consider that a young single mother may be isolated. Older women or professional women who do not have a peer group with children, or people with no extended families, may also be isolated.
- Where possible, some assessment of the parental relationship.
- Any other professional involvement with the child, e.g. social worker — which may lead you to ask about any child protection issues.
- Family and social history. It is useful to draw a family tree, and also ask if the child reminds the parent of anyone.

- *Predisposing:* factors that make the child more vulnerable to the problem
- *Precipitating:* the immediate trigger to the problem and to the family's current presentation
- *Perpetuating:* factors that maintain the problem
- *Protective:* factors that ameliorate the problem

Diagnostic formulation

In medicine, we generally learn that it is best to make one diagnosis that will explain all symptoms, rather than diagnosing more than one problem. This is not always the case when considering emotional and behavioural problems, and it is appropriate to formulate a broader picture. The 'four Ps' (Box 20.4) can help you to draw up your diagnostic formulation.

It is also useful to consider factors that promote change. This is linked to the protective factors, but will also include motivation to change and insight into the problem. The more you can harness that motivation, particularly if the family can find their own solutions, the more likely change will occur. On a practical note, if you make a referral to Child and Adolescent Mental Health Services, the family will generally need to pass the motivation test of returning an opt-in letter.

Management of emotional and behavioural problems

Many parental concerns relate to normal behaviour: for example, food fads in toddlers or night-waking in infants, and it may be adequate simply to provide reassurance. Other concerns relate to difficult behaviour, and you should be able to provide guidance on parenting. Helpful principles are shown in Box 20.5.

Star charts

A useful strategy in overcoming difficult behaviour is using a star chart, which can be adapted to improve and motivate a variety of behaviours, from enuresis to temper tantrums and disruptive behaviour at school. A calendar is drawn up and each day the child has behaved well, a star or smiley face is awarded. A prize can be given when an agreed number of stars have been earned. This can be very effective in reinforcing desirable behaviour, while alleviating focus on the negative.

BOX 20.5 Guidelines for parents in preventing and managing difficult behaviour

- Provide structure and routine in everyday life
- Set clear limits of acceptable behaviour
- Be consistent
- 'Catch your child being good' and reward positive behaviour rather than punishing negative behaviour
- Enforce the above with love and affection
- Star charts and time out are useful strategies

Table 20.1 Behaviour indicative of serious disturbance

Behaviour	Disturbance
Deliberately destructive	Low self-esteem Hostile relationships Possible conduct disorder
Deliberate self-harm	Severe distress Loss of attachment Low self-esteem
Running away	Lack of affection Severe distress
Encopresis	Lack of self-worth Inadequate care
Age-inappropriate sexual behaviour	Sexual abuse

Time out

Time out is a strategy that is useful during an episode of difficult behaviour. The child has to stay in a quiet spot for a fixed short period of time. One minute per year of age is a good guide, and a kitchen timer is a useful way of enforcing the time. This method allows the child (and the parent) time to cool off, and also gives the parent a clear but limited non-violent means of discipline.

Involving other professionals

An important aspect of good management involves arranging a follow-up appointment. Other professionals may also be available to provide support and help for the child. The health visitor is a particular asset for preschool children, as is the teacher for the child at school. More intransigent cases may require referral to Child and Adolescent Mental Health Services. The sort of behaviour that is indicative of serious abuse is shown in Table 20.1. Any of these behaviours may be associated with abuse, and it is also important to consider the presence of child protection issues.

Emotional and behavioural problems presenting in the preschool child

Problems presenting in the preschool child are generally those of self-regulation and routines, and depend on the age and stage of development. They include problems with crying, sleep, feeding, toileting and behaviour. Babies may be communicating to their parents, through, for example, poor sleep patterns, excessive crying, difficulties with feeding, restlessness and gastric disturbance, that they are anxious and tense, distressed or fearful. Parents may not know how to respond to these communications with support and empathy, or may misread a baby's cues because of their own history or previous events in the baby's life, or simply a lack of knowledge of what is normal. Supporting families to provide an appropriate response is essential, in order to reduce the incidence of emotional and behavioural problems and their consequences in later life. Parents may be concerned that there is something wrong with the child, and in some cases there may be a medical problem. Differentiating between normal or abnormal behaviour, as well as knowing when further treatment is necessary, is important.

Crying

This is a common paediatric problem. A normal healthy baby cries for between 1 and 3 hours a day. Parents normally start to notice and pick out different types of crying, such as hunger, pain and boredom, by the time the baby is 1–14 days old.

About 10% of babies may cry excessively, more than 3 hours in 24. Reasons why babies may cry excessively include:

- Temperament and sensitivity to environmental change.
- Prematurity or difficult birth/special care admission.
- Environmental change. Some babies can be more sensitive to changes in their surroundings or care routine.
- New developmental stage in learning or growth.
- Tension. Babies sense when their parents are tense and it can affect their behaviour. This can be a bit confusing, and can become a circular situation.
- Colic. This can cause excessive crying in the first 3 months (Ch. 24).

www.cry-sis.org.uk

General advice to parents with babies who cry excessively, or are sleepless or demanding

Poor sleep patterns

Problem-orientated topic:

a baby who will not sleep

Joanna S. brings her 2-year-old daughter, Melissa, to see you. Joanna says she is exhausted because Melissa will not sleep through the night. She does not settle down to sleep, and when she does eventually go to sleep, she wakes up at some point in the middle of the night. Often mum resorts to bringing Melissa into her bed because she is so tired. She would like some help in establishing a sleep routine.

Q1. What should you ask about in the history?
Q2. Can you give a brief diagnostic formulation?
Q3. What will help you with your assessment?
Q4. What advice can you give?

Q1. What should you ask about in the history?

It is important to obtain a full assessment of the problem, including parental views.

Sleep routines
Ask about daytime sleeps and bedtime routines. Ask about any other children and their routines. Sometimes the advent of a new baby, another significant change at home or conflicting needs of different children will impact on sleep routines.

Parental concerns
What does the mother feel is the main problem? There is a suggestion here that her tiredness is significant. Ask more about this and how it is affecting her. It takes a fair amount of will and energy to address a sleep problem. Are there concerns about the effects of sleeplessness on the child? Ask about sources of support. Is there a partner/grandparents/other support? What are they doing? Are mum and partner in accord about family rules, or is one somehow undermining the other?

Birth and early history/family history
A general paediatric history will help your assessment of whether this is an isolated problem, or whether there are other issues with routines such as feeding or with the child's behaviour. Children with neurodevelopmental problems may be more likely to have sleep

difficulties and may need specialist help. Problems with the birth, illness in the child, or unresolved grief in relation to the death or significant illness of another child or family member may lead to parental anxiety, contributing to difficulty enforcing boundaries or leaving the child to go to sleep.

Medical problems

Are there any factors suggestive of medical problems in the history? In particular, ask about any night-time cough suggestive of asthma, snoring and early morning grogginess suggestive of obstructive sleep apnoea, or itch associated with eczema or scabies. Your examination will then be guided by your assessment of the presence of medical problems.

The child

A healthy child depends on stimulation and attention (whether negative or positive) for survival and development, and therefore it can be viewed as normal for a child to learn when it is possible to control a parent at bedtime to provide this.

You may have an idea from the general history as to whether the child may have a difficult temperament (p. 212), with poorly established circadian rhythms. In some cases the problem may be more that the child is afraid to go to sleep. This may occur in the presence of insecure attachment and separation anxiety, domestic violence or sexual abuse.

On further questioning you find out that Melissa was born by emergency section for fetal distress, and was in Special Care overnight. Joanna admits she was terrified at the time. She says she is still a bit anxious about Melissa. When you ask about the sleep routine, Joanna says she tends not to leave Melissa to go to sleep on her own, and does not like to leave her to cry. Melissa never seemed to settle into routines easily as a baby, but has had no other health problems. Mum says she has come to clinic now because she has become short-tempered with Melissa, and she does not want this to continue. She has given up her job in the media, which involved travelling away from home, to look after Melissa. She says she realizes she has lost touch with her friends and has made an arrangement to meet one of them for lunch. Her husband works a lot of late nights, but he helps with childcare when he is there.

BOX 20.6 Sleep problem: failure to settle as well as night-waking

Predisposing
- Difficult birth history
- Mother–baby separation
- Maternal anxiety for child's health/survival at birth — ?unresolved
- Difficult temperament

Precipitating
- Mother exhausted, has become short-tempered, ?depressed

Perpetuating
- Entrenched pattern between mother and child
- Father not home most bedtimes
- Lack of social support

Protective
- Father supportive when around
- Mother reconnecting with social support
- Mother has insight and is taking responsibility for the problem

---

Q2. Can you give a brief diagnostic formulation?

See Box 20.6.

Promoting change

Joanna has recognized that there is a problem, has thought of some solutions herself, and is also asking for help and advice.

Q3. What will help you with your assessment?

A sleep diary may be helpful to obtain a more detailed picture of Melissa's sleep pattern, and to see what specific factors may be perpetuating the problem, as well as where change can most easily be instituted. Information obtained from the diary will include the child's wake time and mood on waking, any naps during the day, bedtime routines and going to sleep time, as well as times and duration of night-waking. In each case the parent's actions or responses are recorded as well. In some cases filling in the sleep diary may be therapeutic in itself, as parents may gain more insight into the problem.

Depression

It is worth asking more about how the mother feels to see whether she might be depressed. Further GP and/or health visitor involvement may be useful. Depressed mothers are a high risk, as depression may interfere with their ability to tune into their baby's signals and provide a sensitive, emotionally nurturing and care-giving environment. Postnatal depression is linked to an increase in insecure attachment in toddlers, behavioural disturbance at home, less creative play and greater levels of disturbed or disruptive behaviour at primary school, poor peer relationships, and a decrease in self-control with an increase in aggression.

Q4. What advice can you give?

First give an explanation. Parents may find it helpful to know how common sleep problems are and that they can be solved, but that this takes some energy and persistence. Explain that the fact that the problem is getting worse may imply that the treatment is actually working. It may be useful to explain that all children wake up at night, but that some children have not yet learned how to settle themselves back to sleep. Give this advice in the context of support and reassurance. Around 50% of night-wakers like Melissa have a problem settling to sleep. In these cases, the first problem to tackle is the settling to sleep.

Helpful advice for parents
- Learn to read your child's cues of tiredness.
- Choose an appropriate time to enforce the sleep routine.
- Ensure all carers are involved and will agree to be consistent.
- Have a relaxing routine leading up to bedtime, e.g. warm bath, snack, story.
- Set a bedtime, enforce firmly and calmly say goodnight.
- If the child cries, ignore; if that is too much, at least give no positive attention.
- If the child gets out of bed, return him or her promptly and firmly.
- Give positive reinforcement (e.g. star or sticker chart) following good nights.
- Be consistent. Giving in now and again will reinforce the unwanted behaviour.
- Sleep problems can be solved. Get support when problems arise.

(◉) www.cry-sis.org.uk/

For more detailed advice to parents, follow the link to sleep problems

Who else can help?
If you are limited by time constraints, basic advice has not worked or the problem seems more complex, it may be appropriate to involve the health visitor. If the problem still fails to respond or you identify more complex underlying issues, consider referral to a Child and Adolescent Mental Health service.

Tantrums and difficult behaviour

Tantrums are a normal part of childhood development and peak between the ages of 18 months and 3 years. Frustration, anger and tantrums are typical for toddlers, and may involve hitting, biting and other potentially harmful behaviour. Some babies and toddlers may resort to breath-holding (p. 292) as part of the tantrum, and this is often a frightening event to witness. Parents often talk about these episodes in the context of the 'terrible twos'. In some cases, parents feel they are wilful on the part of their children. This is not the case. Children are merely 'testing' how to express and contain their feelings safely and how to assert their developing will and individual personality.

> ## Problem-orientated topic:
>
> ### tantrums
>
> Regina, a 37-year-old mother, brings her 2½-year-old child, Grace, to see you. She is complaining about Grace's behaviour. The child seems to shout and get cross very often, for no apparent reason. This may then be followed by a full-blown tantrum. Mum says she has tried everything to stop this, but with no success. She is worried the neighbours will think she is hurting her child. Sometimes Grace nips or hits her little sister. This has been happening for the last few months. Mum is worried that Grace's younger sister is starting to copy her.
>
> Q1. What further information will help you with your assessment?
> Q2. What advice can you give parents about tantrums?

Q1. What further information will help you with your assessment?

Parental concerns
You have obtained some information about these already. Regina has already told you she is concerned about the impact on her younger child and about the reaction of the neighbours.

Developmental history

It is important to take a full developmental history. Grace was found to have been slow to talk, and to have only just started to say two words together. Delayed speech development may be associated with frustration. Other language or comprehension problems may mean the child does not understand what is expected of him or her. Wider developmental or cognitive difficulties may mean that tantrums may be more severe or persistent. Any family history of deafness or developmental delay may be significant.

General health

Check whether there has been a hearing test, and whether there have been any episodes of otitis media or upper respiratory tract infections. Ongoing or fluctuating hearing loss may be associated with behaviour problems.

Does the child have any symptoms of pain, discomfort or tiredness that may be affecting behaviour? Has the child had a significant head injury?

Ask about any medications. Anticonvulsants or night-time sedatives, for example, may affect behaviour.

Parental factors

Try to assess whether there is consistency of parental discipline from day to day and also between parents.

It is useful to know how other members of the family deal with anger, but this information is difficult to ascertain. A child whose sibling or parent is modelling tantrum behaviour is less likely to learn to deal with frustration or conflict. A child who is experiencing severe anger or witnessing domestic violence is unlikely to respond to simple behavioural measures.

Are there any particular parental stresses or issues of lack of support that make it more difficult to manage the child?

ABC diary

This can be used for almost any type of behavioural problem. Ask the parent to record relevant details of the most recent tantrums according to the following format. It is important that parents understand what the headings mean and the purpose of keeping the diary:

- A — antecedents
- B — behaviour
- C — consequences.

This can also be used to help you with history-taking and in formulating specific management strategies.

Q2. What advice can you give to parents?

The Royal College of Psychiatrists has some useful information designed for parents (also useful for professionals) that is easy to read and evidence-based. There are 36 fact sheets on a variety of emotional and behavioural topics. These can be downloaded or bought as a collected volume.

 www.rcpsych.ac.uk/info

> For advice on dealing with tantrums, follow the links to 'Leaflets for Young People' and then to 'Mental Health and Growing Up', 3rd edn, leaflet 3

The over-active child

Problem-orientated topic:

an over-active child

Ashraf, a 3-year-old boy, is referred by his GP because his parents are concerned that he is hyperactive. They complain that Ashraf will not do as he is told. He talks continually but rarely listens. His mother says he is restless, does not sit still and moves from one thing to another. He does not like to go to sleep, and does not usually to go to bed before 9.00 pm. The only time he does sit still is when watching CBeebies on television, which he can do for hours at a time, and he has a television in his room. Mum would like him to be more like his sister, who she describes as her 'little helper', and who loves to sit and draw. Dad is not too worried because he says he has been told he was like that as a child. The family have a very small garden, and Ashraf does not have any friends who live nearby. He attends nursery part-time, where he is described as having no problems. During the interview, Ashraf explores the workings of your examination light and stethoscope, and opens all the boxes of toys. He is told off eight times. He takes the blocks out and sits absorbed making an elaborate castle, and playing a game that you can hear involves Spiderman. His parents are absorbed talking to you about him and do not appear to notice.

Q1. Is Ashraf hyperactive?

Q2. What advice can you give to his parents?

Q1. Is Ashraf hyperactive?

He is not. Many parents worry that their children have attention deficit hyperactivity disorder (ADHD), when in fact their behaviour is in the range of normal. ADHD is a syndrome complex that requires the child to have specific symptoms of inattention, hyperactivity and impulsivity at home and at school (Ch. 29). When interpreting the criteria, it is essential to take the child's age and developmental stage into account. Many 2–3-year-olds are normally over-active and have a short attention span. If these behaviours are present in a child older than 4 at home and at school, then ADHD may be in your differential diagnosis.

Q2. What advice can you give to his parents?

- Reassure the parents.
- Encourage parental consistency.
- Advise them to 'catch the child being good' and praise him specifically for desired behaviour.
- Talk about how Ashraf can be given more opportunities for energetic play and for play with friends.

If parents want to change the sleep pattern, talk about sleep routines or think about involving the health visitor. Most of the advice is the usual advice about good parenting. Many parents find it useful to have some written information.

www.rcpsych.ac.uk/info

'Mental Health and Growing Up' series, leaflet 2: 'Good Parenting'

Emotional and behavioural problems presenting in the school-age child

Obtaining a history

School life brings its own problems and also affects how the child adjusts to difficulties at home. It is important to find out how the child has made the adjustment to school, and about relationships with teachers and peers, as well as about academic achievement in different areas. It is vital to involve children directly and this starts with taking a history from the children themselves. Having started school, they have their own life.

When speaking to the child, think how you can support his or her attempts to communicate.

Either sit down or position yourself at the same level as the child. Try to talk with the child, rather than at the child. Use simple words and ideas, and check that the child understands you. Start off with a (hopefully) neutral subject. It is sometimes helpful to use drawings and play as a way of getting alongside the child. This also

gives you the opportunity to make an observation about the child's fine motor skills. Let children tell you about their drawing, rather than interpreting this for them.

It is worth remembering that further information can be obtained from school, although of course you should only contact school with the parent's permission.

> **Problem-orientated topic:**
>
> **the child who is struggling at school**
>
> Charlie, age 6, is brought to see you, the school doctor, by his mother. She says his teacher told her on parents' evening that Charlie is having a lot of difficulties at school. He has problems with his writing and is a bit clumsy. He does not pay attention in class. She is concerned and would like some help for him. Charlie has been otherwise healthy and his developmental milestones have been within normal limits. He was happy and had friends in nursery.
>
> Mum says their relationship is quite intense, as there are just the two of them at home. You ask about Charlie's father. Mum says that after dad kept breaking promises to come and see Charlie, she has stopped him seeing his father as he gets too upset. You ask Charlie what he thinks the problem is and he says that there are a group of boys who pick on him at school. He does not want to talk any more. You ask him to draw you a picture. He draws a picture of a boy with spiky hair, that you notice looks a bit like him. You ask him to tell you about his picture. He tells you that this is a picture of the boy they call stupid. You notice his mother looks upset as he says that.
>
> Q1. Can you give a brief diagnostic formulation?
>
> Q2. What is your management plan?

Q1. Can you give a brief diagnostic formulation?

See Box 20.7.

Q2. What is your management plan?

1. Ask mother and Charlie what specific help they would like.

Predisposing
- Difficulties with fine motor skills and clumsiness; may have dyspraxia (Ch. 19)
- Insufficient information about learning abilities in other areas
- Inattentiveness — ?hearing problem or secondary to emotional state
- Parental separation — repeatedly let down by father

Precipitating
- Information from teacher about Charlie's problems
- ?Charlie being bullied at school (not sure if this is new or ongoing)

Perpetuating
- Low self-esteem — Charlie seems to believe he is stupid
- Lack of resolution of relationship with his father
- ?Mother unsupported

Protective
- Mother concerned
- Supportive school
- Mother and school working together

2. If examination confirms evidence of difficulties with fine motor skills and incoordination, consider referral for occupational therapy assessment.
3. Refer for hearing test.
4. Find out from the teacher more about Charlie's abilities and how he is at school. It may be useful to talk to the school special needs coordinator (SENCO), if involved.
5. Talk about the possibility of Charlie being bullied and how you can support mother, if necessary by talking to the school and making an appropriate plan.
6. Discuss Charlie's referral to Child and Adolescent Mental Health Services for work on his self-esteem and relationship with his father. It is important when making such a referral to check that the family want to engage in this process. Further discussion may shed some light on the 'intense relationship' between Charlie and his mother, and whether they need some help with this.
7. Talk to the mother about what support she has, and whether she has work or interests outside the home.
8. Arrange a follow-up appointment.

Recurrent and unexplained symptoms

Children who have recurrent symptoms, such as abdominal pain (Ch. 25) or headaches (Ch. 24) that do not respond to treatment, may have mental health problems. These may occur if the symptoms are primarily functional, or if the child has first had a primary illness. An underlying emotional component is also likely if a child has unexplained symptoms such as complaining of inability to walk in the absence of any abnormal physical signs or demonstrable pathology. In all these cases, help from Child and Adolescent Mental Health Services can be sought. Rarely, recurrent or unexplained symptoms can be a presentation of fabricated or induced illness (Ch. 21), and additional consultation with an appropriate consultant paediatrician and social services will be necessary.

Unwanted habits and behaviour

Parents may complain about a range of behaviours that occur normally. These include thumb-sucking, head-banging, body-rocking, nail-biting, hair-pulling, teeth-grinding, simple tics and masturbation. It is useful to know some simple facts, and to know when reassurance and some simple behavioural tips are appropriate. As is usual when dealing with children's behaviour, it is more helpful for the parent to 'catch the child being good', rather than chastising the child or trying to stop the undesired behaviour, as this may lead to reinforcement. In many cases, children may not be able to control these habits until they grow older.

Masturbation

This is common in both sexes in preschool children. The usual problem is the issue of its social acceptability. If parents wish to limit masturbation, it usually responds to common-sense techniques like ignoring the behaviour or distraction. Alternatively, children can be encouraged to masturbate in private.

Nail-biting and thumb-sucking

About 25% of children between 3 and 6 years of age suck their thumbs or bite their nails. Thumb-sucking is normal in early infancy. However, beyond a certain age, it makes the older child appear immature and may interfere with normal alignment of the teeth. It is a difficult habit to influence, and it is best to ignore it as it resolves over time. The child who actively tries to stop thumb-sucking should be given praise and encouragement.

Nail-biting is a difficult habit to break, unless the child has some motivation to do so. Application of bitter-tasting nail varnish can be helpful. In some children nail-biting is a sign of tension.

Food refusal

Feeding problems are very common in young children. About 10% of young children demonstrate some problem with food refusal between 9 and 15 months of age, and start to refuse food offered to them. It is common for this to be associated with food faddiness. This occurs in association with children's developing sense of self as they assert their autonomy by closing their mouth and turning away. Sometimes it may be associated with coercive or rushed feeding. At later stages, about one-third of 5-year-olds have a mild to moderate eating problem. In all these cases, as long as a child thriving, some common-sense advice about nutrition and behaviour is probably all that is needed. (See also page 29.)

Enuresis

Urinary continence is generally achieved by the age of 3 or 4. Around 10% of 5-year-olds, 5% of 10-year-olds and 2% of teenagers still have enuresis. There is often a family history in children with enuresis. Failure to achieve toilet training or regression to wetting may be a sign of stress. Common precipitating events include the birth of a sibling, a death in the family, a move to a new home and marital conflict. Enuresis may also result from inadequate or inappropriate toilet training. It is fully discussed on page 326.

Encopresis

Encopresis, or the passage of faeces in inappropriate places, usually indicates a serious emotional disturbance. It needs to be distinguished from soiling, which results from leakage of liquid faeces around hard stool when a child is constipated. However, secondary psychological problems can still result when the problem is not recognized or understood. Constipation and soiling are discussed on page 304.

Reference

Spender Q, Salt S, Dawkins J et al 2001 Child mental health in primary care. Routledge, London. This is a comprehensive easy-to-read book for non-mental health practitioners. It contains a useful chapter on behavioural techniques for use by enthusiastic professionals in primary care

Malcolm Levene   Amanda Thomas   Neela Shabde

Child protection in the community

LEARNING OUTCOMES

By the end of this chapter you should:

- Know and understand which children are most susceptible to child abuse
- Know and understand the legal framework protecting children
- Know and understand the roles and responsibilities of the primary care doctor in protecting children
- Know and understand the framework for interagency working
- Know how child abuse and neglect present in primary care
- Know the reporting mechanisms for suspected abuse
- Be familiar with the Child Protection Case Conference and Child Protection Register, if the child is the subject of a child protection plan
- Understand the emotional impact of abuse
- Understand the needs of looked-after children
- Understand how children with emotional abuse and neglect present and are managed.

Introduction

Protecting children from intentional harm is the role of all doctors, whether they work in primary care or as a paediatrician, although their role in protecting children will differ. There is a basic level of knowledge that all such doctors must possess in order to be able to fulfil this function. This chapter describes the basis of child protection from the point of view of a primary care doctor and Chapter 37 describes this from a paediatric trainee's perspective.

These two chapters give an overview of child protection, but in Britain it is a requirement that all paediatric trainees undergo a formal educational programme for doctors, including a training day organized by the Royal College of Paediatrics and Child Health (RCPCH), the National Society for Prevention of Cruelty to Children (NSPCC) and the Advanced Life Support Group (ALSG). These chapters are not intended as a substitute for this formal training but rather as an overview and summary of material that is available through the College.

The responsibility for child protection is not primarily a medical one and the underlying principle of child protection is sharing concerns on a multi-agency basis, developing solutions and maintaining safety networks for children and their families.

What is child abuse?

Child abuse is the description given to a varied set of actions considered to be harmful to children. These can be defined under a number of categories, which are described in more detail both in this chapter and Chapter 37:
- Neglect
- Emotional abuse (includes factitious or induced illness)
- Physical abuse
- Sexual abuse.

Child abuse is most frequent in vulnerable families. Risk factors for abuse include:
- Prematurity, separation and impaired bonding in the neonatal period
- Children with a difficult temperament (behaviour more a consequence than a risk factor)
- Chronic illness/disability in the child
- Poverty/single-parent status/step-parent or cohabitee present
- Male unemployment
- Domestic violence
- Absence of social support
- The carer who was abused in childhood
- History of parental mental health problems/illnesses
- Alcohol and substance abuse
- Large family size.

The legal framework

Child protection in Britain is guided by a legal framework articulated by the Children Act 1989 and 2004. This incorporates principles within the United Nations Convention on the Rights of the Child and the European Convention on Human Rights. Children are protected by multi-agency working, promoting children's welfare and protecting them from abuse and neglect. The Department of Health (1999) document, 'Working Together to Safeguard Children', summarizes all the legislation and sets out principles for professionals working with children. The emphasis is on:
- Focusing on the child and family rather than the injury
- Identifying roles and responsibilities of different agencies and practitioners
- Placing child protection procedures within the remit of a local Area Child Protection Committee (ACPC), which coordinates interagency working
- Describing processes to be followed when there are concerns about a child and actions to be taken to safeguard and promote the welfare of children suffering, or at risk of suffering, significant harm.
- Providing guidance on child protection for children in specific circumstances, such as children living away from home or children with disabilities.

The role of primary care professionals in child protection

The doctor represents an important partner in the network of child protection. The primary care doctor, together with the practice-based health visitor, is in an excellent position to provide a pivotal overview of the child within the family. The first concern about child abuse may arise from the doctor's concerns about injuries, failure to thrive, abnormal behaviour or disclosure by the child. Alternatively his or her concerns for the child may be aroused by evidence of domestic violence, parasuicide attempts, mental illness in the family or the parent's inappropriate emotional response to the child. Doctors must recognize their own role as a cog in the multi-agency wheel that must turn efficiently to protect children (p. 224).

The responsibilities of doctors with regard to child protection are summarized in Box 21.1.

Ability to

- Recognize symptoms and signs of child abuse
- Recognize children in need of support and/or safeguarding, and parents who may need extra help in bringing up children
- Contribute to inquiries about children
- Have access to and be familiar with local child protection procedures
- Access the Child Protection Register (or identify a current need for protection with social services)
- Act upon any child protection concerns that they have about children in accordance with Section 47 of the Children Act (or equivalent)
- Maintain their training in child protection to a level specified by local and national policy

Knowledge of

- The referral pathways to those with specialist paediatric skills to assess children where child abuse is suspected
- How to contact the social services department

The basic principles for doctors involved in child protection are:

- Recognition of the problem
- Reporting of suspicions
- Investigation of the problem.

Table 21.1 summarizes knowledge, skills and attitudes that all doctors must develop in order to discharge their responsibilities in protecting children adequately.

The doctor must be able to balance the needs of the adults against those of the child. Struggling families should be given support to raise their children in a safe environment, but children may need to be protected if their parents are harming them. The needs of the child must be paramount. Parents who themselves have been abused may find it difficult to love and care for their children in an acceptable way. It should be recognized that they may potentially require a range of support. Health visitors are particularly well placed to identify early markers of potential abuse and to introduce services to support the family.

Interagency working — working together

This describes working together and sharing responsibility, which require that agencies and professionals, including paediatricians:

- Share information
- Collaborate and understand each other's roles and responsibilities
- Work in partnership with one another and with children and their families to plan comprehensive and coordinated services
- Recognize vulnerable children and coordinate services from various appropriate agencies, including the voluntary sector
- Work with adult services, particularly mental health
- Work to protect children and cooperate with the criminal justice system in the prosecution of the perpetrator.

The Framework for the Assessment of Children in Need and Their Families provides the foundation for a systematic assessment of children and families. The framework triangle embraces three key areas:

- The child's developmental needs
- The parental capacity
- The wider family and environmental factors.

The process draws on the contribution of a range of agencies in the comprehensive assessment of the child and family. The framework emphasizes that the assessment is a process, not a single event, and that the resulting interventions arise from the conclusions of this.

All NHS trusts should have a named doctor and named nurse for child protection who take a professional lead within the Trust on child protection matters. Their

Table 21.1 Summary of the doctor's role in protecting children*

Stage	Knowledge	Skills	Attitudes
Recognition	Predisposing factors Clinical indicators	Clinical acumen Developmental examination	Acceptance that abuse is prevalent
Reporting	Local reporting arrangements Role appreciation When to intervene	Communication skills Documentation	Principle that protecting the child is paramount Acknowledgment of adverse effects of abuse and neglect
Investigation	Role appreciation Role of others	Communication skills Report writing	Willingness to share information Cooperation with other agencies Coping skills

* Adapted from Bannon MJ, Carter YH 2003 Protecting Children from Abuse and Neglect in Primary Care. Oxford University Press, Oxford.

responsibility includes education, support and supervision. Each local area must have a designated doctor and nurse for child protection who work closely with the named professionals in supporting activities within Trusts.

Presentation in primary care

The basic principles involved in child protection are:
- Recognition and reporting
- Contributing information to the multi-agency investigation and risk assessment
- Providing support for the child and family.

The doctor in primary care has a responsibility to recognize the possibility of child abuse, and if uncertain, to report his or her concerns to others with responsibilities and greater experience in investigating the problem.

Recognition of the problem

'If you don't think, you won't diagnose.'

Presentation of abuse

The child may disclose an incident of abuse in confidence to a doctor. Disclosure to a relative, friend or professional is probably the most common way in which child sexual abuse comes to light. Doctors should be aware of the pitfall of promising confidentiality before being told the child's secret. There is no place for confidentiality where there is suspected abuse or neglect. The child should be informed that the information will be passed on to the social services for his or her protection, as well as for the protection of other children. A doctor should never interrogate a child if she or he has disclosed abuse, as this may compromise the subsequent legal process, but gentle and non-leading questioning may be appropriate. The doctor should have no ethical dilemma as to whether this information should be reported to the statutory agencies for child protection, as the General Medical Council acknowledges that protection of the patient overrides the duty of confidentiality to the patient. Good communication skills with children and young people are very important.

There is no simple diagnostic test for child abuse and in some cases the symptoms are subtle or non-specific. In many cases the diagnosis is straightforward, but in others — for example, where the parent vigorously denies any abuse — the situation is more difficult. The doctor does not need to be certain of the diagnosis to raise concern. The doctor's responsibility is first and foremost to report his or her suspicions and share those concerns with others.

The main presenting features of the different forms of child abuse are discussed below and in Chapter 37. A summary of the major presenting features are:
- Presentation with injury that is inconsistent or unexplained
- Allegations or disclosure of abuse from a child, carer or neighbour
- Pattern of poor and inadequate care of the child
- Presence of individuals in the household who are suspected or known to be a risk to children
- Repeated visits or contacts for minor trivial or unexplained complaints with primary care providers, e.g. GP, accident and emergency department
- Accumulated concerns about the child or family from various members of the primary care team.

Reporting

'Doing nothing in suspected cases is not an option.'

It is the doctor's responsibility to report concerns about an individual child to the appropriate authorities. This usually means a discussion between the doctor and either a local paediatrician or the local social services department, which will provide an out-of-hours service if you feel that there is an urgent risk to the child. The referral should be followed up with written notification. The primary care doctor does not need to be an expert in child protection. Further investigations will be taken forward by an experienced paediatrician. The notifying doctor's responsibility is for vigilance and reporting. Accurate notes written at the time of referral are essential.

Each local Area Child Protection Committee (ACPC, becoming a Local Safeguarding Children Board (LSCB) in 2006) will have developed procedures and published simple guidelines, including names and telephone numbers of useful contacts, as well as specific guidance regarding what to do and say.

Intervention and investigation

'If in doubt, ask for help or advice.'

Intervention is coordinated through social services, who have a statutory responsibility to respond when notified of a child suspected to be suffering, or likely to suffer, from significant harm. The process of investigating a child at risk is summarized in Figure 21.1. An initial assessment will be performed, drawing together sources of information from all relevant sources according to

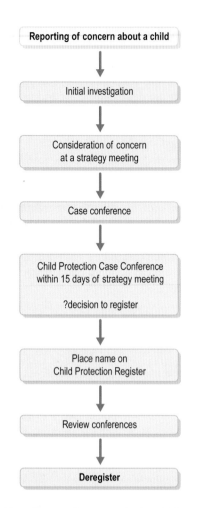

Fig. 21.1 Flow diagram for stages in the child protection protocol

the principles of 'Working Together'. This is referred to as the strategy meeting. At the end of this process a decision is made on whether there is sufficient evidence to proceed to investigation (Section 47 Child Protection).

The Child Protection Case Conference (CPCC)

This multi-professional meeting is convened when the child protection investigation concludes that there is a risk of significant harm to the child. It must be convened within 15 working days of the initial strategy meeting. It is usually chaired by a senior professional, usually from the social services.

The agencies invited to this conference include, where relevant to the case, social services, education, police, health (primary care and hospital as relevant), local authority legal department, probation, housing and voluntary agencies. In addition, the meeting is attended by members of the family, with a supporter

and, as appropriate in some cases when the child is in care, foster carers.

The aim of the CPCC is as follows:
- To share information about the child
- To determine whether the child is at significant risk of harm
- To agree a plan of action to safeguard the child's welfare
- To agree individual responsibilities in carrying out this plan
- To decide whether to place the child's name on the Child Protection Register.

If the conference decides that there is a need for a plan to protect the child from future risk, this fact will be recorded and made available to professionals who need to know. Formal child protection registers will no longer exist after 2006. For children with such a protection plan, a review conference will be arranged, usually within 3 months, to assess the progress of the child protection plan and decide the need for continuing. As a result of subsequent review meetings and when the child is no longer considered to be at risk of significant harm or when he or she has reached the age of 18 years, the plan may be discontinued.

The plan should identify the following:
- The needs of the child, with focused objectives to safeguard the child and promote his or her welfare
- A key worker with overall responsibility for ensuring the protection plan is implemented
- A core group of professionals and family members who will put the plan into practice.

Emotional impact of abuse

Many children who have been abused may show little evidence of psychological problems in childhood, but this represents a 'latent' phase that may manifest later in life as emotional disorder. In adolescence this may take the form of truancy, violence, substance abuse or mental health problems. Those children who are most damaged may themselves show self-damaging behaviour, become drug and alcohol abusers, or turn to prostitution or violence.

Emotional abuse has the most damaging effect in later life, with the inability to form normal relationships and hence the perpetuation of the risk of abuse to the next generation of children. Its long-term effects are greater than in children who have suffered physical abuse alone.

Persistent neglect has a pervasive effect on the child's self-esteem, with consequent effects on intellectual, physical, social and emotional development that are correlated with school failure. These effects may also result in later failure to develop normal relationships. It is suggested that this may result later in life in maternal depression, drug abuse and antisocial or criminal activities.

Looked-after children

A child is looked after when he or she is in local authority care or is being provided with accommodation by the local authority for more than 24 hours. A looked-after child can be accommodated voluntarily with his or her parent's/guardian's agreement or following a court order. Children can be cared for by extended family members, foster carers or another responsible adult or in a residential home/school. At any one time approximately 60 000 are in care and approximately 80% are in care due to abuse and neglect. Looked-after children are particularly vulnerable to further abuse and neglect, are the most socially excluded of all children, and as a group have poor experiences of education and very low educational attainment. Around 67% of looked-after children have mental health problems in later life. About half of the prison population and young people living rough report having been in care.

Children who are looked after should have a health needs assessment (which may include a physical examination), either before their placement or as soon as is reasonably practical after a placement is made. The health needs assessment should be carried out by a registered medical practitioner (ideally, one who is paediatrically trained), who should prepare a report and a future healthcare plan. A review health assessment should be carried out twice yearly if the child is under 5 years and annually for children over 5 years. Health assessments should cover a range of issues beyond those of physical health, which include developmental health and emotional wellbeing. Primary care teams and paediatricians have an important role to play in the identification, recording and coordination of the healthcare needs of looked-after children.

Adoption

Adoption of a child, through an adoption order, transfers all parental responsibility to the adopters. All children require a health assessment prior to adoption, with provision of a report regarding the child. Primary care teams and paediatricians have an important role in provision of health assessments for the adoption panel.

Child neglect

> **Problem-orientated topic:**
>
> **neglect**
>
> Wayne, aged 15 months, is referred because of pallor and delayed development. He is the youngest of four children, and on examination he is dirty and his clothes are unkempt. The mother is an alcoholic and the father is in prison. The three older children attend school sporadically, none is fully immunized and all have speech and language delay.
>
> Q1. What is the most likely cause of Wayne's problems?
>
> Q2. How would you define child neglect?
>
> Q3. How would you assess this case?
>
> Q4. How would you manage this child and family?

Q1. What is the most likely cause of Wayne's problems?

Wayne is most likely to be suffering from a form of abuse referred to as neglect. Neglect may take several forms:

- Neglect of the child's physical needs, e.g. nutrition (Wayne's anaemia arising as a result of a diet low in iron, resulting in pallor)
- Failure to pay attention to the child's personal hygiene, clothing etc. (Wayne is dirty and unkempt)
- Failure to provide stimulation and education (developmental delay in Wayne and frequent school absences in the older siblings)
- Neglect of the child's medical needs (neither Wayne nor his siblings are fully immunized)
- Neglect of supervision and lack of awareness of safety issues
- Neglect of interaction with adults and with other children of the same age
- Failure to provide affection and appropriate nurturing.

Q2. How would you define child neglect?

The Department of Health defines neglect as:

persistent failure to meet a child's basic physical and/or psychological needs, likely to result in the serious impairment of the child's health or development. It may involve a parent or carer failing to provide adequate food, shelter or clothing, failing to protect a child from physical harm or danger, or the failure to ensure access to appropriate medical care or treatment. It may also include neglect of, or unresponsiveness to, a child's basic emotional needs.

Families in whom a child is subject to neglect have been described as those that 'are low on warmth and high on criticism'. Repeated criticism reminds the child that he or she is unloved (emotional abuse), with a consequent risk of neglect or other forms of abuse including either physical or sexual. Another common family trait is a lack of consistency in disciplining the child.

Neglect is the most common reason for putting children's names on the Child Protection Register. Persistent neglect has a pervasive effect on the child's self-esteem, with consequent effects on intellectual, physical, social and emotional development that are correlated with school failure. These effects may also result in later failure to develop normal relationships and to parent one's own child. This may result later in life in maternal depression, drug abuse and antisocial or criminal activities.

Q3. How would you assess this case?

History
- Assess the parent's knowledge and understanding of the child's health and developmental needs.
- Document the family's social history, financial resources and support networks.
- Assess the parent's relationship with the presenting child.
- Is there a history of substance abuse in the family?

Examination
- Is Wayne smelly, dirty or unkempt, and does he have untreated medical conditions, e.g. squint, and infections or infestations?
- Observe parent/child interactions (or the lack of them) during the consultation.
- Assess the child's growth and development. Speech and language are particularly affected. The child may be stunted, underweight or overweight.
- Does the child look pale — anaemia or prison pallor?

Q4. How would you manage this child and family?

- Involve other agencies (primary healthcare, social services, education) and obtain further information on the family. The health visitor or teacher may be particularly well placed to provide this.

- Participate with other agencies in the assessment and treatment plan, including follow-up of the child.
- Identify the child's unmet needs (health, social, developmental, educational).
- Refer for speech and language therapy, if appropriate.
- Request a multi-agency assessment using the Framework for Assessment of Children in Need and Their Families.

Emotional abuse

Problem-orientated topic:

soiling

Robbie is 8 years old and is referred to you with soiling. His attendance at school is erratic, and when he does attend, he is described as aggressive to teachers and pupils and verbally abusive. He has been suspended from school for violence on two occasions. He is reported to have no friends. His mother describes him as 'evil'.

Q1. What do you think is the cause of his problems?

Q2. How would you assess this child and family?

Q3. What management options are available for him?

Q1. What do you think is the cause of his problems?

All children need to be loved and respected within a secure, consistent and emotionally warm environment. Failure to provide this emotional support may cause severe long-term problems and children may be unable to form long-term relationships and achieve successful parenting themselves. This perpetuates the abuse when the child becomes a parent. The long-term adverse effects of emotional abuse are thought to be greater than the effects of physical abuse. Physical and sexual abuse almost invariably involves some component of emotional abuse.

The Department of Health have defined emotional abuse as:

persistent emotional ill-treatment of a child such as to cause severe and persistent adverse effects on the child's emotional development. It may involve conveying to children that they are worthless or unloved, inadequate, or valued only insofar as they meet the needs of another person. It may feature age or developmentally inappropriate expectations being imposed on children. It may involve causing children to feel frightened or in danger, or the exploitation or corruption of children. Some level of emotional abuse is involved in all types of ill-treatment of a child, though it may occur alone.

Harmful behaviour leading to emotional abuse includes:
- Inconsistent parenting
- Exposure to violence between the parents
- Excessive anxiety about a child's health
- Scapegoating
- Induction of fear or insecurity
- Developmentally inappropriate roles and expectations of the child, such as caring for disabled parents
- Rejection
- Isolation of the child in a room alone with little social contact
- Exposure to degrading or humiliating practices
- Ignoring
- Corrupting or encouraging criminality.

Unlike physical or sexual abuse, emotional abuse is readily observable in the consulting room or family home. The primary care doctor and health visitor are well placed to detect emotional abuse through their observations and knowledge of the family situation. Domestic violence and frequent attendance at GP surgeries for stress-related complaints are features suggestive of the fact that a child in the family may be suffering from emotional abuse or neglect.

At-risk children and those families where there is heightened risk include:
- Children who are unwanted, e.g. of the 'wrong' sex
- Disabled/chronically ill children
- Children of vulnerable parents (alcohol or drug abusers, mentally ill, domestic violence).

Q2. How would you assess this child and family?

The presentation may vary, depending on the age of the child.

Babies
- Feeding difficulties, excessive crying, poor sleep patterns
- Failure to relate to care-givers (who may describe them as 'a difficult baby, doesn't feel like he belongs to me' or 'he doesn't love me').

Toddlers and preschool children
- Head banging or excessive rocking
- Aggressive behaviour
- Developmental delay
- Poor growth — failure to thrive.

School-age children
- Wetting and soiling
- Relationship difficulties
- Poor school performance
- Truancy and antisocial behaviour
- Feeling worthless and unloved.

Adolescents
- Depression
- Self-harming
- Substance abuse
- Eating disorder
- Oppositional, aggressive and delinquent behaviour.

Q3. What management options are available for him?

Increasing social support for the family may ease family stress, and recognizing and treating specific problems such as developmental disorders in the child are important. 'Sure Start', where available, may also provide satisfactory intervention for problem families. Interventions to protect mothers from domestic violence are also important. More difficult cases may benefit from referral to Child and Adolescent Mental Health Services.

Factitious or induced illness

This condition, previously known as Munchausen syndrome by proxy, is relatively uncommon in paediatric practice. In this condition, a parent (usually the mother) invents, induces or exaggerates symptoms of an illness in her child to obtain some form of gratification. This may be sympathy, attention, publicity or money.

Features of this condition are shown in Box 21.2.

Presenting features

Clinical features suggestive of factitious or induced illness (FII) include:
- Poisoning with drugs or household items such as salt, in order to induce symptoms.
- Blood added to urine, vomitus or stool.
- An acute unexplained life-threatening event that only occurs when the parent is present. Covert video surveillance in hospital has revealed that the cause is most likely to be deliberate suffocation by the parent.

- Repeated apnoeic attacks or fits never witnessed by others.
- Fever.
- Failure to thrive (milk poured down the sink).

Management

GPs are in a good position to notice if parents are consulting numerous health providers, as they should have appropriate letters etc. The doctor's priority is to ensure that the child avoids ongoing harm. FII may be fatal. Share information with other clinical carers, such as nurses and other specialists. Refer to the social services or police if you have continuing concerns rather than proof of FII.

It is not necessary to share your concerns with the parents if, by doing so, you may put the child at risk. It is important to consider carefully the risk of disclosure of concern to the family before adequate discussions have taken place and protection has been achieved for the child.

Physical and sexual abuse

As well as emotional abuse and neglect, physical and sexual abuses are also common and important conditions. Serious injury and child sexual abuse may present either to primary care or in hospital. They may require specialized forensic skills to diagnose and document for court. These two conditions are discussed in more detail in Chapter 37 and the section below represents a summary of features that are important for doctors in primary care. It should be read in conjunction with Chapter 37 and the RCPCH/NSPCC/ALSG course, 'Safe-guarding children'.

Physical abuse

The doctor must be alert to the varied ways in which physical abuse may present. The common types of injury that may result from physical abuse include:
- Bruising from blows, kicks or beating with objects
- Fractures: for example, from grabbing limbs, direct blows or shaking
- Bites (distinguish between animal and human dental patterns)
- Burns from being held in direct contact with hot objects or scalds from forced immersion
- Intra-oral injuries suggesting forcible insertion of bottles or spoons.

Important features that should arouse suspicion of physical abuse are:
- Multiple superficial injuries of varying type, size and age
- Delay in presentation
- Bruises or marks with characteristic features of inflicting instruments
- Injuries not consistent with the history
- Injuries not consistent with the child's developmental age
- Injuries to an infant's central nervous system.

Important sites for inflicted bruises include the face, lower jaw, ears, neck, buttocks, trunk and proximal parts of limbs. Accidental injury is most commonly found on the bony prominences, e.g. shins, elbows or forehead. Common patterns include fingertip or handslap marks, pinch marks, localized petechiae, e.g. around the neck, and marks of implements, e.g. belt, strap, stick or shoe.

A thorough medical examination, including assessment of growth, development and behaviour, is essential in all cases of suspected child abuse. It is essential to document carefully the number, distribution and pattern of all bruises and injuries. Up to a half of all mobile children have at least one bruise and many have more than one, although more than ten are suspicious.

Burns and other thermal injuries occur commonly in childhood and often present to primary care doctors. A relatively small number are due to child abuse, but are known to be under-recognized. Thermal injury includes burns and scalds that may be caused by hot water, food or steam, cigarettes, lighters or matches, friction from being dragged across a carpet, electrical shocks, hot metal objects such as an iron or radiator, or chemical burns. Cigarette burns cause deep circular craters 0.5–1 cm in diameter, which scar. Accidental brushed contact causes superficial injury roughly circular but with a tail.

Child sexual abuse

Sexual abuse in children will not be recognized if it is not considered by the clinician. A high index of suspicion must exist and healthcare professionals must acknowledge that child sexual abuse may occur in any family. The abuser is most commonly a member of the household, an extended family member or a family friend. In the vast majority of cases the child knows the abuser, who may be either male or female. Sexual abuse of children by strangers is uncommon.

Child sexual abuse has both short- and long-term effects.

- Short-term:
  - Behavioural problems
  - Difficulties forming friendships
  - School failure and truancy
  - Difficulty in forming trusting relationships
- Long-term:
  - Sexual relationship difficulties
  - Mental health problems
  - Social dysfunction
  - Greater likelihood of patients abusing their own children.

There are very few pathognomonic signs of sexual abuse and the diagnosis is usually made by piecing together a jigsaw of information from many sources (Fig. 21.2).

Diagnosis may be suspected from the following features:

- *Disclosure.* This is the most common way in which the condition is diagnosed and children rarely fabricate disclosure of sexual abuse. If a child discloses in confidence, he or she must be told that the information will be passed on for his or her protection, as well as for the protection of other children. The doctor should have no ethical dilemma as to whether this information should be disclosed, as the General Medical Council acknowledges that protection of the patient overrides the duty of confidentiality to the patient.
- *Vaginal discharge or urinary symptoms.* A vulval swab and urine culture should be taken. Do not insert the swab into the vagina but take the specimen from the labia in a prepubertal child. If a vulval swab identifies a sexually transmitted disease,

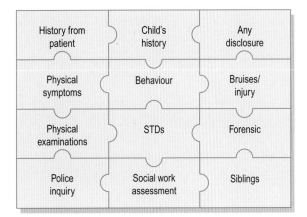

Fig. 21.2 **The jigsaw of sexual abuse**

immediate referral to a child protection team should be made.
- *Rectal or vaginal bleeding.*
- *Behavioural disturbances.* These are a common result of child sexual abuse and may include self-harm, mutilation, aggression and sexualized behaviours.
- *Pregnancy.*

If a doctor suspects child sexual abuse, this information must be passed on to social services. Discussion with a named paediatrician may be useful if further advice is required. The primary care-giver should be informed of the referral, unless there is any concern that the abuser may be warned and evidence may be destroyed or pressure put on the child to withdraw disclosure or change his or her story.

The doctor must keep careful and accurate contemporaneous notes of the interview and any examination findings. All paediatricians should be familiar with the Royal College of Physicians document, 'The Physical Signs of Sexual Abuse in Children'.

Acknowledgments

We are very grateful to Dr Chris Hobbs for helpful advice.

Reference

Bannon MJ, Carter YH (eds) 2003 Protecting children from abuse and neglect in primary care. Oxford University Press, Oxford

MODULE FOUR

Edited by Malcolm Levene

Common Problems in Primary Care

MODULE FIVE

Mary Rudolf

Growth: normal and abnormal

LEARNING OUTCOMES

By the end of this chapter you should:

- Know when a child's growth is of concern
- Know how to diagnose the common and important conditions responsible for poor growth
- Know the causes of poor weight gain in young children and babies
- Appreciate the stresses of having a child with weight faltering (failure to thrive), especially if there are eating difficulties, and be able to advise carers on management
- Know how to advise a child who is suffering from obesity
- Be able to weigh and measure a baby and child accurately
- Be able to plot measures on a growth chart, correcting for prematurity when appropriate
- Be able to calculate body mass index (BMI).

MODULE FIVE

The basic science of growth

Normal growth occurs as a complex interplay between:
- Genetic influences
- Hormonal factors
- Nutritional availability
- Environmental exposure.

Poor growth may result from endocrine abnormalities, disease or poor environment.

Factors influencing growth

There are important differences between the factors influencing normal prenatal and postnatal growth.

Fetal growth

www.sciencedirect.com

Follow links to Gluckman PD, Hanson MA 2004 Maternal constraint of fetal growth and its consequences. Seminars in Fetal and Neonatal Medicine; 9:419–425

Growth before birth occurs as an interaction between genetic and environmental influences. A landmark study of mating large male Shire horses with small female Shetland ponies showed that maternal size was a major constraining factor in the prenatal growth of the foal. This has obvious evolutionary advantages in ensuring that the fetus does not grow too large

235

to obstruct labour, predisposing to the death of the mother.

The factors affecting normal fetal growth are as follows.

Environmental factors

In normal pregnancies environmental factors have the major influence on fetal growth. 'Maternal constraint' limits fetal growth, which is a complicated relationship between uterine capacity and the ability of the placenta to provide sufficient nutrients. In multiple pregnancy the total weight of the babies is more than that of a singleton, although the individual weight of the babies is less than that of a singleton. This suggests that the availability of transplacental nutrients is a greater factor than uterine capacity.

Hormonal factors

Assuming sufficient supply of nutrients from the placenta, the hormonal milieu is important in determining embryonic and fetal growth. Insulin and insulin-like growth factors (IGFs) are the major prenatal trophic hormones. It appears that IGF-2 is particularly important in embryonic growth, and IGF-1 in later fetal and early infant linear growth. Insulin stimulates fat deposition (Ch. 48). Growth hormone has no effect on early human growth.

Placental factors

Normal placental function is essential for prenatal growth (Ch. 46) and the most common cause for intrauterine growth restriction is placental insufficiency. The placenta not only provides all the fetal nutritional needs, but also contributes to the fetal hormonal milieu necessary for normal growth. Maternal diet can influence nutritional availability to the fetus, which has major implications for pregnancy in developing countries where the maternal diet may be poor (Ch. 38).

Genetic factors

Genetic factors have a minor effect on fetal growth and the paternal genomic contribution has virtually no effect in determining birth size. Maternal environmental effects override fetal genetic contribution to prenatal growth.

Childhood growth

Genetic factors

Genetic factors largely account for final adult height, which generally can be anticipated to lie between the midparental centiles (average of parents' height (cm) + 7 (if boy), − 7 (if girl) = mid parent corrected height). The genotype is also a major determinant of final height.

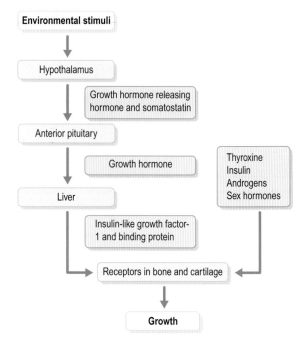

Fig. 22.1 **Hormonal factors influencing growth**

The Y chromosome controls the major genetic effects, as evident by males (XY) being taller than females (XX). Turner's syndrome (XO) females are shorter than XX females, and males with the XYY pattern tend to be taller than average XY males. Males with Klinefelter's syndrome (XXY) are no shorter on average than normal XY males.

Hormonal influences (Fig. 22.1)

Human growth hormone (hGH) is secreted by the anterior pituitary and is expressed in two main forms by at least five genes on chromosome 17. hGH regulates protein synthesis and fat breakdown for energy use. It is particularly important for cartilaginous development within the epiphyses and consequently influences height. The production of hGH is stimulated by growth hormone releasing factor (GRF) from the hypothalamus. A growth hormone release-inhibiting factor (somatostatin) is also produced by the hypothalamus as well as other tissues and inhibits hGH release as well as acting on its remote receptor sites. The influence of higher brain centres on hypothalamic function may explain why adverse emotional factors may affect growth.

Insulin and IGFs, also termed somatomedins, are produced in liver and other organs and circulate in the blood. They have the effect, like insulin, of stimulating protein synthesis and depressing catabolism.

Other pituitary-derived hormones, such as thyroid and parathyroid hormone, have an important effect on maturation and growth, and hypothyroid children grow poorly. Sex hormones regulate the onset of puberty and are responsible for the adolescent growth spurt (see below). They also ultimately cause fusion of the epiphyseal centres and so cause linear growth to cease. Adrenal hormones have an influence on growth and excess corticosteroids have a profound suppressant effect (Ch. 35).

Nutrition

The availability of adequate nutritional substrate is essential for normal growth, and starvation inhibits growth in children. Malnutrition also delays the onset of puberty, which can have an important effect on final height.

Environmental factors

Factors known to affect growth include:
- *Socioeconomic status*. Adult height is on average 4.5 cm greater in socioeconomic class I, compared with class V.
- *Disease*. Any chronic disease can cause stunting of growth.
- *Emotional environment*. An adverse emotional environment can slow growth. This is probably mediated through hypothalamic factors.
- *Altitude*. This is probably mediated through lower oxygen saturation levels.

Periods of growth

Growth in infancy

At birth, a baby's weight and length are influenced mainly by intrauterine factors. The rate of growth in the first year of life is more rapid than at any other age. Between birth and 1 year of age, children on average increase their length by 50% and triple their birth weight. Head circumference increases by one-third. Crossing centiles is initially common, but by the age of 2 most children have attained their genetically destined centile, and the baby has changed in shape to take on the appearance of the lean and more muscular child.

Growth in the preschool and school years

In the preschool years a child continues to gain weight and height steadily. Beyond the age of 2 or 3 years until puberty, the growth rate is steady at about 3–3.5 kg and 6 cm per year, and centile crossing is not usually seen.

Growth in adolescence

Adolescence is characterized by a growth spurt, which occurs under the influence of rising sex hormone levels. During the 3 or 4 years of puberty boys grow about

25 cm and girls 20 cm, and it is normal for centiles to be crossed until final height is achieved, which usually is located midway between the parental centiles.

Growth in adverse circumstances and catch-up growth

During a period of illness or starvation the rate of growth is slowed. After the incident the child usually grows more rapidly so that catch-up towards, or actually to, the original growth curve occurs. The degree to which catch-up is successful depends on the timing of the onset and the duration of slow growth. This is particularly important in infants who have suffered intrauterine growth retardation and who may have reduced growth potential.

In nutritionally compromised children, weight falls before height is impaired and head growth is the last to be affected. If growth has been slowed for too long or into puberty, complete catch-up is not achieved. There are important therapeutic implications in the early detection of children with abnormal growth velocity patterns, as early treatment is more likely to ensure that acceptable adult height is achieved.

Head growth

Although there is a tendency for large babies to have large heads and small babies smaller heads, head size is largely independent of body size. Head growth is driven by the growth of the brain, and if for any reason the brain fails to grow normally, the head will be small, so that it is common to find that children with developmental problems have microcephaly. Rapid head growth is a cause for concern and may result from raised intracranial pressure, when the sutures become pushed apart. So saying, pathological causes of unusual head size are uncommon and the most common explanation for both small and large heads in otherwise normal individuals is familial.

Short stature

See also Chapter 35.

Problem-orientated topic:

a short child

Jeannie is 12 years old. She attends her doctor's surgery because she is short. She is in general good health, but has recently become rather withdrawn and is

Continued overleaf

having a difficult time at high school, where she has been recurrently teased about her height. Her father is 5′ 6″. Her mother is 5′3″ and had menarche at the age of 15 years.

Jeannie's height is 127 cm (below 0.4th centile) and her weight is 26 kg (0.4th centile) (Fig. 22.2).

Q1. When should one become concerned about short stature?

Q2. What is the likely cause of Jeannie's short stature?

Q3. What other conditions should be considered?

Q4. What should you look for in your clinical evaluation?

Q5. What investigations might be appropriate?

Q6. When is referral indicated?

Q1. When should one become concerned about short stature?

Given the social disadvantage of being short, especially for a man, it is not surprising that short stature commonly causes concern. Box 22.1 provides some guidance as to when growth in childhood may be of concern.

Q2. What is the likely cause of Jeannie's short stature?

Jeannie's parents are both relatively short and her mother had menarche late, so familial short stature and maturational delay are likely explanations. However, it is important to exclude organic problems. A good clinical evaluation and a growth chart should help you decide if the cause is pathological rather than physiological.

Q3. What other conditions should be considered?

It is important to exclude organic problems, particularly if there is a falloff in growth over time (p. 242). The causes of short stature are shown in Box 22.2.

Q4. What should you look for in your clinical evaluation?

Key points
- A good history and physical examination will identify most pathological causes of short stature.

BOX 22.1 Guidelines for concern beyond the age of 2 years

The short or tall child
Height or weight beyond the dotted lines on the growth chart (> 99.6th or < 0.4th centile) is outside the normal range and pathology is more likely to be found. Many children whose height or weight lies in the shaded areas are normal but an evaluation needs to be considered.

Crossing of centiles
As a rule of thumb, one should be concerned if two centile lines are crossed.

Discrepancy between height and weight
There is a great deal of variation as regards leanness and obesity. The child who is very thin or overweight may have a problem.

Discrepancy with parental heights
A child should be evaluated if there is a large discrepancy between the child's height centile and the midparental centile. The child of tall parents who has a growth problem should not wait until he or she falls below the second centile to be evaluated.

Parental or professional concern
A good clinical evaluation should be carried out in any child when the parents or other professionals are concerned about growth.

- The child's height must be related to the parents' heights.
- Emotional and social *consequences* of the short stature should be identified.

History
Your history needs to focus on symptoms suggestive of underlying conditions, such as intracranial pathology, hormone deficiency, chronic illness and gastrointestinal symptoms.
- *Medical history*. Headache, diarrhoea and abdominal pain, constipation, cough, wheeze and fatigue are particularly relevant. Chronic conditions such as asthma, arthritis or diabetes may be significant, as is any chronic medication.
- *Family history*. A child's growth cannot be interpreted without reference to parental and siblings' heights. Ask about parental onset of puberty, as maturational delay is common and often familial. Maternal menarche after the age of 14 years is suggestive. Onset of paternal puberty is harder to identify.
- *Birth history*. Low birth weight is significant. A child born severely preterm or small for gestational age (SGA) may have reduced growth potential,

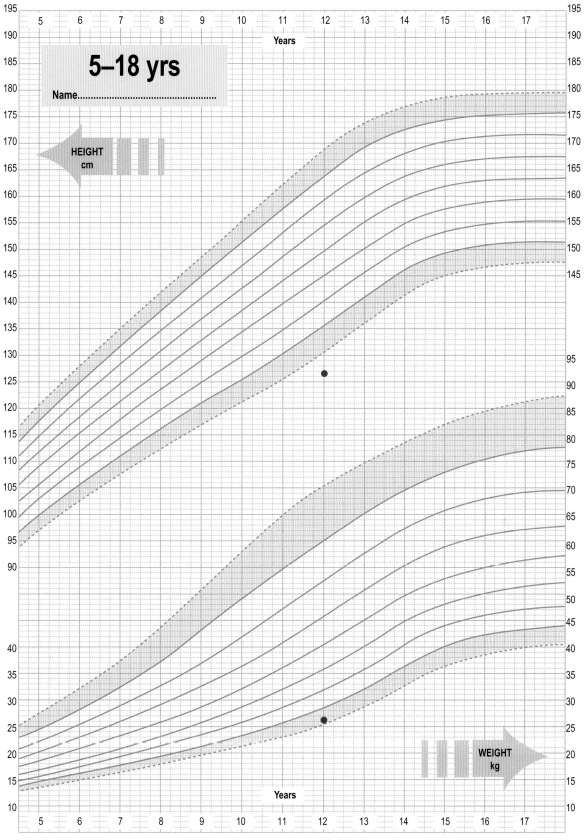

Fig. 22.2 Jeannie's growth chart

Physiological causes

- Normal variant (often familial, also known as 'constitutional short stature')
- Maturational delay (often familial)

Pathological causes

- Endocrine:
  - Hypothyroidism
  - Corticosteroid excess
  - Growth hormone deficiency
- Chronic illness:
  - Inflammatory bowel and coeliac disease; chronic renal failure may be occult
- Genetic:
  - Turner's syndrome
  - Other genetic syndromes
  - Skeletal dysplasias
- Intrauterine growth retardation
- Psychosocial

particularly if height as well as weight is affected.

- *Psychosocial history.* Psychosocial factors can severely stunt a child's growth, and you must be alert to the possibility of emotional neglect and abuse. When assessing any short child you should also find out about any social or emotional difficulties *resulting* from his or her stature.

Examination

A very thorough examination is required, focusing particularly on the following:

- *Pattern of growth.* Where possible, you should review previous growth measurements, as they provide important clues to the aetiology of the condition. Falloff in growth usually indicates a medical condition requiring treatment.
- *Anthropometric measures.* Take careful measures of weight and of length (to age 24 months) or height and plot them on a growth chart.

- *General examination.* Signs of hypothyroidism, body disproportion, and signs of Turner's syndrome (Ch. 35) and dysmorphism are particularly important to identify. Examine each organ system in turn, looking for evidence of occult disease.

Q5. What investigations might be appropriate?

Your clinical evaluation should guide any investigations. If you find a decrease in growth velocity, investigations are always required (Table 22.1).

Q6. When is referral indicated?

If a physiological cause — namely, constitutional short stature or maturational delay — is likely, the child can be followed in primary care. The growth rate needs to be periodically checked, and the family should be reassured that there is no underlying pathological problem. In addition it is important to address any psychosocial difficulties the child is having, and occasionally psychological counselling is required.

Reduction in growth rate is a definite indication for paediatric assessment (p. 242). Boys with maturational delay may benefit from testosterone. The use of growth hormone in children with physiological short stature is controversial and probably confers little benefit on final adult height.

Causes of short stature (Box 22.2)

Physiological causes of short stature

Normal variant short stature

Stature is largely genetically determined, and short parents tend to have short children. In normal variant short stature, the history and physical examination are normal, and the bone age is appropriate for age. Often reassurance is all that is required. Social difficulties are common in the adolescent years, particularly for boys, and occasionally children need psychological support at this time.

Table 22.1 Investigations in a child with short stature

Investigation	Relevance
Blood count, plasma viscosity or erythrocyte sedimentation rate	Inflammatory bowel disease
Urea and electrolytes	Chronic renal failure
Coeliac antibodies	Screening test for coeliac disease
Thyroxine and thyroid-stimulating hormone	Hypothyroidism
Karyotype (in girls)	Turner's syndrome
Growth hormone tests	Hypopituitarism, growth hormone deficiency
X-ray of the wrist for bone age (Fig. 22.3)	Delayed bone age suggests maturational delay, hypothyroidism, growth hormone deficiency or corticosteroid excess. A prediction of adult height can be made from it

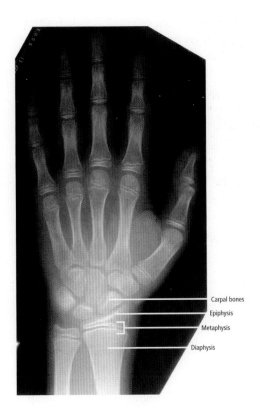

Fig. 22.3 X-ray of the left wrist taken for bone age.
The development of the various bones is assessed to give an estimate of the child's skeletal maturity.

Carpal bones
Epiphysis
Metaphysis
Diaphysis

Maturational delay

Children with maturational delay are often called 'late developers' or 'late bloomers'. The biological clock operates more slowly than usual. Children in this circumstance are short and reach puberty late, their final height depending on their genetic constitution, which may be normal. A family history of delayed puberty and menarche is often obtained, and the bone age is delayed.

Most families simply require reassurance that final height will not be affected, but occasionally teenage boys find the social pressures to be so great that it is helpful to trigger puberty artificially with testosterone, thus causing an early growth spurt. This treatment does not have an effect on final height.

Endocrine causes of short stature

(See also Chapter 35.)

Hypothyroidism

Hypothyroidism may be congenital or acquired as autoimmune thyroiditis (Hashimoto's syndrome), which occurs particularly in girls. Thyroid deficiency has a profound effect on growth, and may present as short stature. Other features include a falloff in school performance, constipation, dry skin and delayed puberty. Investigations include a low T4, high thyroid-stimulating hormone (TSH) and antithyroid antibodies. Treatment is lifelong replacement of thyroid hormone.

Corticosteroid excess

Cushing's syndrome and disease are extremely rare in childhood, growth suppression from exogenous steroids being much more common. In children requiring long-term high-steroid therapy, the deleterious effects on growth can often be minimized by giving the steroids on alternate days.

Growth hormone deficiency

Growth hormone deficiency is a rare cause of short stature. It may occur secondary to lesions of the pituitary such as tumours or cranial irradiation, or can be isolated, when it may or may not be accompanied by deficiency of other pituitary hormones.

The diagnosis is made by growth hormone testing. Brain imaging is needed to identify any underlying pathology. Deficiency is treated with daily subcutaneous injections of synthetic growth hormone until the child stops growing.

Other causes of short stature

Chronic illness

Any chronic illness can lead to stunting of growth. However, chronic illnesses rarely present as short stature because the features of the illness are usually all too evident. Chronic conditions that may present with poor growth, in advance of other clinical features, include inflammatory bowel disease, coeliac disease and chronic renal failure.

Turner's syndrome (Ch. 35)

Turner's syndrome (gonadal dysgenesis) is an important cause of short stature and delayed puberty in girls. It is a genetic disorder caused by the absence of one X chromosome. The resulting phenotype is female, with gonads that are merely streaks of fibrous tissue. Intelligence is usually normal, and characteristic features include webbing of the neck, shield-shaped chest, wide-spaced nipples and a wide carrying angle. Some girls are only diagnosed in adolescence when puberty fails to occur.

Girls with Turner's syndrome should be followed in an endocrinology clinic, where they are generally given hormonal treatment to promote growth. Puberty must be initiated and maintained by oestrogen therapy.

Table 22.2 **The differential diagnosis of short stature**

Diagnosis	Growth pattern	History	Physical examination	Bone age
Constitutional short stature	Steady growth below the centile lines	Short parents	Normal	Normal
Maturational delay	Usually short, with falloff of growth in early teens	Family history of delayed puberty/menarche	Delay in developing secondary sex characteristics	Delayed
Endocrine disorders (hypothyroidism, Cushing's, growth hormone deficiency)	Falloff of growth	Symptoms of hypothyroidism, on inhaled or oral steroids, symptoms of brain tumour	Signs of hypothyroidism or Cushing's, rarely signs of brain tumour	Very delayed
Chronic illness	Falloff of growth	Symptoms of inflammatory bowel disease, malabsorption, fatigue	Ill-looking, symptoms of underlying illness, although inflammatory bowel disease and chronic renal failure may be occult	Delayed ±
Genetic syndromes	Slow growth below centiles	–	Signs of Turner's or other dysmorphism	Variable
Intrauterine growth retardation	Short from birth	Small for gestational age	Normal but small	Normal
Psychosocial	Variable depending on social circumstances	Adverse circumstances	Unhappy, signs of neglect or abuse	Usually normal

Other genetic syndromes

Short stature is a common feature in many genetic syndromes. Dysmorphic features are usual and learning disability is common.

Skeletal dysplasias

The skeletal dysplasias are a group of disorders where body disproportion occurs, resulting in shortened limbs. The most common of these is achondroplasia, which is inherited as an autosomal dominant trait.

Intrauterine growth retardation

Intrauterine growth retardation can result from a variety of causes (Ch. 46). The impact on postnatal growth depends on which stage of the pregnancy the growth retardation occurred. If the insult occurred early in gestation, the baby is born not only underweight but also short and often with a small head. If length is short, newborns may have reduced growth potential and remain short throughout life. If catch-up growth occurs, it does so in the first 2 or 3 years.

Psychosocial causes of short stature

Adverse psychosocial factors can severely affect a child's growth. In the young child it is referred to as failure to thrive (p. 244). The true incidence of psychosocial poor growth is unknown, but it is likely that it is quite common. On being placed in foster care, children often have a growth spurt, even when growth has previously been apparently normal.

The differential diagnosis of short stature is given in Table 22.2.

Plateauing in growth

Problem-orientated topic:

a child with plateauing growth

Jane is 8 years old. Her mother is concerned, as she does not seem to be following the same growth pattern as her brother and sister did. She brings you the height measures she has taken each year on Jane's birthday (Fig. 22.4). Jane is not short, but she seems to have crossed centiles.

Q1. Should you be worried?

Q2. What conditions might cause a falloff in growth?

Q3. What should you do?

Q1. Should you be worried?

Measurements made at home are likely to be very inaccurate; however, Jane's growth since she was measured by the school nurse at school entry suggests that there has indeed been reduced growth velocity.

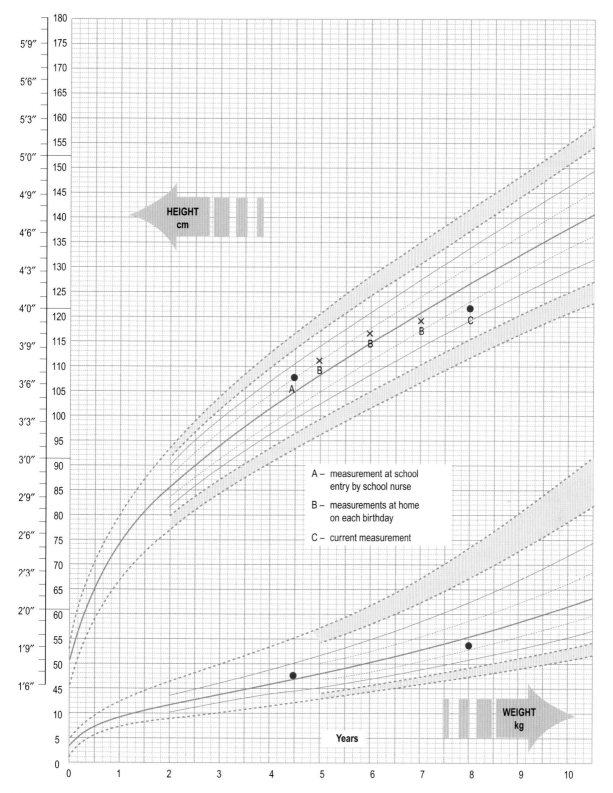

Fig. 22.4 **Jane's growth chart**

A – measurement at school entry by school nurse

B – measurements at home on each birthday

C – current measurement

- Endocrine:
  - Hypothyroidism
  - Corticosteroid excess
  - Growth hormone deficiency
- Chronic illness:
  - Inflammatory bowel and coeliac disease; chronic renal failure may be occult
- Psychosocial

You should therefore be concerned. Falloff in growth is always worrying and merits investigation. If initially tall, the child may not be short in relation to peers.

Q2. What conditions might cause a falloff in growth?

The causes of falloff in growth are shown in Box 22.3.

Q3. What should you do?

The clinical approach and management of falloff in growth are the same as those described in the previous section, but the chance of finding pathology is higher. Any child with plateauing of growth needs a referral to a paediatrician or paediatric endocrinologist.

Tall stature

Tall stature is only rarely pathological and is usually simply a variant of normal. Tall women often encounter social difficulties and tall girls may present for help. Obese children tend to be tall for their age but on the whole reach puberty early, and so their final height is usually in the normal range.

Rapid growth can very rarely be a sign of hormonal disturbance such as giantism (growth hormone excess) or precocious puberty. These are discussed in Chapter 35.

Faltering growth and failure to thrive

Problem-orientated topic:

a child with faltering growth

James is 15 months old. He started life on the 50th centile but at 12 weeks his weight started dropping off (Fig. 22.5). He has had a series of ear infections but no serious illnesses. He is developing normally but has become difficult to feed. His mother is desperately anxious, and meals are now taking up to 1 hour in length.

Q1. Does James have a growth problem?

Q2. How should one define failure to thrive and growth faltering?

Q3. What are the possible causes for James's growth pattern?

Q4. What clinical pointers should you look for in your clinical evaluation?

Q5. What investigations are indicated?

Q6. What strategies and advice might be useful in James's situation?

Q1. Does James have a growth problem?

Infants commonly cross centiles during the first 2 years of life. When they cross down this often causes concern, although it is usually physiological and due to the baby moving to its genetically intended centile. However, poor weight gain can also be an indication of psychosocial or (more rarely) medical problems. Expertise is required to differentiate the normal infant from the one who is failing to thrive.

Q2. How should one define failure to thrive and growth faltering?

Failure to thrive implies both a failure to grow and a failure of emotional and developmental progress. The term is sometimes considered pejorative and is being replaced by growth or weight 'faltering'. Both terms usually relate to poor weight gain in a toddler or baby, although they may also be used in reference to an older child, and may also refer to height.

There are no established criteria for defining failure to thrive. However, the following can act as guidelines as to when a clinical evaluation is advisable:
- Weight below the 2nd centile
- Height below the 2nd centile
- Crossing down two centile channels for height or weight.

Q3. What are the possible causes for James's growth pattern?

The causes of weight faltering are listed in Box 22.4.

In the past children were classified as having organic (OFTT) or non-organic failure to thrive (NOFTT). Children more often than not do not fall simply into one category or the other, but fail to gain weight well for a combination of reasons. It is important to identify all the factors involved.

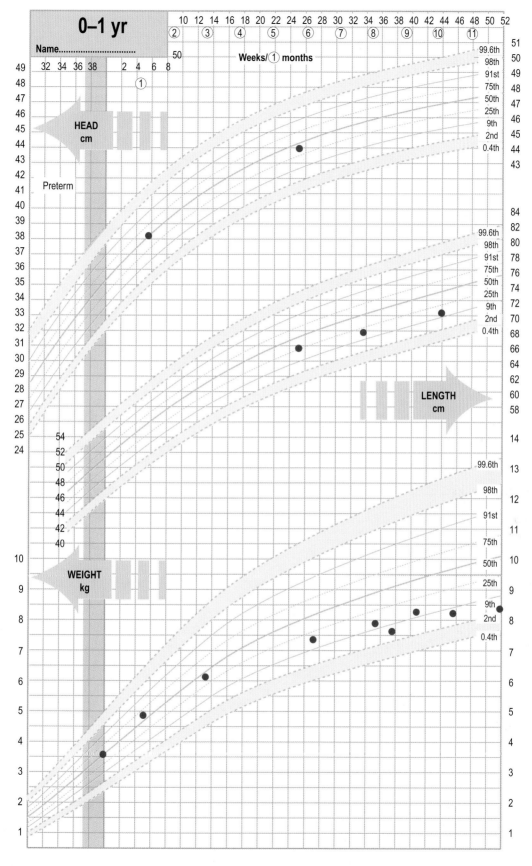

Fig. 22.5 James's growth charts.
(a) 0–1 years

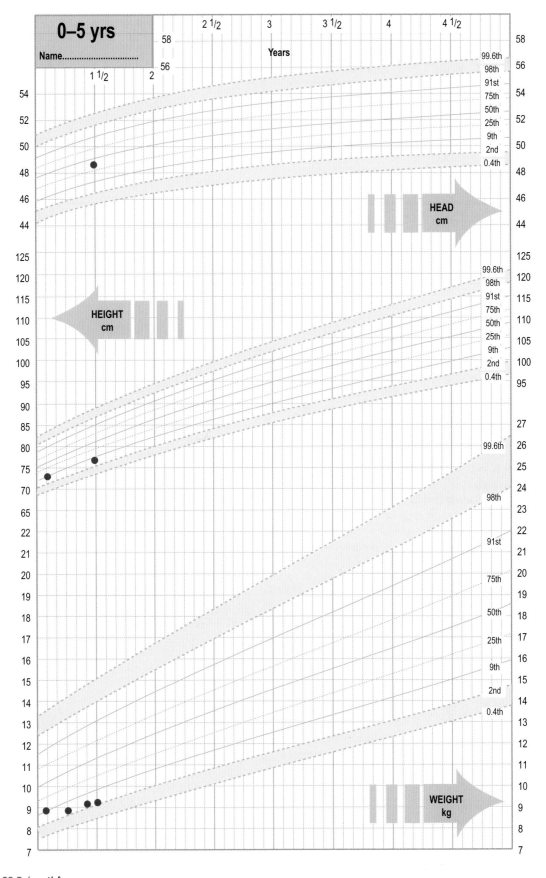

0–5 yrs

Name..............................

Years

HEAD
cm

HEIGHT
cm

WEIGHT
kg

Fig. 22.5 (*cont'd*)
(b) 0–5 years.

Q4. What clinical pointers should you look for in your clinical evaluation?

Key points
- You must differentiate the normal baby who is crossing centiles from the baby who is failing to thrive.
- Identify any symptoms and signs that suggest an organic condition.
- Only perform laboratory investigations if there are clinical leads in the history and physical examination.
- Identify psychosocial problems that might be affecting the baby's growth.

It is very distressing for the family when a young child fails to thrive, so your evaluation needs to be carried out sensitively. The purpose of the evaluation is first to differentiate the child demonstrating normal growth faltering from the child with a problem, and then to identify the contributing factors, whether organic or non-organic.

History
- *Nutritional history.* Obtain a good dietary history. Include questions about any feeding difficulties, which may have been present from birth but often develop at weaning and in the toddler years. Eating difficulties may be the *cause* of the failure to thrive, or may be generated from the anxiety that naturally occurs when a baby grows poorly because of other causes. It is helpful to ask the mother to keep a food diary for a few days, recording all that the baby has eaten.

- *Review of symptoms.* Most organic conditions are identifiable by history. Diarrhoea, colic, vomiting, irritability, fatigue and chronic cough are the most important features to elicit.
- *Past medical history.* The birth history is important. A low birth weight may indicate adverse prenatal conditions that affect growth potential. Recurrent illness of any nature may affect growth.
- *Developmental history.* This is needed for two reasons. Firstly, failure to thrive may affect a baby's developmental progress and, secondly, the child who has neurodevelopmental problems from any cause often has associated eating difficulties that may be limiting nutritional intake.
- *Family history.* Relate the child's growth to that of other family members. Medical problems affecting other children in the family may suggest a diagnosis. A good social history should identify psychosocial problems that may be causing or at least contributing to the problem.

Examination
You need to carry out a full physical examination to complement the history. Occasionally clinical signs alone can indicate a cause for the poor growth.
- *General observations.* The baby's appearance is important. The healthy small baby will look very different from the neglected or ill child. The child who is malnourished for whatever reason will appear thin, with wasted buttocks, a protuberant abdomen and sparse hair. A neglected child may look unclean and uncared for. Observations must also extend to the mother and how she relates to the baby, which can provide valuable clues to maternal–infant attachment difficulties.
- *Growth.* Plot growth on a growth chart and compare current measurements with previous. The pattern of growth can be very helpful in the diagnostic process. Figure 22.6 shows growth charts that are illustrative of common conditions.

Q5. What investigations are indicated?

There is good evidence that 'fishing' for a diagnosis by carrying out multiple investigations is a futile exercise. Investigations should only be carried out if clues to a problem are obtained from the history and physical examination. The only exception is a blood count and ferritin level, as iron deficiency is extremely common in this group of children, and can affect both development and appetite. Other investigations that may be helpful, if clinically justified, are shown in Table 22.3.

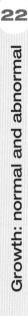

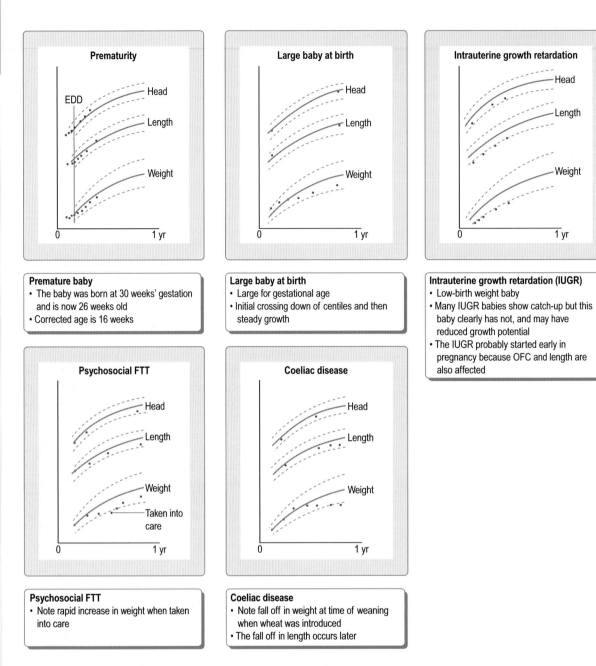

Premature baby
- The baby was born at 30 weeks' gestation and is now 26 weeks old
- Corrected age is 16 weeks

Large baby at birth
- Large for gestational age
- Initial crossing down of centiles and then steady growth

Intrauterine growth retardation (IUGR)
- Low-birth weight baby
- Many IUGR babies show catch-up but this baby clearly has not, and may have reduced growth potential
- The IUGR probably started early in pregnancy because OFC and length are also affected

Psychosocial FTT
- Note rapid increase in weight when taken into care

Coeliac disease
- Note fall off in weight at time of weaning when wheat was introduced
- The fall off in length occurs later

Fig. 22.6 Growth charts illustrating five common conditions in infancy. (EDD = expected delivery for dates; OFC = occipito-frontal circumference.)

Q6. What strategies and advice might be useful in James's situation?

The ability to nurture a baby is perhaps the most basic attribute of parenting. When a child fails to thrive it usually causes extreme distress, anxiety and feelings of inadequacy. It is important therefore that a normal, healthy but small baby is not wrongly labelled as having a problem. On the other hand, it is important that both organic and psychosocial problems are identified and addressed, as failure to thrive has important consequences on the child's developmental progress as well as growth. A thorough clinical evaluation, together with information from the health visitor, can usually sort out the problem. Helpful advice regarding the young child with eating difficulties is shown in Box 22.5. Occasionally admission to hospital for observation may be required.

Causes of failure to thrive (Box 22.4)

Non-organic weight faltering

The most common causes for weight faltering are psychosocial. The problems include difficulties in the

Table 22.3 Investigations to consider in the evaluation of failure to thrive

Investigation	What you are looking for
Full blood count, ferritin	Iron deficiency is common in failure to thrive and can cause anorexia
Urea and electrolytes	Unsuspected renal failure
Stool for elastase and fat globules	Pancreatic insufficiency and malabsorption
Coeliac antibodies, jejunal biopsy, sweat test	Coeliac disease and cystic fibrosis are causes of malabsorption
Thyroid hormone and thyroid-stimulating hormone	Congenital hypothyroidism causes poor growth and developmental delay
Karyotype	Chromosomal abnormalities are often associated with short stature and dysmorphism
Hospitalization	Hospitalization can be a form of investigation. Observation of baby and mother over time can provide clues to the aetiology

---

BOX 22.5 Helpful advice for a child with eating difficulties

Dietary advice
- Offer meals and snacks frequently to stimulate the appetite
- Start with food that the child likes
- Give only small amounts to start with and offer more if food is eaten
- Increase caloric intake naturally rather then by supplements, e.g. full-fat milk, cheese, yoghurt and butter added to mashed potato, pasta etc.
- Reduce fluid intake if > 1 pint per day, as this can reduce appetite
- Limit use of a dummy to encourage food intake and language development
- Never force-feed

Mealtimes
- Make mealtimes relaxed social events
- Let the child touch and play with food and encourage independent eating
- Limit mealtimes to 30 minutes, as little extra is gained by longer meals
- Praise the child for eating but pay little attention to aversive behaviour

---

home, limitations in the parents, disturbed attachment between the mother and child, maternal depression/psychiatric disorder and eating difficulties. Neglect is the underlying factor in only a few children.

Clinical features

Weight gain is usually first affected, but a reduction in linear growth and head circumference may follow and the child's developmental progress may be delayed. The family circumstances may range from the child from a caring home who is well looked after, with parents who are anxious and concerned and interact well with the child, to the neglected child. Eating difficulties, where the child has a minimal appetite or refuses to eat, are common. Meals are very stressful

and the parents may be drawn into excessive measures (sometimes force-feeding) to persuade the child to eat. At the other end of the spectrum is the neglected child who shows physical signs of poor care and emotional attachment. In this case the problem is often denied and compliance with intervention is poor.

Management

Management must be tailored to fit the problem. Most families can be helped by appropriate intervention, usually consisting of dietary advice and psychological support. Practical support can ease the stress, and nursery placement can be very helpful in this regard, as well as helping to resolve eating difficulties. In those cases where neglect is the cause and the family are not amenable to help, social services must be involved.

Prognosis

With appropriate intervention, the problem usually resolves or at least stabilizes. A few children need to be removed from their homes.

Genetic and organic causes

Gastro-oesophageal reflux

Vomiting and possetting are common complaints in a baby, and usually do not deleteriously affect growth. However, occasionally reflux can cause failure to thrive, particularly if associated with oesophagitis, which causes pain and anorexia.

Malabsorption

Malabsorption is an important cause of failure to thrive. Symptoms of diarrhoea and colic are usually present as diagnostic clues. The most common causes of malabsorption in childhood are coeliac disease and cystic fibrosis. In the former, the growth curve characteristically shows a falloff in weight coincident with the introduction of gluten to the diet.

Chronic illness

Children and babies with any chronic illness can fail to thrive. They rarely present as a diagnostic dilemma,

Table 22.4 The differential diagnosis of weight faltering/failure to thrive

Diagnosis	Growth pattern*	History	Physical examination
Constitutional	Steady growth below centiles, or 'catch-down' for larger baby	Short parent(s)	Normal
Psychosocial	Crossing down of centiles at any age	Eating difficulties common, maternal depression may be present	Usually normal but poor or disturbed maternal–infant attachment may be evident
Coeliac disease	Crossing down of centiles classically occurring at introduction of wheat solids	Frequent stools or diarrhoea, irritability	Distended abdomen, wasted buttocks
Cystic fibrosis	Crossing down of centiles	Appetite often fine, chest infections, diarrhoea	Poorly child Protuberant abdomen, decreased muscle mass, chest signs possible
Gastro-oesophageal reflux	Crossing down of centiles early in life	Vomiting, irritability, occasionally apnoea	Normal
Intrauterine growth retardation	Low birth weight with subsequent poor weight gain, length and head circumference may be reduced	Possible placental insufficiency, difficult pregnancy, smoking, alcohol	Small normal, look for signs of intrauterine infection (TORCH — *to*xoplasmosis, *rubella* cytomegalovirus, *herpes* simplex virus)
Neglect	Crossing down of centiles, catch-up if removed from home	Difficult or troubled family circumstances	Poorly cared for, nappy rash, developmental delay common

* Refers to weight in the first instance.

as the manifestations of the disease are usually evident. However, organic failure to thrive may be compounded by psychosocial difficulties and these need to be addressed. Very rarely, chronic disease can be occult and present as failure to thrive.

Genetic constitution
Small parents tend to have small children and the small healthy normal child of short parents should not arouse concern. Usually in this case growth is steady along the lower centiles, but the large baby born to small parents may cross down centile lines before settling on the destined line.

Intrauterine growth retardation
If a fetus experiences adverse uterine conditions its growth may be retarded. When this occurs early in gestation, length and head circumference in addition to weight can be affected. In this circumstance the potential for postnatal growth may be jeopardized. The cause of the intrauterine growth retardation should, where possible, be identified.

Genetic syndromes
Dysmorphic syndromes are not uncommonly associated with short stature. If dysmorphic features are present, the diagnosis can be suspected. An important syndrome causing shortness is Turner's syndrome (Ch. 35).

Endocrine dysfunction
Congenital hypothyroidism causes failure to thrive and developmental delay. Most cases are detected through neonatal screening.

The differential diagnosis of weight faltering/failure to thrive is given in Table 22.4.

Unusual head growth

The head grows rapidly in the first 2 years of life and then slows down, but continues to grow throughout childhood. In the early years the sutures are open, and then fuse around the age of 6 years. Prior to fusion they can separate in response to raised intracranial pressure. The posterior fontanelle usually closes by 8 weeks of age, and the anterior by 12–18 months.

Head size is not directly proportional to body size, but large children are more likely to have large heads, and vice versa. As in body growth, it is not unusual for head circumference measurements to cross centiles in the first year. However, when this occurs, clinical assessment is needed to exclude pathological causes.

The large head

(See also p. 290–1.)

Problem-orientated topic:

a child with a large head

The health visitor measures Jason's head at the 8-week check. She notes that the head circumference has crossed centiles since the

Continued overleaf

newborn examination (Fig. 22.7). Jason has been developing normally and is smiling and able to lift his head in the prone position. His parents describe him as easygoing and have no concerns.

Q1. Is this a worrying pattern of head growth?

Q2. What symptoms and signs should you look for in your clinical evaluation that might suggest hydrocephalus?

Q3. How do you advise the parents and health visitor?

Q1. Is this a worrying pattern of growth?

A large head is usually a normal variant, and often is a familial feature. An unusually large head may indicate hydrocephalus, in which case evidence of raised intracranial pressure may be present. Large heads may also be a feature of certain genetic syndromes. The causes of a large or enlarging head are shown in Box 22.6.

Q2. What symptoms and signs should you look for in your clinical evaluation that might suggest hydrocephalus?

Key points
- An enlarging head is a greater cause of concern than a steadily growing large head.
- Parental head size is helpful in deciding if this is a normal variant.
- Assess the baby's developmental skills.
- Evidence of raised intracranial pressure indicates hydrocephalus or subdural collection of fluid.

History
- *Is the baby developing normally?* Abnormal developmental progress in a child with a large head is strongly indicative of pathology.
- *Are there symptoms of raised intracranial pressure?* The baby with hydrocephalus or subdural effusion is likely to be irritable and lethargic, have a poor appetite and vomit.

Examination
- *Growth measures.* The pattern of head growth is important. Crossing of centile lines is a greater cause of concern than steady growth of a large head. Length and weight indicate whether the head is disproportionately large (Fig. 22.7).

BOX 22.6 Causes of a large or enlarging head
- Normal variation (often familial)
- Hydrocephalus
- Subdural effusion or haematomas
- Feature of certain dysmorphic syndromes

- *Signs of hydrocephalus.* The child with hydrocephalus has characteristic features (see below).
- *Development.* A developmental examination should accompany the developmental history.

Q3. How do you advise the parents and health visitor?

Frequent measurements of head circumference can generate anxiety, and should not be performed if the head size is considered to be a variant of normal. When raised intracranial pressure is suspected, immediate investigation is required, along with referral to neurosurgery. If the anterior fontanelle is still open, a cranial ultrasound can be performed to detect hydrocephalus, effusions or haemorrhage. If the fontanelles are closed, computed tomography (CT) or magnetic resonance imaging (MRI) scans are required to delineate underlying pathology.

Pathological causes of a large head

Hydrocephalus

Hydrocephalus may result from a congenital abnormality of the brain such as aqueductal stenosis, or be acquired as a result of intracranial haemorrhage, infection or tumour. Premature babies with severe intracranial haemorrhage are particularly at risk. Hydrocephalus is commonly associated with neural tube anomalies and occurs in 80% of babies with spina bifida (Ch. 28).

Clinical features
Clinical features include irritability, lethargy, poor appetite and vomiting. In infants, the anterior fontanelle is wide open and bulging, the sutures are separated and the scalp veins are dilated. The forehead is broad and the eyes deviated down, giving the 'setting sun' sign. Spasticity, clonus and brisk deep tendon reflexes are often demonstrable. In older children the signs are more subtle, with headache and a deterioration in school performance.

Management
Cranial ultrasound, CT and MRI scans provide information that determines the appropriate neurosurgical procedure.

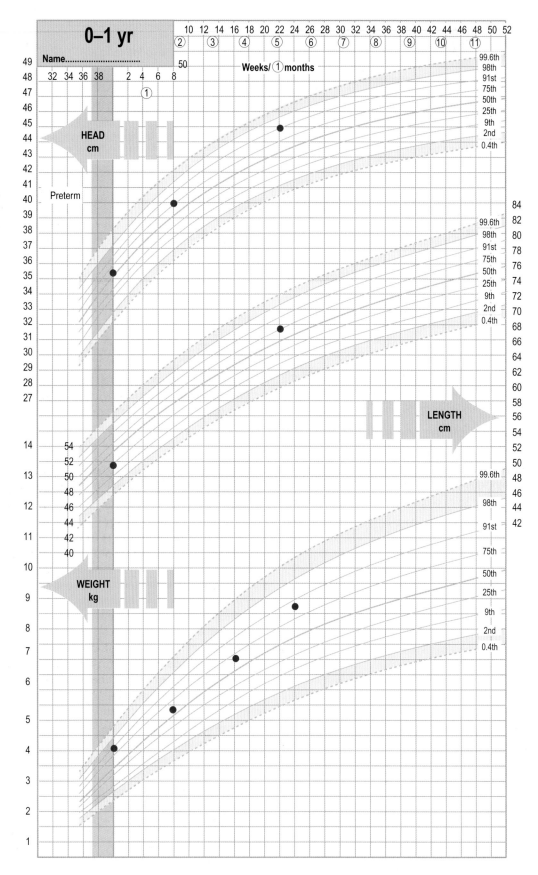

0–1 yr

Name................................

Preterm

HEAD cm

LENGTH cm

WEIGHT kg

Weeks/①months

Fig. 22.7 Jason's growth chart

Prognosis

Children with hydrocephalus are at increased risk for a variety of developmental disabilities and learning difficulties, particularly related to performance tasks and memory. Visual problems are also common. For these reasons it is important that they receive long-term follow-up.

Subdural effusions and haematomas

A subdural haematoma is a collection of bloody fluid under the dura. It results from rupture of the bridging veins that drain the cerebral cortex. Although any form of head trauma may produce subdural bleeding, a physically abused infant who is forcibly shaken is particularly susceptible to this injury (Ch. 37). Subdural haematomas may be acute or chronic, in which case they may eventually be replaced by a subdural collection of fluid. Subdural haematomas can lead to blockage of cerebrospinal fluid flow and hydrocephalus.

Clinical features

Although an enlarging head is a feature, the infant is more likely to present with fits, irritability, lethargy, vomiting and failure to thrive. Signs of raised intracranial pressure and retinal haemorrhages are common. Diagnosis is made by radiological imaging.

Management

Management is neurosurgical. All cases of subdural haematoma should be evaluated thoroughly for the possibility of abuse.

Prognosis

The prognosis for recovery is variable and depends on the associated cerebral insult.

The small head (microcephaly)

Problem-orientated topic:

a child with a small head

Julia is a 9-month-old baby. She was born small for gestational age and her growth has always been borderline, with her weight, length and head circumference now all between the 0.4th and 2nd centiles (Fig. 22.8). There are no dysmorphic features. Julia has just now achieved sitting with support and she has reasonable head control. She began to reach out for objects at 7 months and has just started transferring from hand to hand. She vocalizes with vowel but not consonant sounds.

Q1. Does Julia have microcephaly?

Q2. What do you need to focus on in your clinical evaluation?

Q3. Does Julia need to be investigated?

Q1. Does Julia have microcephaly?

By definition microcephaly is a head circumference below 2 standard deviations (below the 2nd centile). Julia therefore does have microcephaly; the question is whether this is of concern. A small head can be familial, in which case it can be quite normal. However, a small head may indicate limited brain growth, which can result from a number of perinatal insults. Very rarely poor head growth occurs as a result of premature fusion of cranial sutures (craniosynostosis). The causes of microcephaly are shown in Box 22.7.

Q2. What do you need to focus on in your clinical evaluation?

Key points

- Determine whether the child is developing normally.
- Check parental head size.

History

- *Is the baby developing normally?* If a baby is developing normally, it is unlikely that the head size is a cause for concern. If developmental delay is present, the baby needs to be evaluated for perinatal insults or genetic syndromes.
- *Past medical history.* The perinatal history may throw light on factors such as infection, alcohol or hypoxic–ischaemic events that may have affected brain growth.

Examination

- *Growth measures.* Length and weight of the baby indicate whether the head size is disproportionately small. The pattern of head growth is important. Crossing of centile lines is a greater cause of concern than steady growth of a small head.

BOX 22.7 Causes of microcephaly or poor head growth

- Normal variant (often familial)
- Limited brain growth:
  - Perinatal insult to the brain, e.g. hypoxic–ischaemic insult
  - Genetic syndromes usually associated with learning disability
  - Neurodegenerative conditions
  - Craniosynostosis (p. 255)

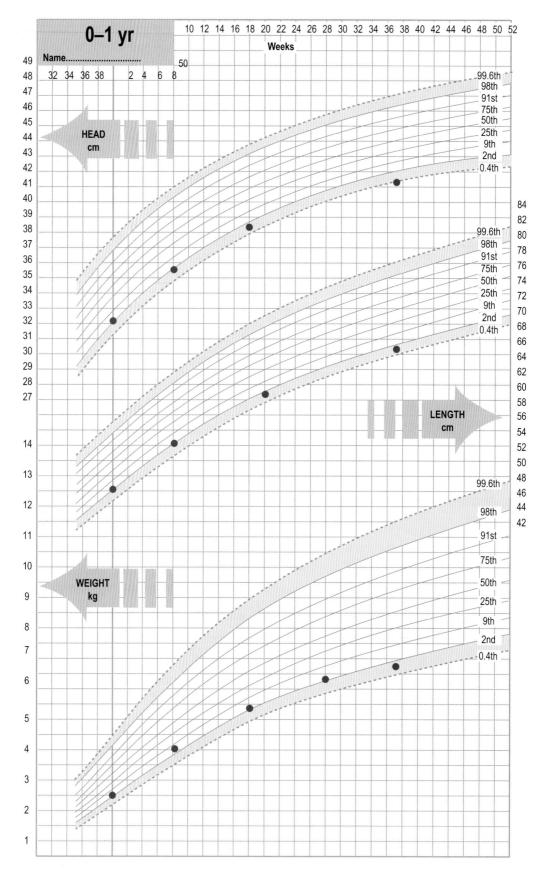

Fig. 22.8 **Julia's growth chart**

- *Parental head size.* Microcephaly in normal individuals is often familial.
- *Developmental skills.* Confirm the developmental history by carrying out a good developmental assessment.
- *Dysmorphic features.* Dysmorphic features suggest the diagnosis of a genetic syndrome.

Q3. Does Julia need to be investigated?

Julia has microcephaly and developmental delay, so she does merit investigation. If she did not have delay, there would be less concern. The level of developmental delay merits a good developmental evaluation and she should be referred to a developmental paediatrician. A karyotype and neurometabolic screen are indicated if a neurodegenerative or dysmorphic syndrome is suspected. An MRI might be helpful to determine underlying pathology. A skull X-ray is unlikely to be helpful unless craniosynostosis is suspected, in which case premature fusion of the sutures is seen.

Pathological causes of microcephaly

Cranial insults

A variety of insults to the developing brain can affect brain growth detrimentally and lead to microcephaly. These include:
- Hypoxic–ischaemic encephalopathy (Ch. 48)
- Congenital infections (Ch. 48)
- Genetic disorder or syndrome
- Toxins, such as alcohol
- Malnutrition
- Meningitis.

Developmental disorders

Many dysmorphic syndromes are accompanied by microcephaly. The most common of these is Down's syndrome.

Craniosynostosis (craniostenosis)

In this rare condition premature fusion of the sutures occurs. Very rarely all the sutures are involved, so restricting growth of the skull and, as a consequence, growth of the brain. This results in a rise in intracranial pressure. The diagnosis is made on plain skull X-ray and urgent neurosurgical intervention is required.

Obesity

Obesity is increasing as a problem in childhood. The vast majority of overweight children have nutritional obesity, and this diagnosis can be simply made on the basis of the clinical evaluation. The importance of identifying the obese child is principally in order to provide support and advice and to attempt to prevent the complications of obesity later in life. Although there is a folk belief that obesity is caused by a child's 'glands', this is very rarely the case.

Basic science of weight control

Body weight depends on the interaction of many genes, and twin studies have shown that 50–90% of BMI variability is genetically determined. The individual's response to high caloric intake is subject to strong genetic influence. Weight gain in children is a normal process, but its control is complicated and not yet fully understood.

There are four important factors:
- Food intake
- Signals from adipose tissue
- Central control
- Satiety signals.

Signals from adipose tissue

Under normal circumstances the amount of body fat influences food intake, requiring hormonal signals to be sent from fatty tissue to the brain to modify appetite. The most important appetite control hormone is leptin, although insulin also has a role. Increased adipose tissue causes increased blood leptin levels, which stimulate receptors within the hypothalamus and reduce appetite. Conversely, food deprivation reduces plasma leptin levels, stimulating appetite. Elevated leptin stimulates the release of hypothalamic melanocyte-stimulating hormone (MSH) and corticotrophin-releasing hormone (CRH) to reduce appetite. Low leptin levels stimulate hypothalamic release of neuropeptide Y (NPY), which increases appetite. High blood leptin levels inhibit NPY release (Fig. 22.9).

Satiety

A meal causes upper bowel distension and stimulates the brain to stop eating; this is mediated through hormones such as cholecystokinin (CCK), released by the bowel. The neurotransmitter serotonin is a primary satiety factor within the brain, and when released, reduces food intake.

 www.sciencedirect.com

Follow the links to English PJ, Wilding PH 2002 Applied physiology: the control of weight. Current Paediatrics 12:130–137

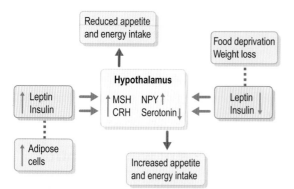

Fig. 22.9 Physiological mechanisms involved in appetite control

Common
- Nutritional

Rare
- Hypothyroidism
- Cushing's syndrome or disease
- Hypothalamic damage (tumours)
- Syndromes: Prader–Willi, Down's

- Calculate the BMI and plot it on a BMI growth chart.
- Assess the child for early complications resulting from obesity.
- Obtain a clear picture of the child's lifestyle, focusing on physical activity and diet.
- Find out about emotional and behavioural problems.

Weight alone is not a measure of obesity in childhood, but must be related to the child's height. Your clinical evaluation should firstly focus on excluding the rare endocrine and genetic causes of obesity. As all of these are accompanied by poor growth, they can be excluded on clinical grounds fairly easily. You then need to assess those aspects of the child's lifestyle that predispose to obesity and any emotional and behavioural difficulties the child is having.

Problem-orientated topic:

obesity

Kirsty is 10 years old. She comes to see you with her mother as she is troubled by her weight. As you can see from her growth chart (Fig. 22.10), she was always a big girl, and started to put on weight significantly when she was 3 years old. The family are concerned that she has a glandular problem causing her obesity.

Q1. Might there be a hormonal cause for Kirsty's obesity?
Q2. What should be included in your clinical assessment?
Q3. Should Kirsty have any investigations?
Q4. What treatment options are there?
Q5. What are the major complications of obesity?

Q1. Might there be a hormonal cause for Kirsty's obesity?

The best guide to whether there might be a medical cause for Kirsty's obesity is her growth chart. Children with nutritional obesity tend to be tall for their age, whereas those with a hormonal or syndromic cause are short or grow poorly (Fig. 22.11). The causes of obesity are shown in Box 22.8.

Q2. What should be included in your clinical assessment?

Key points
- Exclude rare causes of obesity, remembering that most of these children will be growing poorly.

History
- *Diet*. Ask what the child and family eat on a normal day, bearing in mind that this may be a sensitive issue. Nevertheless it can form a basis for advice.
- *Lifestyle*. Ask about physical activity during the day and also about sedentary activities.
- *Sleep problems*. Sleep apnoea is a common complication of obesity, so ask about snoring and about lethargy or tiredness during the day
- *Complications*. Musculoskeletal symptoms are common due to the increased load on the joints. It is rare for diabetes or cardiovascular disease to develop in childhood, although there may be biochemical indicators present.
- *Emotional and behavioural problems*. Social and school problems are very common. Children may be bullied or be bullies, or may suffer from significant depression.
- *Learning difficulties*. Children with a genetic syndrome associated with obesity are likely to have special educational needs.
- *Physical symptoms*. Ask about any physical symptoms that might suggest hypothyroidism or Cushing's disease (Ch. 35) as a cause.

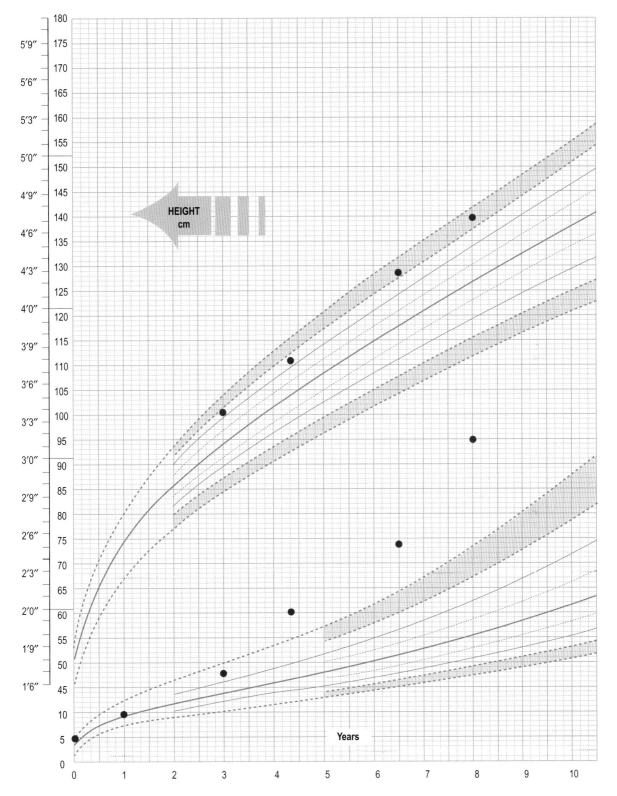

Fig. 22.10 **Kirsty's growth chart**

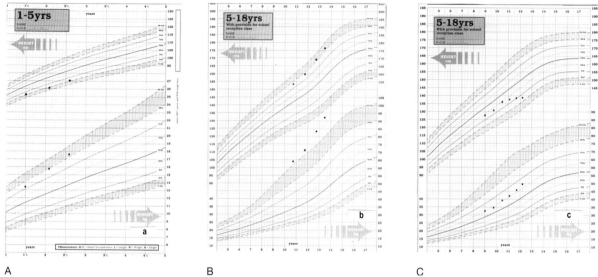

Fig. 22.11 Growth charts illustrating different causes of obesity.
(A) Obesity with short stature suggests a syndromic or hypothalamic cause; (B) obesity with tall stature suggests nutritional obesity; (C) obesity with falloff in growth suggests a hormonal cause.

Table 22.5 **Investigations that may be indicated in the obese child**

Aim	Investigation	Relevance
Looking for a cause	T4, TSH	Low T4 and high TSH are found in hypothyroidism
	Urinary free cortisol	High in Cushing's disease
	Karyotype and DNA analysis	Genetic syndrome
	MRI of the brain	Hypothalamic cause
Looking for consequences of obesity	Urinary glucose, fasting glucose and insulin or an oral glucose tolerance test	Diabetes
	Fasting lipid screen	Hyperlipidaemia
	Liver function tests	Fatty liver

- *Family history.* As obesity is a familial condition (genetically and environmentally), a family history is important. It is important to ask about any family members who have developed, or died from, diabetes or early heart disease.

Examination
- *Growth.* This is the most important indicator of a non-nutritional cause. In nutritional obesity, the child is relatively tall. With pathological causes, the child either is short or demonstrates a falloff in height as the weight increases (Fig. 22.11). You should also calculate the BMI and plot this and waist circumference on the appropriate charts (Fig. 22.12).
- *Signs of an endocrinological cause.* In the child with poor growth, look for signs of hypothyroidism (goitre, developmental delay, slow return of deep tendon reflexes, bradycardia) and steroid excess (moon face, buffalo hump, striae, hypertension, bruising).

- *Signs of dysmorphic syndromes.* Certain dysmorphic syndromes are characterized by obesity. These children are invariably short. Look in particular for microcephaly, hypogonadism, hypotonia and congenital anomalies.
- *Signs of complications.* Check the blood pressure and look for acanthosis nigricans (a dark velvety appearance at the neck and axillae), as this is a sign of insulin resistance.

Q3. Should Kirsty have any investigations?

Investigations (Table 22.5) are required if you are concerned that there is a non-nutritional cause for the obesity, particularly if the child is short, is dysmorphic, is demonstrating a falloff in height or has learning difficulties. In this case thyroid function tests, diurnal cortisol levels and genetic studies are indicated. If the child is very obese, investigation for heart disease, diabetes and steatohepatitis may be needed.

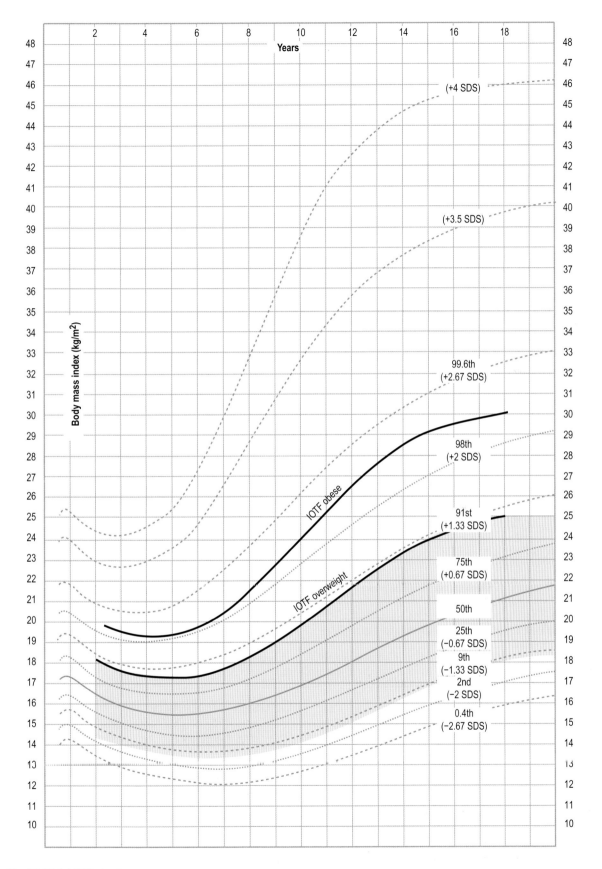

Fig. 22.12 (a) BMI chart

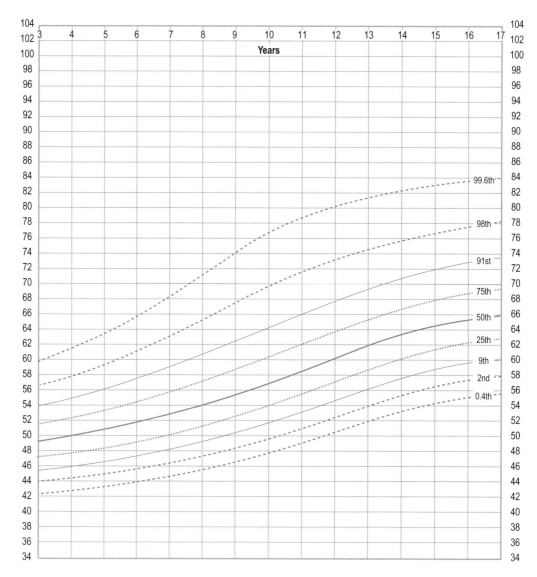

Fig. 22.12 *(cont'd)* **(b) waist circumference chart**

Q4. What treatment options are there?

Lifestyle management is the mainstay of treating obesity (as discussed below). At present there are no medications licensed for use in children.

Q5. What are the major complications of obesity?

Complications of obesity include:
- Psychological problems
- The metabolic syndrome: hyperinsulinism, hyperlipidaemia and hypertension
- Diabetes mellitus
- Cardiovascular disease
- Respiratory disorders, including obstructive sleep apnoea

- Musculoskeletal problems
- A predisposition to polycystic ovary syndrome.

Causes of obesity

Nutritional obesity

The metabolic factors that predispose some individuals to becoming obese have yet to be determined. The correlation between nutrient intake and development of obesity is not simple.

Clinical features

Nutritionally obese children tend to be tall for their age but develop puberty early, so that final height is not usually excessive. Boys' genitalia may appear deceptively small if buried in fat. Knock-knees are common. Obese children have a high incidence of emotional and behavioural difficulties.

Management

Obese children are often the victims of teasing by peers and psychological disturbance is common. If this is not addressed, it is unlikely that lifestyle change will be achieved. Even if weight control is not successful, continuous support is necessary to help these children cope with their condition. In advising on lifestyle it is essential that the family as a whole is engaged rather than targeting the child. Increasing physical activity is key. Reducing sedentary activity is especially important, and walking to school or swimming may be more acceptable than organized sports. In planning a diet, basic nutritional needs must be met. Rapid decreases in weight should not be attempted and during the growing years maintenance of weight, while the child increases in height, is a reasonable goal.

Prognosis

Despite medical intervention, reduction of obesity once it is well established is difficult. Psychological difficulties may well persist into the adult years. Society deals harshly with the obese and studies show that obesity is a handicap later in life. In childhood overt medical complications are few, although metabolic markers for cardiovascular disease, diabetes and fatty liver are common. Obese children are more susceptible to musculoskeletal strain and slipped capital femoral epiphyses. Rarely, insulin-resistant diabetes mellitus develops in childhood. For obese adults, morbidity is significant, with diabetes and hypertension common, leading to early mortality from ischaemic heart disease and strokes. Gallstones and certain cancers are also more prevalent.

Prevention

As in most conditions, prevention is better than cure. There is some evidence that breastfeeding in infancy is protective and promotion of good nutrition in the early years, when food habits are developing, is important. Physical activity needs to be encouraged in all children, not simply the obese. There is a need for these health issues to be addressed in school, particularly during adolescence, when high intake of high-fat foods and decrease in exercise are common. If intervention is provided early in the course of obesity, weight control is likely to be more successful.

Heart and lung disorders

MODULE FIVE

LEARNING OUTCOMES

It is important for primary care clinicians to have a structured approach to common respiratory and cardiac problems. By the end of this chapter you should be able to:

● Formulate a differential diagnosis for the common cardiac and respiratory problems that present to primary care

● Undertake an initial assessment and instigate the appropriate treatment for these illnesses

● Decide on when it is appropriate to refer to secondary/tertiary care services for further assessment of common respiratory and cardiac disorders.

Introduction

In the UK, respiratory illness remains one of the most common reasons for parents to take their child to the GP and for attendance at the accident and emergency department with a medical problem. Although the mortality from respiratory illness in developed countries is low, acute respiratory illness remains one of the leading causes of childhood death world-wide.

Unlike in adults, acquired cardiovascular disease in children is very rare in the UK. Congenital cardiac malformations are much more common, affecting up to 6 per 1000 live births.

Murmurs

(See also Ch. 41.)

BOX 23.1 Features of innocent ejection murmurs

- Systolic
- Soft blowing (pulmonary area) *or*
- Short buzzing (aortic area)
- Symptom-free
- Sign-free: normal pulses (palpable femoral pulses), no palpable thrills or heaves, heart sounds normal, no radiation of murmur and no signs of cardiac failure

Q1. What further features on history and examination would be important?

Although children with structural cardiac defects often have murmurs on clinical examination, the majority of murmurs heard in childhood are innocent. It is common for primary care physicians to detect murmurs in children, particularly in those presenting with a febrile illness, when the cardiac output is increased. It is therefore important to identify features that would discriminate between innocent and pathological murmurs.

There are two main types of innocent murmur:

- *Ejection murmurs.* These are caused by turbulent blood flow through the main outflow vessels of the heart. They are heard loudest in the aortic and pulmonary areas (Box 23.1).
- *Venous hum.* A continuous, low-pitched rumbling murmur is heard below the clavicles. It is caused by turbulent blood flow through the major head and neck vessels. The murmur will disappear when the child lies supine.

Q2. Would you refer this boy for further assessment?

Children with abnormal features on history or examination should be referred for further assessment. Murmurs detected in infancy need particular attention. It is now common practice in many centres for murmurs detected in the neonatal period to be referred for cardiology assessment, as the proportion of pathological murmurs is much higher within this group.

Chest pain

(See also Ch. 41.)

Q1. What further features of the history and examination would be important?

Chest pain is a common problem, particularly in the older child. Parents are often anxious and concerned that chest pain is caused by cardiac disease. However, it is unusual for cardiac conditions to present with chest pain in children and studies have estimated the incidence of cardiac-related disorders in children presenting with chest pain at around 1%. It is therefore important to distinguish features from both history and examination that will discriminate between benign chest pain and more significant pathology.

Q2. What causes of chest pain should you consider in your assessment?

See Table 23.1.

Table 23.1 **Causes of chest pain in children**

Type of pain	Associated features
Musculoskeletal	Local tenderness, pain exacerbated by inspiration or exercise Possible history of trauma
Respiratory	Acute onset of pleuritic pain, often unilateral with symptoms and signs of respiratory disease ± scoliosis Exercise-induced pain with wheeze or dyspnoea
Gastrointestinal	Burning retrosternal pain, epigastric tenderness

Cardiac
  Ischaemic pain
 	
  Pericardial
	
	Gripping, crushing ± radiation to neck, jaw and arms
	Dyspnoea and pallor ± palpitations
	Central sharp pleuritic pain, worse when supine

Psychogenic	History of stress factors, hyperventilation or panic attacks
Others	Shingles, nerve compression, mediastinal tumours, fibrocystic breast disease Gynaecomastia

Musculoskeletal causes

This is by far the most common cause of chest pain in children. Most children will experience short-lived lateral chest wall discomfort in relation to exertion that disappears on resting. This is what is commonly referred to as a 'stitch'. Trauma and muscular strains are also frequent innocent causes of chest pain. The presence of localized tenderness is almost always secondary to a musculoskeletal cause.

Central chest pain with associated tenderness along the costochondral margin is common with costochondritis. This is often a short benign self-limiting illness that responds to simple analgesia and avoidance of strenuous activity.

Precordial catch syndrome is a common childhood condition associated with stabbing left-sided anterior chest wall pain in the absence of respiratory and cardiac disease.

Coxsackie B viral infection (Bornholm disease) causes pleuritic chest pain (pain exacerbated by normal respiration) and chest wall tenderness in association with an upper respiratory tract infection and fever. Resolution often occurs within 1 week.

Respiratory causes

Asthma is a common condition that can cause mild chest discomfort and tightness on exertion. A history of wheeze and atopy supports the diagnosis. Symptoms should improve with inhaled bronchodilators.

Children who have pneumonia will frequently experience chest pain and discomfort secondary to muscular strain caused by excessive coughing.

Involvement of the pleura, as seen with a pleural effusion or empyema, will result in localized pain that is often worse on inspiration. There should be signs of acute illness and respiration is often shallow in an attempt to reduce pain. Air entry will be reduced on auscultation and resonance is dull on percussion. There may also be associated scoliosis in an attempt to reduce movement on the affected side.

Spontaneous pneumothoraces are occasionally seen in children with asthma or Marfan's syndrome and occasionally in healthy normal children. On auscultation air entry is reduced on the affected side, but the percussion note is increased.

Children with sickle cell disease (Ch. 43) can develop an 'acute chest syndrome' as a complication of their condition. Pneumonia and vaso-occlusion of the pulmonary arterioles result in chest pain associated with tachypnoea and signs of consolidation. This is a serious and potentially dangerous complication that needs urgent inpatient assessment.

Deep venous thrombosis and pulmonary embolism are extremely rare during childhood.

Gastrointestinal causes

Gastro-oesophageal reflux can cause oesophageal irritation and burning retrosternal pain, often with food contents or acid being regurgitated into the mouth. Symptoms are often exacerbated when the child lies supine.

Epigastric tenderness in association with chest pain is suggestive of peptic ulcer disease. However, this is an unusual cause of chest pain in children.

Diaphragmatic irritation in association with a number of gastrointestinal disorders (e.g. pancreatitis) can cause chest pain in children. Other features on history and examination that suggest a gastrointestinal cause will almost always be present.

Cardiac causes

Cardiac chest pain is the result of either myocardial ischaemia or pericardial disease.

Ischaemic chest pain is often described as gripping or tight. There may be radiation to the neck, jaw or arm. Pallor, shortness of breath and palpitations are common. Ischaemic pain may occur in children with coronary artery disease (Kawasaki's disease, anomalous coronary arteries, familial hypercholesterolaemia) or in association with tachyarrhythmias (supraventricular tachycardia, ventricular tachycardia).

Pericardial pain is often a central sharp stabbing pain that is exacerbated particularly in the supine position and by normal respiration. Pain may radiate to the shoulder or back. A pericardial rub may be detected (pericarditis) or the heart sounds may be decreased (pericardial effusion).

Aortic dissection should always be considered in children with chest pain and Marfan's syndrome.

Psychogenic causes

Around 30% of all chest pain in children, particularly the older child, is secondary to stress and anxiety. Episodes of pain are commonly associated with hyperventilation and panic attacks. It is important to identify possible triggers and situations in which symptoms arise (e.g. bullying).

Q3. When would you refer a patient for further assessment? (Box 23.2)

In the majority of cases, chest pain will be benign in nature. A detailed history and examination should help distinguish those who need further assessment. For the majority of children, simple analgesia and reassurance are all that is required.

Palpitations

Problem-orientated topic:

a child having palpitations

Susan is a 14-year-old girl who is concerned about episodes where she becomes aware that her heart is thumping and fast. She is extremely worried by these episodes and often hyperventilates.

Q1. What further features on history and examination would be important?

Q2. What are the common causes to consider?

Q3. What investigations would you perform?

Q4. How would you manage this patient's care?

Q1. What further features on history and examination would be important?

It is not unusual for children to become aware of their heart beat, particularly during periods of excitement or anxiety. In the majority of cases this is a normal phenomenon.

It is important to note the general health and emotional state of the child during the episode. Anxious children may experience palpitations associated with hyperventilation and discomfort within stressful situations.

Children who present with episodes of recurrent palpitations need careful assessment. It is important to highlight any family history of arrhythmias or sudden death. Palpitations that start and stop suddenly are more suggestive of a cardiac arrhythmia. Episodes associated with pallor, chest pain, dyspnoea or syncope will need further investigation for a possible cardiac cause.

Q2. What are the common causes to consider?

These include:
- Fever
- Anxiety/exercise
- Anaemia
- Hyperthyroidism
- Cardiac arrhythmia (Ch. 41).

Q3. What investigations would you perform?

When a cardiac arrhythmia is suspected, it is important to arrange a paediatric assessment and a 12-lead ECG. It is particularly important to assess the PR and QT corrected (QT_c) interval of the ECG.

The PR interval may be short in children with accessory electrical pathways between the atria and ventricles. This is often associated with episodes of supraventricular tachycardia (SVT). SVTs are the most common arrhythmias seen during childhood and are associated with very fast (> 210 beats per minute) regular tachycardias.

The QT interval is variable and dependent on the child's heart rate. This can be corrected for and most ECG machines will report the QT_c. Children with prolonged QT syndrome have QT_c intervals > 440 ms and are prone to episodes of ventricular tachycardia (VT) and sudden death. There is often a significant family history.

A normal PR and QT_c will not exclude paroxysmal arrhythmias. It is often difficult to detect arrhythmias when episodes are infrequent. A prolonged ambulant ECG recording is useful, but is dependent on episodes occurring during the period of monitoring.

Q4. How would you manage this patient's care?

The management is dependent on the likely cause. The case should be discussed with a paediatrician or paediatric cardiologist if there are concerns that the episode may be a possible arrhythmia (Ch. 41). Children experiencing anxiety-related palpitations should be reassured and offered support with any major stressors (e.g. bullying).

Syncope

(See also p. 291.)

Problem-orientated topic:

a child with syncope

Jane is a 12-year-old girl who has presented to the surgery after collapsing in assembly. She remembers feeling dizzy initially before falling to the floor and blacking out.

Q1. What further features on history and examination would be important?

Q2. What differentials should be considered?

Q3. How would you manage this symptom?

Q1. What further features on history and examination would be important?

Syncope or 'fainting' is a frequent occurrence during childhood. It is commonly benign and often neurally mediated. Serious and life-threatening causes are rare. Investigations are often normal and are not routinely required.

A careful history, examination including blood pressure (standing and supine) and an optional ECG are useful if there is any worry that this is not a simple faint.

Episodes that occur when the child lies supine or in relation to exercise should raise alarm bells. Likewise,

---

BOX 23.3 Differential diagnosis of syncope

Vasovagal syncope 'faint' (p. 291)

- Neurally induced bradycardia and hypotension
- Common particularly in older children (9–14 years)
- Occurs when upright; may be triggered by pain, emotional stimuli or prolonged standing
- Associated dizziness, nausea, blurred vision or pallor
- Secondary anoxic seizures can cause stiffening or fine twitching
- Recovery often rapid after lying down

Reflex anoxic seizures — 'pallid breath-holding spells' (p. 291)

- Young children (6 months to 3 years)
- Neurally induced transient asystole that occurs in response to pain or emotional stimuli
- Marked pallor, secondary anoxic seizures common

Cardiac

- Rare
- May be associated with palpitations, dyspnoea or chest pain
- Family history of sudden death

Epilepsy

- Uncommon to have isolated collapse without tonic or tonic–clonic phases
- Recovery is often slow — 'post-ictal phase'

Factitious

- Unwitnessed episodes
- Inconsistent story and inappropriate parental or child response

---

a family history of sudden unexpected death would cause concern.

Q2. What differentials should be considered?

See Box 23.3.

Q3. How would you manage this symptom?

Parents are often worried that there is a serious and life-threatening cause. It is important to reassure the child and family. Vasovagal syncope tends to improve with age. Increased water and salt intake may help those with frequent episodes.

Systemic
- Viral: influenza, viral exanthems (chickenpox, rubella, measles)
- Bacterial: meningococcal septicaemia, staphylococcal toxic shock
- Inflammatory: Kawasaki's disease

Upper respiratory tract
- Common cold, pharyngitis, tonsillitis, otitis media

Lower respiratory tract
- Pneumonia, bronchiolitis

Renal
- Urinary tract infection, pyelonephritis

Gastrointestinal
- Gastroenteritis, appendicitis

Neurological
- Meningitis

Musculoskeletal
- Septic arthritis, osteomyelitis

Persistent fever
- See Chapter 44

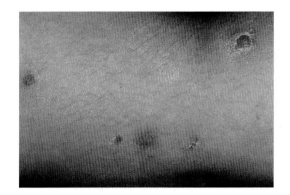

Fig. 23.1 **Chickenpox**

Respiratory tract infections

Problem-orientated topic:

febrile respiratory illness

Joseph is a 4-year-old boy who has been unwell with fever and cough for 3 days. He looks unwell and has a temperature of 39.5°C. He is tachypnoeic and grunting.

Q1. What are the main differential diagnoses to be considered?

Q2. What investigations should you consider?

Q1. What are the main differential diagnoses to be considered?

Infective or inflammatory disorders are most likely and these are listed in Box 23.4.

Q2. What investigations should you consider?

An infection screen is important, which as a minimum in primary care includes a throat swab and urine for culture and sensitivity. If there are concerns about meningococcal septicaemia, then immediate antibiotic treatment should be given (Ch. 44). In hospital, blood cultures and lumbar puncture are necessary if Joseph shows signs of altered consciousness or a stiff neck, or has a purpuric rash.

Non-specific viral illness

Febrile illnesses, with non-specific features of malaise, headache, nausea, cough and myalgia, are often caused by viral infections such as influenza. There are no specific clinical findings on examination and it is important to exclude clinically other causes of these symptoms. Management should be aimed at symptomatic relief with analgesia and antipyretics.

Viral exanthems

Chickenpox and other viral exanthems (measles, rubella etc.) present with features similar to influenza early on in the illness, before the onset of their characteristic rashes.

Chickenpox

Chickenpox is a common infection that is spread by droplet inhalation of the varicella zoster virus from contacts with either chickenpox or shingles (Fig. 23.1). The majority of children have a relatively mild illness when they contract it at an early age. Those who escape childhood infection are at a greater risk of developing the associated complications of chickenpox. Children who have impaired immunity (long-term corticosteroids, immunosuppressant therapy and treatment for malignancy) are at a significant risk of severe and fatal disease. Babies born to mothers who have developed chickenpox between 5 days before and 2 days after delivery are also at increased risk of severe neonatal varicella.

Clinical features

The incubation period between contact and disease is 14–21 days. Spots appear in crops initially on the face and trunk. What initially begins as a macule quickly progresses into a papule, followed by vesicle formation. New crops continue to develop, whilst the earlier crops form pustules before finally crusting over. The rash often causes intense itching. Constitutional symptoms are variable, ranging from mild fever and upset to signs of toxicity in those with more severe disease. The child remains infectious from 48 hours before the onset of the rash until all the crops have crusted over.

Complications

- Secondary bacterial infection
- Encephalitis (typically post-infectious with cerebellar involvement and ataxia)
- Pneumonia
- Disseminated haemorrhagic chickenpox
- Arthritis, hepatitis, pancreatitis, nephritis and thrombocytopenia.

Scarring and secondary bacterial (*Staphylococcus aureus* and *Streptococcus*) infection of the lesions are common complications. Other complications are less common in children.

Management

Immunocompetent children with chickenpox require symptomatic treatment only. Calamine lotion and cool baths are soothing. Oral antihistamines may help ease the itching. Immunocompromised children and babies with peripartum exposure should receive zoster immunoglobulin (ZIG) within 96 hours of contact. Those who develop features of chickenpox despite ZIG should receive intravenous aciclovir.

Vaccination against varicella is common in the US but at present this has not been routinely adopted in the UK.

Upper respiratory tract infection (URTI)

In children, the majority of respiratory infections affect the upper respiratory tract (ears, nose and throat). Viruses are by far the most common pathogen.

The most common URTIs include:
- Common cold
- Pharyngitis
- Tonsillitis
- Otitis media.

Pharyngitis

Children often present with sore throat and fever. The oropharynx is inflamed and erythematous. Pharyngitis is most commonly due to viral infection.

> **BOX 23.5 Indications for adenotonsillectomy**
> - Recurrent severe tonsillitis
> - Glue ear (with grommets)
> - Obstructive sleep apnoea

Tonsillitis

Tonsillitis can cause children to present with sore throat, fever, malaise, vomiting or meningism. On inspection the throat and tonsils are inflamed, often with pus on the surface of the tonsils. Cervical lymphadenopathy is a common feature.

Group A β-haemolytic streptococci and Epstein–Barr virus (EBV, glandular fever) are common causes. Clinically it is difficult to distinguish between bacterial and viral infections of the pharynx and tonsils. For most children treatment should be symptomatic, with prescriptions of analgesia, an antipyretic (paracetamol) and regular oral fluids. It would not be unreasonable to prescribe antibiotics to children with marked constitutional disturbance and high fever or those with pus on the tonsils. Oral penicillin V would be the treatment of choice in this situation. Amoxicillin should be avoided in children with tonsillitis, as it can precipitate a generalized erythematous rash in those with EBV infection.

Recurrent viral pharyngitis is common and often prompts parents to request adenotonsillectomy inappropriately (Box 23.5). Recurrent URTI and large tonsils are not an indication for routine tonsillectomy. Children often have large normal tonsils which later regress in size.

> **BOX 23.6 Common conditions predisposing to acute otitis media**
> - Down's syndrome
> - Cleft lip and palate
> - Other craniofacial abnormalities
> - Immunodeficiency

Acute otitis media (AOM) (see also Ch. 32)

AOM is very common, with approximately 1 in 4 children having had at least one episode in the first decade of life (Box 23.6). Otitis media occurs more frequently in children with associated structural abnormalities of the upper airway that affect the drainage of the Eustachian tube and aeration of the middle ear. Common pathogens include viruses, *Pneumococcus*, *Haemophilus*, *Moraxella catarrhalis*, β-haemolytic streptococci and *Strep. pyogenes*.

Clinical features

Young children with acute otitis media often present with non-specific features of fever, irritability and vomiting. All children who present with fever should have their ears examined, particularly children who are noted to be pulling at their ears.

The eardrum in AOM may appear injected or bulging, often with loss of normal light reflection. If perforation has occurred, the view may be obscured by purulent discharge.

Complications of AOM (mastoiditis and meningitis) are uncommon. Recurrent otitis media predisposes to glue ear and conductive hearing loss.

Management

The use of antibiotics in AOM has been subject to large reviews by both the American Academy of Paediatrics (AAP) and the Scottish Intercollegiate Guideline Network (SIGN). Both generally agree that the majority of children (older than 2 years) presenting to primary care with AOM will improve spontaneously, without the need for oral antibiotics. Instead of being prescribed antibiotics initially, children should be given paracetamol analgesia and a policy of delayed antibiotic prescription should be adopted (antibiotics to be collected at the parent's discretion after 72 hours, if the child has not improved). Children older than 2 years with severe AOM (moderate to severe otalgia and fever > 39°C) should be prescribed early antibiotics. Broad-spectrum antibiotics such as amoxicillin (± clavulanic acid) should be prescribed for 5 days initially.

At present there is little evidence for the correct management of children under the age of 2 years presenting with AOM; the AAP recommends antibiotics for all cases of certain AOM in this age group.

http://adc.bmjjournals.com/

Archives of Disease in Children: Education and Practice. Follow links to 'Comparison of Two Otitis Media Guidelines', and to 'Community-acquired Pneumonia in Children: a Clinical Update'

www.sign.ac.uk

SIGN. Follow links to guidelines on 'Diagnosis and Management of Childhood Otitis Media in Primary Care'

Glue ear (see also Ch. 32)

Glue ear is defined as the persistence of fluid in the middle ear in the absence of signs of active inflammation. It is the most common cause of conductive hearing loss in children. It is associated with an increased risk of speech and learning difficulties in affected children. It occurs commonly following AOM, although the majority of children with AOM and middle ear effusion will resolve spontaneously within 3 months. Like AOM, it is more common in children with structural ear, nose and throat (ENT) abnormalities.

Assessment

- Inspection of tympanic membrane (retracted drum and loss of light reflection)
- Hearing assessment appropriate to child's age
- Tympanometry.

Management

Glue ear will spontaneously resolve after 3 months in most children. Those cases persisting beyond 3 months need further assessment. There is little evidence of significant short-term and long-term effects of medical therapy for glue ear (decongestants, mucolytics, anti-histamines, antibiotics and systemic steroids). Children with glue ear and significant hearing loss will require insertion of aeration tubes (grommets). This is often combined with adenoidectomy for better resolution of symptoms.

Chronic suppurative otitis media (CSOM)

CSOM is a condition of chronic middle ear infection associated with perforation of the eardrum and intermittent or persistent ear discharge. Children with CSOM should be referred for ENT assessment.

There are two broad groups:
- 'Safe' CSOM. Perforation occurs in the central aspect of the eardrum.
- 'Unsafe' CSOM. Perforation occurs in the margins of the eardrum or severe retraction of the drum. This is associated with increased risk of VII cranial nerve palsy, abscess formation and intracranial complications.

Lower respiratory tract infection (LRTI)

Infections of the lower respiratory tract are commonly caused by viruses. *Pneumococcus*, *Haemophilus* and *Mycoplasma* are important pathogens in bacterial pneumonia.

The common LRTIs are:
- Pneumonia
- Bronchiolitis.

Community-acquired pneumonia (CAP)

Pneumonia (Box 23.7) occurs more frequently in children under 5 years of age. Viruses alone account for up to one-third (14–35%) of all childhood CAP. A good proportion (8–40%) of CAP represents mixed infection.

Respiratory viruses
- Respiratory syncytial virus (RSV)
- Adenovirus
- Influenza
- Parainfluenza
- Metapneumovirus

Mixed
- Common viruses plus bacteria

Bacteria
- Common: *Streptococcus pneumoniae, Mycoplasma, Haemophilus influenzae*
- Others: *Chlamydia trachomatis, Bordetella pertussis, Staphylococcus aureus, Mycobacterium tuberculosis* (TB)

Age is a reasonable predictor of likely pathogen; children under the age of 5 are more likely to have a viral cause, although *Strep. pneumoniae* is important.

Viruses are less common in children over the age of 5, and when a bacterial cause is found, it is most commonly *Strep. pneumoniae* or *Mycoplasma* infection.

Clinical features

Fever, dyspnoea and cough are common symptoms reported in children presenting with pneumonia. Feeding difficulties associated with respiratory distress are particularly common in small children. Older children with pneumonia occasionally present to surgeons with abdominal pain secondary to diaphragmatic irritation.

Signs of pneumonia include:
- Fever
- Tachypnoea
- Recession and nasal flaring
- Grunting
- Cyanosis
- Decreased chest expansion
- Dullness to percussion
- Decreased air entry
- Crepitations
- Bronchial breathing (consolidation).

Tachypnoea and fever are good indicators of pneumonia, although both can be present in other conditions such as asthma. Chest signs may be unilateral (lobar pneumonia) or bilateral (bronchopneumonia).

Mycoplasma infection can often cause wheeze, cough and bilateral chest signs, making the distinction between *Mycoplasma* infection and asthma difficult. It is therefore important to consider *Mycoplasma* infection

in older children with wheeze that fails to respond to conventional asthma therapy.

No one sign on its own is diagnostic of pneumonia. It is the combination of signs that will aid the clinician in the consideration of a possible diagnosis of pneumonia. The absence of all signs is probably of more use in excluding pneumonia. However, pneumonia should still be considered in all acutely ill children under 5 years of age who present with fever of > 39°C with no alternative cause, even in the absence of respiratory symptoms or chest signs.

Complications

Complications of CAP affect only a small proportion of children. They include:
- Pleural effusion and empyema
- Septicaemia
- Lung abscess
- Secondary sepsis: osteomyelitis, septic arthritis.

Investigations

The ideal investigation will confirm the diagnosis of pneumonia and distinguish between bacterial and viral causes. Unfortunately there is no rapid and reliable test that can fit both of these criteria.

- *Blood tests.* Acute phase reactants (erythrocyte sedimentation rate, white cell count and C-reactive protein) are unreliable in distinguishing between bacterial and viral pneumonia. The yield from blood cultures in children with pneumonia is low and results can take up to 48 hours before they are available. Thus they have little impact on the initial decision to treat or not to treat with antibiotics. Routine collection of blood cultures should be reserved for children who require admission to hospital for suspected pneumonia.

  Paired serology for *Mycoplasma* infection is useful in cases of pneumonia that are not responding to treatment. Again it has no impact on the initial decision to treat or not to treat because of the delay in receiving results.

- *Nasopharyngeal aspirate (NPA).* This is recommended to identify respiratory viruses in children < 18 months of age.

- *Chest X-ray (CXR).* Consolidation on the CXR is the most consistent sign of infection and is considered the most reliable method of confirming the diagnosis of pneumonia (Figs 23.2 and 23.3). More subtle changes are subject to large differences in interpretation, reflecting the differences in opinion amongst clinicians and radiologists. Radiological findings may lag behind clinical signs, so a negative CXR does not always exclude pneumonia when there are clear clinical signs. Secondly, studies suggest that radiological

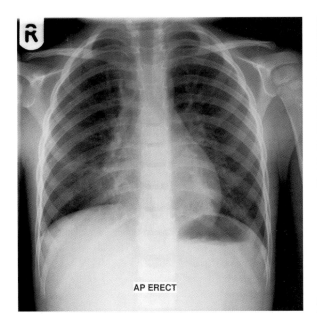

AP ERECT

Fig. 23.2 **Chest X-ray in right middle lobe pneumonia**

consolidation alone cannot be used to assume bacterial infection.

Routine CXR is not required to confirm the diagnosis of pneumonia in children who are well enough to be managed at home. The CXR is useful for confirming the diagnosis and identifying any complications (pleural effusions) in those

admitted for hospital treatment. Interpretation of radiological signs should always be taken in context of the child's age and clinical status (Box 23.8 and Fig. 23.4).

Management

Young children with mild features of infection do not require investigation or treatment with antibiotics. For all other children, antibiotic treatment is recommended.

The majority of children in the community will respond to oral antibiotics prescribed for 5–7 days. Amoxicillin is a good first choice of antibiotic for children with CAP. In the under-5s it is effective against

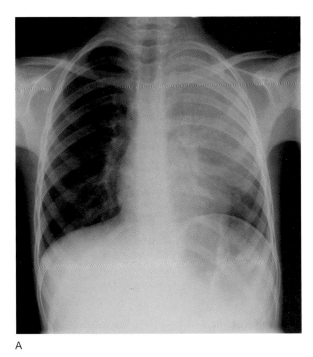

A

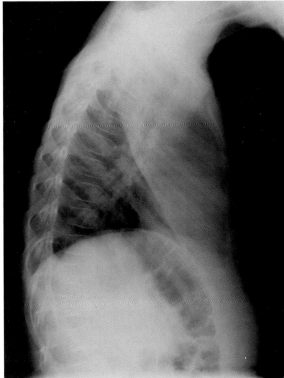

B

Fig. 23.3 **Chest X-ray in left upper lobe pneumonia.**
(A) PA sitting; (B) lateral.

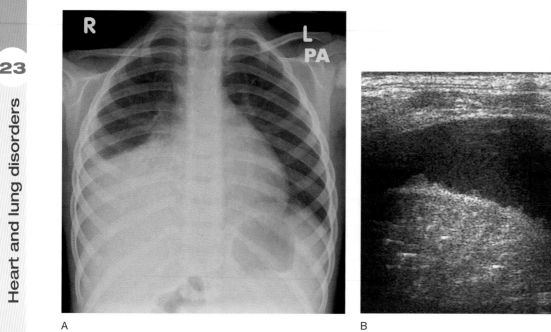

A   B

Fig. 23.4 Right-sided pleural effusion secondary to chest infection.
(A) PA X-ray; (B) ultrasound showing fluid collection above the right diaphragm.

most bacterial pathogens. Macrolide antibiotics (erythromycin, clarithromycin) are good first-line treatments in older children when *Mycoplasma* or *Chlamydia* infection is suspected. If *Staph. aureus* is suspected, then a combination of flucloxacillin and amoxicillin should be prescribed.

The child well enough to be cared for at home on oral antibiotics should be reviewed by the GP if there are any signs of deterioration or if there is no improvement after 48 hours of treatment.

Intravenous antibiotics should be used in the treatment of pneumonia in children who are unable to absorb oral antibiotics or those with features of severe disease. In such circumstances the total (intravenous and oral) course of treatment should be extended to 10 days.

Criteria for admission are as follows:
- The child is vomiting and unable to tolerate oral medication.
- There are signs of severe disease (Box 23.9).
- There are social concerns about the parents' ability to monitor the child effectively.

Wheeze

Problem-orientated topic:

a wheezing child

Samantha is a 3-year-old girl who attends the GP clinic with a 1-day history of noisy

> **BOX 23.9 Signs of severe disease**
>
> - Oxygen saturations < 92% on air
> - Respiratory rate > 70/min in infants
> - Respiratory rate > 50/min in older children
> - Chest recessions, nasal flaring, grunting and apnoea
> - Feeding < 50% normal fluids
> - Signs of dehydration

breathing. On examination she is coryzal, her temperature is 36.8°C and the respiratory rate is 32, and on inspection she has mild respiratory distress. On auscultation of the chest she has good air entry but has widespread bilateral wheeze.

Q1. What differential diagnoses should be considered with a child who presents with wheeze?

Q2. What further history and examination would be useful?

Q1. **What differential diagnoses should be considered with a child who presents with wheeze?**

See Box 23.10.

BOX 23.10 Causes of wheeze in children

Asthma

- Recurrent episodes of cough and wheeze, responsive to inhaled bronchodilators
- Cough, often worse at night
- History of atopy in child or other family members
- Triggers: smoke, pollution, animal dander, house dust mite, cold weather, viral infections, stress and exercise

Bronchiolitis

- Majority of cases < 9 months
- Occurs in winter epidemics
- Coryza, cough, dyspnoea and difficulty in feeding; apnoeas in small babies; poor response to bronchodilators
- Crackles and wheeze on auscultation
- CXR: hyperinflation, patchy perihilar changes ± collapse
- 80% RSV-positive on NPA

Viral-induced wheeze

- Wheeze with infection
- Often past history of bronchiolitis
- Variable response to treatment; may progress to asthma

Mycoplasma pneumoniae

- Older children with wheeze and cough that fail to respond to conventional asthma therapy

Inhaled foreign body

- Toddler with history of choking
- Rapid onset of wheeze and cough
- CXR shows hyperinflation or segmental collapse
- Poor response to inhaled bronchodilators

Heart failure

- Crackles and wheeze on auscultation
- Murmur and hepatomegaly are common
- Enlarged heart on CXR

Q2. What further history and examination would be useful?

At 3 years of age Samantha is too old for bronchiolitis, and an inhaled foreign body would also be unlikely at this age. She had mild bronchiolitis as a baby but was never troubled by her breathing until 3 months ago. Her father had asthma as a child. On examination she has eczema. There were no murmurs or hepatomegaly detected. This makes asthma the most likely diagnosis.

Asthma

Children who are genetically predisposed to asthma develop inflammation and hyper-reactivity of the small airways in response to infection, environmental triggers or exercise. Symptoms are the consequence of small airway obstruction secondary to mucosal oedema, excess mucus production and bronchoconstriction.

The diagnosis of asthma is based on history and response to conventional treatment in the absence of features suggesting alternative diagnoses. Children with asthma have recurrent episodes of cough, wheeze and dyspnoea. Exercise-induced symptoms are common. The reversibility of airway obstruction with inhaled bronchodilators and steroids is an essential feature of asthma. Atopy, the tendency to have eczema, hay fever, allergy and allergic rhinitis, is common amongst asthmatics and their family. One-third of asthmatic children suffer from eczema and almost a half have allergic rhinitis.

Management

The treatment of asthma can be divided into two areas:

- Acute treatment
- Preventing exacerbations/minimizing impact of disease on lifestyle.

Management of acute exacerbation in primary care

The immediate treatment of asthma in primary care depends on the presence or absence of severe or life-threatening features (Box 23.11).

Mild to moderate attacks that show no features of severe or life-threatening asthma can be managed with inhaled β_2-agonists (salbutamol or terbutaline) delivered via a large-volume spacer device. Children aged < 3 years will require a spacer with a face mask rather than a mouthpiece. Children > 3 years should be assessed on an individual basis.

Two to four puffs of salbutamol regularly according to clinical response might be sufficient for mild attacks. Up to ten puffs may be needed initially for more significant exacerbations. Children with acute asthma in primary care who have not improved after receiving an initial dose of ten puffs of inhaled β_2-agonist should be referred to hospital for further assessment. Further doses of inhaled bronchodilator should be given if a nebulizer is unavailable whilst awaiting transfer.

The early use of oral steroids for acute asthma can reduce the need for hospital admission and prevent relapse of symptoms (Table 23.2). There is no evidence to support the use of inhaled steroids as alternative or additional treatment to oral steroids for the treatment

BOX 23.11 Clinical features of severe and life-threatening asthma

Acute severe
- Cannot complete sentences in one breath or too breathless to talk or feed
- Pulse > 120 bpm in children aged > 5 years
- Pulse > 130 bpm in children aged 2–5 years
- Respiration > 30 breaths/min in children aged > 5 years
- Respiration > 50 breaths/min in children aged 2–5 years

Life-threatening
- Silent chest
- Cyanosis
- Poor respiratory effort
- Hypotension
- Exhaustion
- Confusion
- Coma

Table 23.2 Prednisolone dose

Age	Dose
< 2 years	10 mg
2–5 years	20 mg
> 5 years	30–40 mg

of an acute exacerbation. The effects of oral steroids start to become apparent within 3–4 hours of commencing treatment.

Severe or life-threatening asthma requires urgent referral for inpatient care. Nebulized bronchodilator therapy with salbutamol or terbutaline should be commenced prior to arrival of the paramedic team. If no nebulized therapy is available, then inhaled bronchodilators should be administered through a large-volume spacer.

Preventing exacerbations/minimizing impact of asthma on lifestyle

The aim of asthma therapy is to:
- Achieve good symptom control
- Minimize restriction of activities and exercise
- Have a minimal need for reliever therapy
- Reduce exacerbations
- Improve lung function (peak flow > 80% of predicted)
- Avoid side-effects of therapy.

In order to monitor the success of asthma therapies, it is important to assess regularly:
- Frequency and severity of cough, breathlessness and wheeze
- Any sleep disturbance
- Usual exercise tolerance

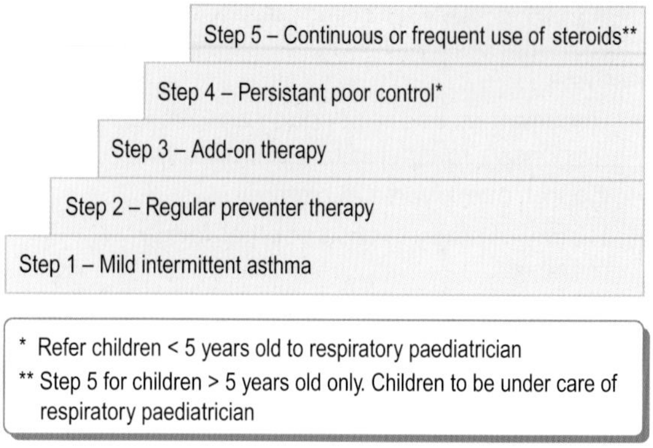

Step 5 – Continuous or frequent use of steroids**

Step 4 – Persistant poor control*

Step 3 – Add-on therapy

Step 2 – Regular preventer therapy

Step 1 – Mild intermittent asthma

* Refer children < 5 years old to respiratory paediatrician
** Step 5 for children > 5 years old only. Children to be under care of respiratory paediatrician

Fig. 23.5 **Stepwise management of asthma in children**

- Avoidance of activities/exercise because of symptoms
- Number and severity of exacerbations over past 6–12 months
- Number of days missed from school because of asthma
- Any chest deformity/Harrison sulci (poor control)
- Growth.

The stepwise management of asthma is illustrated in Figure 23.5. Patients should commence therapy at the step most appropriate to the severity of their asthma. In order to achieve control, stepping up the treatment may be required, in the same way as treatment should be stepped down when asthma has been well controlled and stable. This model stresses the importance of regular monitoring and review of medication.

Step 1: Mild intermittent asthma

Children with mild symptoms should be prescribed inhaled bronchodilators with β_2-agonists (salbutamol/terbutaline) as required.

Step 2: Regular preventer therapy

Regular inhaled corticosteroids should be considered in children who are symptomatic or using β_2-agonists more than three times per week, waking one or more night per week with asthma or having significant exacerbations. In children a reasonable starting dose would be 200 µg/day of budesonide equivalent split over two doses. (*N.B. 100 µg of inhaled budesonide is equivalent to 100 µg of beclomethasone. 50 µg of inhaled fluticasone is equivalent in efficacy to 100 µg of budesonide or 100 µg of beclomethasone.*) Children older than 12 would start at 400 µg/day. If steroids are not acceptable to the family, then a leukotriene receptor antagonist would be an acceptable alternative.

Step 3: Add-on therapy

Children who are still symptomatic after step 2 should receive additional therapy. This is very dependent on the child's age:

- *< 2 years*. Go to step 4 and refer to a paediatrician with a respiratory interest.
- *2–5 years*. Give a trial of an oral leukotriene receptor antagonist (e.g. Singulair).
- *> 5 years*. Use a long-acting bronchodilator (LABA) with β_2-agonist (e.g. salmeterol):
  - If there is a good response, then continue LABA.
  - If there is a partial response but control is still poor, continue LABA and increase the dose of inhaled corticosteroids to 400 µg/day (if 5–12 years) or 800 µg/day (if >12 years) of budesonide equivalent.
  - If there is no response, stop LABA. Increase the daily dose of inhaled corticosteroids to 400 µg/day (if < 12 years) or 800 µg/day (if > 12 years) of budesonide equivalent and consider an oral leukotriene receptor antagonist or oral theophylline.

Step 4: Persistent poor control

It is important to question the diagnosis of asthma in those children with persistent poor control. Children younger than 5 years should be referred to a paediatrician with a respiratory interest for further assessment. Children older than 5 years should have their inhaled corticosteroids increased to 800 µg/day of becotide equivalent and referral should be considered.

Step 5: Oral steroids

Children older than 5 years may be considered for regular or intermittent oral prednisolone. This should be under the direct supervision of a paediatrician with a respiratory interest.

Key point

- Before stepping therapy up and down, always check inhaler technique, compliance and possible elimination of trigger factors.

Inhaler devices

- *Metered-dose inhalers (MDI)*. See Figures 23.6–23.9.
- *Breath-actuated MDIs*. See Figures 23.10 and 23.11.
- *Dry powder inhalers*. See Figures 23.12 and 23.13.

The choice of drug delivery for stable asthma should be based on patient preference and an assessment of correct usage. Many patients may struggle to use an MDI without spacer correctly and it is better to suggest a dry powder device, MDI with spacer (± mask) or breath-actuated MDI inhaler. It is important to consider prescribing more than one device. An MDI with spacer is as effective as a nebulizer for treating mild to moderate exacerbations of asthma, but many children will not carry a spacer on their person and will need a smaller device for ease of

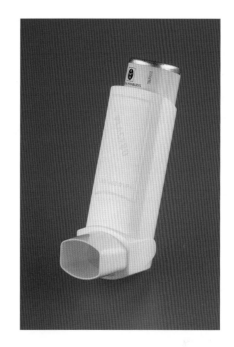

Fig. 23.6 **Pressurized aerosol metered-dose inhaler (MDI)**

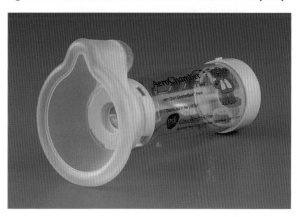

Fig. 23.7 **AeroChamber spacer device**

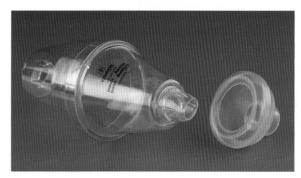

Fig. 23.8 **Volumatic spacer inhaler**

access to treatment. It would be good practice to give every child a spacer and MDI for acute exacerbations as well as their preferred choice of inhaler.

Generally, breath-actuated and dry powder devices are for children older than 5 years of age. Children

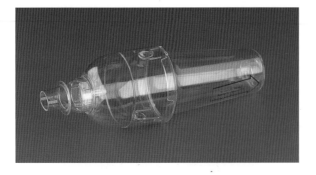

Fig. 23.9 **Nebuhaler spacer inhaler**

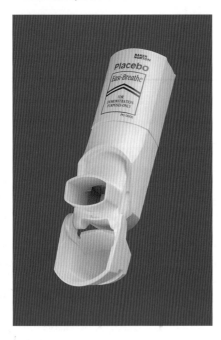

Fig. 23.10 **Easi-Breathe aerosol inhaler**

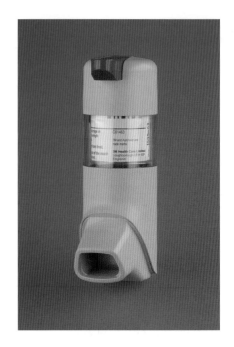

Fig. 23.11 **Autohaler aerosol inhaler**

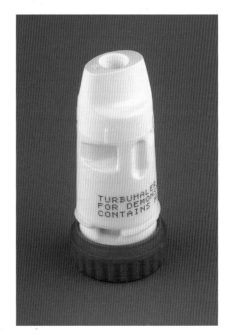

Fig. 23.12 **Turbohaler powder inhaler**

under 5 years should have a spacer device. The aerochamber with mask is better for small children. Often from about 3 years children will be able to start using a large-volume spacer or blue aerochamber with mouthpiece, which improves drug delivery.

When to refer

See Box 23.12.

www.brit-thoracic.org.uk/

British Thoracic Society (BTS). Follow links to guidelines on BTS/SIGN 'British Guideline on the Management of Asthma' and 'Guidelines for the Management of Community-acquired Pneumonia in Children'

Bronchiolitis

Bronchiolitis (Box 23.13) is a common viral respiratory tract infection occurring in annual winter epidemics. It affects children under the age of 18 months, although the majority of cases occur in those who are less than 9 months of age.

RSV accounts for 75–80% of cases, the remainder being caused by adenovirus, influenza and parainfluenza viruses. It is one of the most common reasons for acute presentation to primary and secondary care during the winter period.

There is currently no vaccine against RSV infection. High-risk infants (those with congenital heart disease

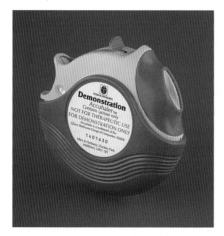

Fig. 23.13 **Accuhaler (dry powder for inhalation)**

BOX 23.12 Indications for referral to secondary care

- Diagnosis unclear or in doubt
- Symptoms present from birth or perinatal lung problem
- Excessive vomiting or possetting
- Severe upper respiratory tract infection
- Persistent wet cough
- Family history of unusual chest disease
- Failure to thrive
- Unexpected clinical findings, e.g. focal signs in the chest, abnormal voice or cry, dysphagia, inspiratory stridor
- Failure to respond to conventional treatment (particularly inhaled corticosteroids above 400 µg/day or frequent use of steroid tablets)
- Parental anxiety or need for reassurance

---

and ex-premature infants with chronic lung disease) are offered passive immunity with monoclonal antibodies to RSV. This is given as monthly intramuscular injections during the winter months.

Investigations

Pulse oximetry is essential in all bronchiolitic children with signs of respiratory distress. NPAs are sent for immunofluorescence to RSV and other common respiratory viruses. In most children bronchiolitis is a clinical diagnosis and routine CXR adds little benefit. Where the clinical features are atypical (high fever, unilateral signs, prolonged illness) or when the child shows signs of severe respiratory distress, a CXR and basic blood parameters (full blood count, urea and electrolytes and blood cultures) may be useful if secondary bacterial infection is suspected.

BOX 23.13 Clinical features of bronchiolitis

History
- Coryzal illness, cough, dyspnoea and poor feeding
- Apnoea in small babies

Examination
- Tachypnoea and tachycardia
- Hyperinflated chest
- Intercostal and subcostal recession
- Wheeze and crepitations
- Pale or cyanosed

Investigations
- Pulse oximetry
- NPA: RSV and respiratory viruses
- CXR (not required for straightforward cases):
  - Hyperinflation (flat diaphragms and horizontal ribs)
  - Patchy collapse and consolidation

Management

The majority of children with bronchiolitis will be managed safely in their own home, with reassurance and advice to parents on when to return. Indications for admission include low oxygen saturations, signs of severe respiratory distress, apnoeas, poor feeding, parental anxiety and infants who have risk factors for more severe disease.

Children admitted with bronchiolitis and poor feeding will often require either nasogastric or intravenous fluids. Humidified oxygen is delivered by head box. Handling of the infant should be kept to a minimum. Routine antibiotics are not prescribed unless there is evidence of secondary infection. Ribavirin is rarely used in most UK centres. Inhaled and oral steroids are of no benefit in the treatment of bronchiolitis.

Complications

Most children will recover from bronchiolitis within 1–2 weeks. A high proportion of children will develop wheeze with subsequent viral infections in the first few years following bronchiolitis.

Bronchiolitis obliterans is a rare complication of bronchiolitis infection. Most cases occur with severe viral infection, most commonly adenovirus. Chronic inflammation of the airway is associated with more permanent damage to the small airways.

Inhaled foreign body

Foreign body inhalation must always be considered in children presenting with acute respiratory difficulties or pneumonia that is failing to respond to treatment.

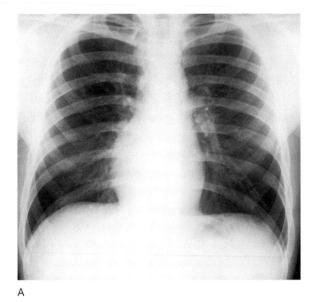

A

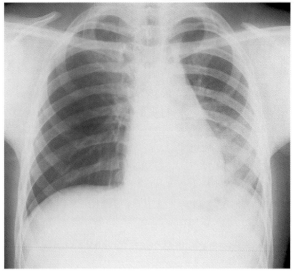

B

Fig. 23.14 Inhaled foreign body.
(A) Inspiratory X-ray film; (B) expiratory X-ray film.

Mobile toddlers who place everything into their mouth are at the greatest risk of inhaling small objects such as peanuts or beads. Thankfully the death rate from inhaled foreign body in childhood has fallen in recent years, partly related to increased public awareness.

Clinical features
The clinical features following inhaled foreign body are related to the position of lodgment. The most common place for lodgment of a foreign body in children has been shown to be the right main bronchus, accounting for 42%, whereas 17% will become lodged in the larynx or trachea.

Wheeze is a common feature if the main stem bronchus is involved, stridor can occur with high obstruction and chronic cough occurs with segmental collapse. The wheeze associated with foreign body inhalation is often fixed and sometimes unilateral, and the response to bronchodilator therapy is poor. Children with recurrent pneumonia, where there is failure of a collapsed lobe to re-expand, may have a distally lodged foreign body. Children with undiagnosed foreign body aspiration are at long-term risk of bronchiectasis in the affected lobe.

Often, but not always, there will be a history of choking associated with rapid onset of breathing difficulties, but there is often a delay between the choking episode and presentation. A careful history is essential to avoid overlooking this important diagnosis.

Diagnosis
The diagnosis of inhaled foreign body is supported by radiological changes on CXR (Fig. 23.14).

Management
If foreign body aspiration is strongly suspected, rigid bronchoscopy should be performed under general anaesthesia.

Cough

Problem-orientated topic:

a child with recurrent disturbing cough

John is a 6-year-old boy who presents to his local surgery for the second time with a history of disturbing cough over the past 3 weeks. When he first presented to the surgery he was prescribed oral amoxicillin for a presumed lower respiratory tract infection.

The cough is not associated with any fever or productive sputum. He has not travelled recently and there has been no infectious contact. The family did not notice any choking before the onset of symptoms. Although his cough is worse at night, he has never been particularly troubled in the past and there is no associated wheeze.

John has been previously fit and well. There is no history of atopy. Both parents are smokers.

Continued overleaf

Clinical examination is unremarkable. His height and weight are on the 50th centile. His peak flow is 98% predicted for his height.

John and his mother are increasingly concerned about the duration of his symptoms.

Q1. What differential diagnoses should be considered in a child with recurrent cough?

Q2. What do you think is the most likely diagnosis?

Q1. What differential diagnoses should be considered in a child with recurrent cough?

See Box 23.14.

Asthma is a common cause of chronic cough in children. Although John has a cough that is worse at night, the fact that he has never been troubled previously, the absence of wheeze, the lack of family history of atopy, and the normal peak flow readings would go against asthma as a likely cause of his symptoms. It would be unusual for cystic fibrosis or primary ciliary dyskinesia to present at this age in a child who is otherwise well and thriving. Likewise, there is nothing in the history to suggest recurrent infections and immune deficiency. It would be unusual for a 6-year-old to inhale a foreign body and without a significant history this would be extremely unlikely. The lack of fever, foreign travel or contact with TB would rule out TB as a likely cause.

BOX 23.14 Causes of recurrent or persistent cough in children

- Prolonged infection (viral, *Mycoplasma*, pertussis, TB)
- Postnasal drip (rhinitis)
- Gastro-oesophageal reflux
- Asthma
- Inhaled foreign body
- Cystic fibrosis
- Primary ciliary dyskinesia
- Immune deficiency
- Habit
- Smoking (including passive)

Q2. What do you think is the most likely diagnosis?

In John's case, the most likely cause of cough is prolonged infection with *Mycoplasma*, pertussis or viral pathogens. It would be appropriate to reassure John and his parents that it is not unusual for a cough to last several weeks before disappearing. A 7–10-day course with a macrolide antibiotic (erythromycin or clarithromycin) would be appropriate if *Mycoplasma* or pertussis infection were suspected.

It is well recognized that parental smoking is a significant risk factor for recurrent episodes of cough and wheeze during childhood. It may be appropriate to highlight the risks and offer smoking cessation support.

Pertussis (whooping cough)

Whooping cough is an infection characterized by paroxysms or spasms of cough associated with vomiting and inspiratory whoop. The majority of children affected by the disease are under the age of 5 years, with those under 12 months being more severely affected. In small children the typical whoop is often absent. However, apnoeas and cyanotic episodes are more frequent. The paroxysmal stage is often preceded by an early catarrhal stage associated with rhinorrhoea, malaise, conjunctivitis and fever. The paroxysmal stage can typically last up to 10–12 weeks.

Complications
- Pneumonia
- Encephalopathy
- Bronchiectasis (late).

Complications of pertussis are rare but there still remains a significant mortality associated with the disease, particularly under the age of 1. Small children with cyanotic or apnoeic episodes require hospitalization during the worst stages of the illness.

Diagnosis
Diagnosis of whooping cough is confirmed by culture of the bacterium *Bordetella pertussis* on per nasal swabs. Per nasal swab culture can take several days or weeks to confirm the diagnosis.

Management
Children should be prescribed oral erythromycin in order to eradicate organism carriage and reduce spread amongst other family members. Unfortunately erythromycin does not alter the course of the illness in those with active infection. Current vaccination programmes in the UK provide up to 90% protection

Table 23.3 Important causes of stridor in children

Diagnosis	Feature
Croup	Most common cause of acute stridor Peak age 1–2 years old Barking cough, hoarse voice, low-grade fever Often mild illness, although can occasionally be severe and need referral to paediatric intensive care unit (PICU)
Epiglottitis	Rare since vaccination against *Haemophilus influenzae* type B Often 1–7 years old Toxic, drooling saliva, dysphagia, soft muffled voice, no cough and quiet stridor Paediatric emergency
Bacterial tracheitis	Uncommon Usual organism *Staph. aureus* Toxic sick child with stridor, often requires intubation and IV antibiotics
Anaphylaxis	Acute stridor with swollen lips and/or urticaria following allergen exposure
Inhaled foreign body	Toddlers with history of choking Sudden onset of symptoms
Laryngomalacia	Noted in first few weeks of life, often from birth Floppy larynx that collapses inwards on inspiration Chronic stridor worse with crying, feeding, lying supine and infection (acute on chronic) Often resolves spontaneously by 1–2 years
Structural abnormalities	Uncommon, often < 4 months of age Children with multiple cavernous haemangiomas may have subglottic lesions Ex-preterm infants may have subglottic stenosis from endotracheal intubation

against pertussis infection after all three primary immunizations.

Stridor

Problem-orientated topic:

13 **a child with a loud barking cough**

Ben is a 1-year-old boy with a 2-day history of cough and noisy breathing. On examination he has a loud barking cough. His respiratory rate is 34 breaths per minute. He has significant tracheal tug and inspiratory stridor at rest. His temperature is 38.1°C. His parents have tried steam but there has been no improvement.

Q1. What important causes must you consider?

Q2. What therapies do you think may be effective?

Q3. When should you refer to hospital?

Q1. What important causes must you consider?

See Table 23.3.

Viral croup (laryngotracheobronchitis)

Viral croup is the most common cause of acute stridor in children. The peak age is around 1–2 years of age.

Common pathogens include parainfluenza virus, RSV and rhinovirus. Inflammation and partial obstruction of the upper airways (larynx, trachea and bronchi) result in stridor and cough. Small children are particularly at risk because of the relative small size of their upper airways.

Unlike the relatively rare conditions such as epiglottitis and bacterial tracheitis, croup has a more insidious onset over a few days. Systemic toxicity and fever are considerably less. Children with croup have a typical barking or seal-like cough, often associated with a hoarse voice, stridor and low-grade fever. Symptoms last 3 days on average and, as in many respiratory conditions, symptoms are often worse at night.

The majority of children with croup will have a mild illness that can be managed at home. Children with significant respiratory distress and stridor at rest will require treatment and reassessment. Those who show significant improvement following treatment may be considered for discharge home. There should be a low threshold for admission in children under the age of 12 months, all children with marked respiratory distress or oxygen requirement at presentation, and cases where parents remain concerned or anxious about discharge. Parents of children not requiring admission should receive clear instructions when to return (chest wall recession, tracheal tug, tachypnoea, colour change, inability to feed and decreased level of consciousness).

Spasmodic croup

Some children can develop recurrent short-lived episodes of croup, particularly at night, without the typical coryzal prodrome that is seen in classical viral croup. A history of atopy and episodic stridor is common in children with spasmodic croup. However, there are large numbers of children who have recurrent episodes of croup with features of both viral and spasmodic croup. It is more likely that these two presentations are opposite ends of a spectrum of a single illness.

Q2. What therapies do you think may be effective?

Simple measures
In all cases of stridor, it is very important to keep the child and parents calm. Direct inspection of the throat can be dangerous and may result in complete obstruction of the airway. Likewise, routine lateral neck X-rays are no longer useful and carry the risk of further upset and deterioration.

Humidification
Steam inhalation for croup is widely used but of little proven benefit. The perceived benefit (placebo effect) reported by many families probably relates to the presence of the carer in a warm calming environment. There is little reason to discourage the use of steam at home, provided it is done safely. A steamy bathroom with the hot water tap running and the plug open is acceptable, but any use of kettles or bowls of hot water should be discouraged because of the risk of scalding.

Adrenaline (epinephrine)
Nebulized adrenaline is very effective in severe croup; the alpha-mediated vasoconstriction results in decreased mucosal oedema. The duration of action is between 20 minutes and 3 hours. Adrenaline is used in the most severe cases when intubation is considered. The waning pharmacological effects of adrenaline result in a return to the pre-treatment baseline rather than a true rebound. For a considerable number of children with severe croup, the period of improvement on adrenaline is long enough to allow the steroid treatment to start working.

Steroids
Approximately 1–5% of croup cases required endotracheal intubation before the introduction of steroid therapy. The use of corticosteroids has been shown to improve clinical parameters, decrease admission rate, decrease the duration of hospital stay, and reduce the need for rescue nebulized adrenaline in children with croup. Nebulized budesonide or oral dexamethasone have been shown to be equally effective in treating children with mild, moderate and severe croup. Studies comparing oral dexamethasone with nebulized

budesonide showed no significant difference in duration of onset.

Intubation
A small number of children will still require endotracheal intubation for severe croup. The decision to intubate should be based on worsening airway obstruction with signs of exhaustion or impending respiratory failure. Children with epiglottitis and bacterial tracheitis require specialist care, with input from senior ENT and anaesthetic staff. Intravenous antibiotics and intubation are often required. Steroids and adrenaline have minimal effect on these conditions.

Q3. When should you refer to hospital?

Most children with acute stridor will have viral croup. Those with mild croup (no signs of respiratory distress at rest) may be managed at home, with parental observation. Children with significant respiratory distress or those showing atypical features should be referred for acute paediatric assessment.

Ben has a typical history suggestive of viral croup. His significant inspiratory stridor at rest with marked tracheal tug would require acute paediatric assessment.

Worrying signs in children with stridor are listed in Box 23.15.

Snoring

Problem-orientated topic:

a boy who snores

Mohammed is a 6-year-old boy who has been brought to the surgery by his mother. His mum is concerned that he is difficult to wake in the morning and tires easily during the day. General physical examination is unremarkable apart from grossly enlarged tonsils.

Continued overleaf

On further questioning, his worried mum comments that he snores very loudly.

How would you assess this problem?

How would you assess this problem?

Sleep-disordered breathing is a spectrum of disorders ranging from primary snoring to obstructive sleep apnoea. Snoring can occur in as many as 10–25% of children. However, less than 10% of these may have obstructive episodes of apnoea during sleep. The prevalence of behavioural disorders (aggression and hyperactivity) and cognitive impairment is increased in children who have significant sleep-disordered breathing.

Children with a history of significant snoring or obstructive episodes during sleep should be screened using overnight oximetry. Children who have obstructive sleep apnoea will often demonstrate significant periods of desaturation associated with periods of obstructed breathing (30–45 seconds). Adenotonsillectomy can often lead to a dramatic improvement in children with primary obstructive sleep apnoea.

Allergic rhinitis

Allergic rhinitis is a common paediatric problem that is often dismissed as trivial or minor. Sufferers may complain of nasal discharge, itchy nose, sniffling, nasal congestion and excessive sneezing. Postnasal drip and cough are common, as are nosebleeds and middle ear effusions (glue ear) with associated hearing loss. It is not unusual for parents and teachers to become annoyed by the child's symptoms. Mouth breathing and snoring are also common. Sleep disturbance and school absence trouble the more severely affected cases.

Inflammation of the nasal mucosa in allergic rhinitis is usually mediated through the IgE inflammatory response to inhaled allergens. Perennial (all-year-round) symptoms are often triggered by house dust mite and animal dander, whereas seasonal rhinitis is often associated with pollens. Chronic inflammation of the nasal mucosa results in increased reactivity to non-allergenic stimuli such as heat and cold.

Allergic rhinitis is more common in children with a history of asthma, eczema or food allergy. Rhinitis is occasionally a feature of other conditions. Nasal polyps are uncommon in allergic rhinitis, so their presence would raise the suspicion of an alternative cause.

Cystic fibrosis and primary ciliary dyskinesia (Ch. 42) are probably the most important disorders to consider when polyps are detected.

Investigations

Routine investigations are not always required. IgE and radioallergosorbence testing (RAST) to common allergens may be useful to identify triggers, although not essential.

Management

Inhaled nasal steroids are safe and effective in the treatment of children with allergic rhinitis. The newer non-sedating antihistamines are useful adjuncts. Topical and systemic decongestants are of limited use in allergic rhinitis and should be avoided. All children should be given routine advice regarding house dust mite measures and avoidance of trigger factors.

Epistaxis

Epistaxis or nosebleed is common in childhood. More than 90% of bleeds occur anteriorly and arise from Little's area, where the venous plexus forms on the septum. These bleeds often provide a constant ooze of blood loss. Bleeding is often associated with local trauma from nose picking.

Investigations

Children with a history of recurrent nosebleeds and abnormal bruising/bleeding or a significant family history of bleeding disorders should be screened for coagulation disorders, along with a full blood count to exclude thrombocytopenia (leukaemia).

Bleeding associated with an offensive discharge should raise the suspicion of retained foreign body. Systemic hypertension rarely causes nosebleeds in children.

Management

It is often easy to control bleeding by applying local pressure (5–30 minutes) over the soft part of the nose. A nasal pack can be inserted if this fails. Cauterization of a bleeding point may also be performed for recurrent significant bleeding.

www.clinicalevidence.com

Follow the links to the child health section: asthma, acute otitis media, bronchiolitis, croup and nosebleeds in children

Arnab Seal   Gillian Robinson

Brain and movement disorders

LEARNING OUTCOMES

By the end of this chapter you should:

- Know how to assess and manage pain in children
- Know how to assess a crying baby and be aware of common causes
- Know how to assess children with headaches, recognizing common causes and danger signs
- Know how to assess children with abnormalities of head shape and size and how to distinguish normal variants from pathological conditions
- Know how to evaluate the child with episodic strange movements
- Know how to differentiate epileptic disorders from other paroxysmal disorders
- Know how to assess febrile seizures and be able to counsel parents
- Know how to assess and manage a child with a limp and recognize underlying common causes
- Know how to assess and manage a child with back pain.

MODULE FIVE

Recognition, assessment and management of pain in children

Painful conditions and procedures are common in babies and children. Recognition, assessment and management of pain are important, as unrecognized and inadequately managed pain can have negative physical and psychological consequences. In children this is particularly challenging due to their difficulties in expressing their pain to adults in ways that are recognized and clearly understood. At different ages and from child to child, children vary greatly in their

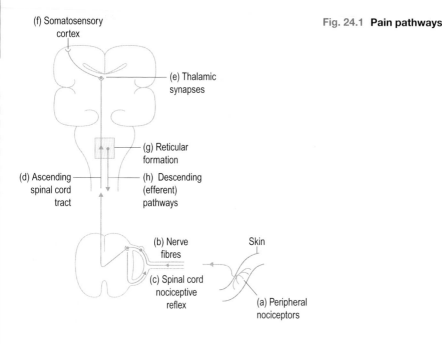

Fig. 24.1 **Pain pathways**

(f) Somatosensory cortex

(e) Thalamic synapses

(g) Reticular formation

(d) Ascending spinal cord tract

(h) Descending (efferent) pathways

(b) Nerve fibres

Skin

(c) Spinal cord nociceptive reflex

(a) Peripheral nociceptors

emotional and cognitive development, as well as their response to pain. It is also important to appreciate the effect of cultural factors, which may affect pain perception. This leads different children to prefer different strategies when managing their pain.

It is difficult to assess pain and distress separately. As pain perception increases with escalating distress, this also needs to be addressed. Measures include explanation to both the parents and the child, addressing their anxieties, comforting the child and providing distraction in addition to pain relief.

Basic science of pain

Pain evokes both a neurological and an emotional effect. The neurological pain pathways are shown in Figure 24.1. Pain is detected in peripheral nociceptors, or pain receptors (a), which are afferent nerve endings of myelinated A-delta and unmyelinated C nerve fibres (b). These synapse at the spinal cord, where a nociceptive reflex (c) exists that prompts withdrawal from painful stimuli before conscious perception of pain occurs. Pain impulses then ascend the spinal cord (d) to the somatosensory cortex (f) via subcortical connections in the thalamus (e).

Pain perception is modulated both in ascending pathways and in brainstem areas that affect descending (efferent) pathways (h) in the reticular formation (g) and inhibit pain stimuli, thus reducing pain perception and awareness in the injured tissue. Endogenous opioids such as endorphins and enkephalins have an important role in this effect.

Pain assessment

Pain needs to be assessed with techniques appropriate to the child's age and cognitive ability (see also p. 106). Pain can be assessed by:
- The child reporting pain
- The parent reporting pain on the child's behalf
- A change in a child's appearance, behaviour and activity level
- A change in physiological parameters: heart rate, blood pressure and respiratory rate
- Knowledge of the underlying medical condition and how it affects children.

There are a number of validated pain assessment and self-reporting tools available. Self-reporting tools can be reliably used for children over the age of 4 years. Pain assessment tools, which have a behavioural and a physiological basis, can be used from birth onwards. It is important to use a pain assessment tool that is appropriate to the child's developmental level, personality and condition. Examples include:
- Objective pain scale (OPS) for neonates and toddlers, which uses blood pressure, crying, movement, agitation and a verbal evaluation of body language indicators
- 'Faces' for 3–7-year-olds, which uses a set of cartoon-style faces in various stages of pain (Fig. 10.2, p. 106)
- Linear analogue scales for children over 3 years, which use a vertical or horizontal line with verbal, facial or numerical anchors on a continuum of pain intensity.

Holistic pain assessment should include the child's self-report using a validated pain assessment tool, and the parent or carer's report, together with the assessment of appropriately trained staff.

Pain management

Where pain is identified and its severity is assessed, measures are needed for its control. The management of pain involves identifying and addressing the cause of the pain, adequate analgesia and comfort. Children's distress may be helped by the presence of their usual carer, feeding, distraction or play therapy. The choice of analgesic and route of administration depends on the pain severity and cause. Opioids are of choice in severe pain, whilst paracetamol and ibuprofen are useful for mild to moderate pain. The route of administration and the dosage should be tailored to the needs of the individual child. There is little risk of adverse events if the correct dosage is used. Patient-controlled analgesia in children over 6 years and parent-controlled analgesia have been shown to be effective in the control of severe pain.

The use of local anaesthetic agents, either topically, e.g. local anaesthetic cream prior to venepuncture (p. 117), or by local infiltration or by regional techniques is a safe and effective method of controlling procedural pain in children. Topical anaesthetic cream (Emla, Amitop) needs to be applied under an occlusive dressing some 45–60 minutes before the painful procedure.

An accurate assessment of pain intensity, a combination of pharmacological and non-pharmacological measures to control pain and distress, and adequate counselling of the child and family are effective in pain management in babies and children.

Post-operative pain relief is discussed in Chapter 49.

🌐 www.rcn.org.uk/resources/guidelines.php

The recognition and assessment of acute pain in children

The crying baby

Problem-orientated topic:

a baby who will not stop crying

Mum brings Joe, a 3-month-old baby, to you, her GP, as she is concerned that he has been crying and inconsolable for the last 18 hours. He has always been an unsettled baby, especially in the early evenings.

Q1. What is normal crying?
Q2. What is the most likely cause of Joe's crying?
Q3. What other causes should be considered?
Q4. What should you look for in your clinical evaluation?
Q5. Which investigations are useful?
Q6. When should referral to hospital be considered?

Q1. What is normal crying?

Babies cry to communicate their needs to their carers. Parents soon recognize different cries as signalling hunger, discomfort from a dirty nappy, a need for company and tiredness. Parents find the crying child that cannot be comforted stressful and worrying. A normal baby's crying increases from birth to a maximum at 2 months, averaging 2–2.5 hours a day, with a peak between 6 and 12 p.m. Excessive crying is most frequently a symptom of a problem with the child, but it may also reflect a problem within the environment being sensed by the baby; tense anxious parents will often have tense anxious babies.

Q2. What is the most likely cause of Joe's crying?

Three-month-old Joe's inconsolable crying, especially in the evenings, is likely to be a form of infantile colic. Colic is used to describe babies in the first months of life who have episodes of inconsolable crying, accompanied by drawing up of the knees, which occur a number of times a day, particularly in the evening. To date no cause has been identified. Useful strategies to manage this include:

- Providing a routine and avoiding over-stimulation
- Holding the baby and walking with him or her, or gently jogging the infant up and down
- White noise, such as the washing machine
- Visiting family and friends, and allowing trusted carers to help with the baby
- In the absence of a trusted carer and if the crying is intolerable, leaving the baby safely in cot or crib while the carer has some time away from the noise.

Q3. What other causes should be considered?

Abnormal or unusual crying in babies can be due to a variety of conditions. Asking parents about the nature of the cry and assessing whether the baby appears well or not help in diagnosis (Fig. 24.2).

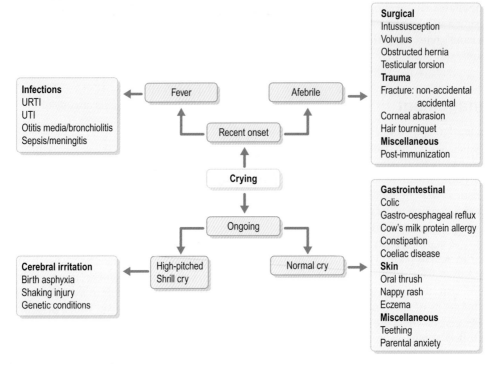

Fig. 24.2 The crying baby: differential diagnosis.
(URTI = upper respiratory tract infection; UTI = urinary tract infection.)

Q4. What should you look for in your clinical evaluation?

A good history and physical examination will identify most pathological causes of excessive crying (Box 24.1).

History
Ask the carers about:
- Recent change in cry, feeding or general alertness (meningitis, sepsis, shaking injury)
- Recent temperature (infections)
- Vomiting and whether bilious (bowel obstruction)
- Frequency and nature of baby's stool (constipation, gastroenteritis, intussusception)
- Timing of last immunization
- Whether the baby is moving all four limbs normally (trauma, non-accidental injury)
- Social history: how many other children there are in the family, social support available.

Examination
Assess the following:
- Temperature, perfusion, skin for rashes, including nappy area or bruising
- Coryzal symptoms: runny nose
- Respiratory system: respiratory rate, work of breathing
- Examination of ears and throat for signs of infection

BOX 24.1 Clinical evaluation of the crying baby

Ask yourself:
- Does this baby 'handle well' or is it an unwell baby?
- Are the parents coping and is there enough support for them at home?

- Abdominal examination: including mouth for thrush, any tenderness or masses, hernial orifices and testes
- Cardiovascular examination: including peripheral pulses
- Central nervous system examination: fontanelle, alertness, tone, ability to be comforted
- Limbs: swelling, localized tenderness, pain on limb movement
- Digits: ensure no hair or fabric tourniquet
- Eyes: fluoroscein — corneal abrasion; fundi — any retinal haemorrhages.

Q5. Which investigations are useful?

If the history and examination point to a particular cause, then specific investigation should be undertaken to confirm this, e.g. abdominal ultrasound for suspected intussusception.

Any irritable, unwell baby with fever needs to have clean-catch urine taken for urinalysis and microscopy culture and sensitivity. If this fails to demonstrate a cause, a septic screen should be considered, which could include full blood count (FBC), C-reactive protein (CRP), chest X-ray and lumbar puncture.

In the absence of any pointers in a well baby, reassurance with or without a period of observation is the correct management strategy. Always offer parents the opportunity to return if they have further concerns.

Q6. When should referral to hospital be considered?

- Baby appears systemically unwell
- Baby is febrile without a clinical focus
- Baby has bilious vomiting
- Baby cries, with episodes of pallor
- Baby has hernia or swollen testes
- Baby is of socially isolated carers
- Baby appears to have limb pain or there are concerns about child abuse (Ch. 21).

Headache

Problem-orientated topic:

a child with intermittent headache

Jasmine is a 12-year-old girl who, over the last 6 months, has been complaining of intermittent headache. She describes the headaches as being over both sides of her forehead, starting suddenly and being severe and throbbing. They make her feel sick. If she lies down in a dark room for a few hours the headache goes away. The headaches used to occur around once a month, but they are starting to become more frequent. Jasmine has been sent home early from school on a number of occasions due to her headaches. At school she is a popular girl and manages well with her school work. Apart from the headaches, she is in good health. Her mother remembers having similar headaches as a teenager. Jasmine is growing well and her examination is unremarkable.

Q1. What conditions should be considered?
Q2. What is the likely cause of Jasmine's headaches?

Q3. What are the important features to elicit in the clinical assessment?
Q4. When is referral indicated?
Q5. What investigations would you consider?
Q6. What management options should be considered?

Q1. What conditions should be considered?

Headache is a common symptom in school-age children. Severe acute headache can be a symptom of meningeal irritation or raised intracranial pressure, but it is more commonly associated with a viral 'flu-like illness. Recurrent and chronic headache can also stem from raised intracranial pressure, but is more commonly due to tension headache or migraine. Figure 24.3 is a simple clinical guide to approaching a child with headache.

Q2. What is the likely cause of Jasmine's headaches?

Intermittent severe frontal throbbing headaches associated with nausea suggest a diagnosis of migraine. This is supported by the absence of adverse social or academic factors, a positive family history, normal growth and clinical examination.

Q3. What are the important features to elicit in the clinical assessment?

A detailed history is key to identifying the cause of headaches.

History
- How often do the headaches happen? Is this changing?
- Onset of the headache: sudden or gradual?
- Is there any aura?
- Severity and duration of the headache
- Site of the headache
- Any pattern associated with the headaches
- Are there any associated features?
  - E.g. nausea, visual symptoms, weakness, seizures or altered behaviour
- Are there any precipitants?
  - E.g. foods, smells, stress or light
- Are there any factors that relieve the headache?
- Are there any other illnesses?
  - Does the child have a ventriculoperitoneal shunt in situ?
  - Any recent sinus, teeth, ear or visual problems?

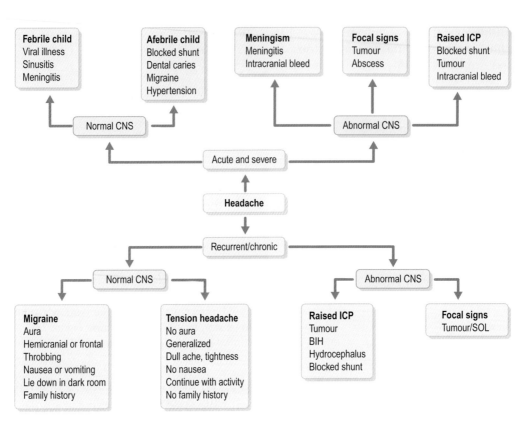

Fig. 24.3 A clinical approach to a child with headache.
(BIH = benign intracranial hypertension; ICP = intracranial pressure; SOL = space-occupying lesion.)

- Is there any family history of note, particularly migraine?
- Psychosocial history:
  - What has been the impact of the headaches on the child at school and at home?
  - Have there been any difficulties at home or school?
  - How is the child managing with school work?
- Drug history.

Examination

What should you look for on examination? A thorough clinical examination focuses on:
- Growth, particularly short stature or falling off centiles
- Neurological examination, in particular fundi, coordination, gait
- Local causes, particularly ears, throat, teeth, sinus pain
- Blood pressure.

Q4. When is referral indicated?

Referral is indicated if there is:
- Acute severe headache with signs of meningeal irritation
- Acute or chronic headache in a child with an intracranial shunt

> **BOX 24.2 Danger signs associated with raised intracranial pressure**
>
> **Symptoms**
> - Morning headaches ± vomiting
> - Increasing frequency or severity
> - Recent onset or worsening seizures
> - Weakness
> - Diplopia
> - History of regression
> - Deteriorating school performance
>
> **Signs**
> - Papilloedema
> - Deteriorating coordination
> - VI nerve palsy
> - Decreased conscious level

- Headache associated with altered consciousness, e.g. drowsiness
- Any of the danger signs shown in Box 24.2.

Q5. What investigations would you consider?

There is no routine investigation indicated in the evaluation of recurrent headache. Neurological imaging

Table 24.1 **Criteria of diagnosis of migraine (International Headache Society)**

Type	Grade	Criteria
Migraine without aura	A	At least five attacks fulfilling B to D below
	B	Headache lasting 4–72 hours (2–48 hours in children)
	C	Headache characterized by at least two of the following: 1. Unilateral location 2. Pulsating quality 3. Moderate or severe intensity (inhibits or prohibits daily activity) 4. Aggravated by climbing stairs or similar routine physical activity
	D	Headache accompanied by at least one of the following: 1. Nausea or vomiting, or both 2. Photophobia and phonophobia
Migraine with aura	A	At least two attacks fulfilling B below
	B	Presence of at least three of the following: 1. One or more fully reversible aura symptoms indicating focal cerebral cortical dysfunction or brainstem dysfunction or both 2. At least one aura symptom develops gradually over more than 4 mins, or two or more symptoms occur in succession 3. No aura symptom lasts more than 60 mins. When more than one aura symptom is present, accepted duration is proportionally increased 4. Headache follows aura with a symptom-free interval of less than 60 mins (it may also begin before or simultaneously with aura)

should be considered in children with an abnormal neurological examination or other physical findings suggesting central nervous system disease.

Q6. What management options should be considered?

Acute treatment is adequate analgesia with paracetamol, ibuprofen and/or codeine. If vomiting is prominent, domperidone may be useful. For children over 12 years, sumatriptan nasal spray is effective if used at the onset of symptoms.

Preventative strategies should address avoidance of known precipitating factors. Drug therapy should be considered if there is social or academic disruption. Propranolol, clonidine or pizotifen may be tried, although results may be variable.

Common causes of chronic intermittent headache in childhood

Migraine

Migraine occurs in 10% of children aged 5–15 years. Migraines are slightly more common in boys during childhood, but in teenage years girls predominate with a ratio of 3:1. Menarche is associated with this increased prevalence and symptoms may relate to the menstrual cycle. The diagnosis of migraine is based on criteria set down by the International Headache Society, which have been modified for children (2nd edition, Table 24.1).

www.i-h-s.org

Follow the links to guidelines

Management

Most episodes of migraine can be managed with symptomatic treatment using paracetamol, ibuprofen and/or codeine. If vomiting is prominent, domperidone may be useful. For children over 12 years sumatriptan nasal spray is effective if used at the onset of symptoms.

Tension headaches

This is the most common type of primary headache. It was initially considered to be psychogenic in origin, but there is increasing evidence in adult studies of a neurological basis, especially in severe or chronic cases. Tension headaches are divided into episodic and chronic subtypes. The episodes of headache last minutes to days and the pain is bilateral with a pressing or tightening quality. It has a mild to moderate intensity and does not worsen with activity. There is no nausea but photophobia or phonophobia may be present. Physical and neurological examination are essentially normal, apart from pericranial tenderness in some cases. Investigations are not indicated; when performed, they are normal. Simple analgesia with paracetamol and ibuprofen, head massage and relaxation techniques are effective forms of treatment.

Local causes

Painful ears (otitis externa or otitis media), sinusitis, painful eyes (conjunctivitis, corneal abrasion, glau-

289

Table 24.2 Causes of abnormal head shape

Head abnormality	Definition	Causes
Microcephaly (p. 253)	Head circumference less than 2nd centile	Idiopathic Familial Infection — cytomegalovirus (CMV) Antenatal alcohol exposure After cerebral injury Associated with learning difficulties Craniosynostosis (p. 255)
Macrocephaly	Head circumference greater than 98th centile	Familial Increased fluid – Hydrocephalus (Ch. 28) – Subdural collections due to shaking injury (Ch. 37) Increased brain matter – Megencephaly, e.g. mucopolysaccharidoses, tumours Increased bone of skull – Syndromes, e.g. achondroplasia – Chronic haemolytic anaemias
Plagiocephaly	Normal head circumference, abnormal shape	Abnormal moulding Craniosynostosis (p. 255) Neuromuscular disorders Genetic disorders, e.g. Down's syndrome

coma) and dental pain can all cause headache. This is best managed by addressing the primary cause and prescribing analgesia.

Raised intracranial pressure (ICP)

Raised ICP may present with one or a combination of the clinical features described in Box 24.2. Conditions presenting with raised ICP include blocked intracranial shunt, benign intracranial hypertension and space-occupying lesions; these are dealt with in detail in Chapter 28.

Hypertension

Hypertension (Ch. 40) is an important but uncommon cause of headache in children. In young children hypertension is usually secondary to acute or chronic renal disease. Primary hypertension becomes more common in obese adolescents, but is unlikely to be severe enough to cause headache or encephalopathy.

Abnormalities of head shape

Abnormalities of head shape and size are common. Many are benign or familial, but may reflect an underlying abnormality of cerebral ventricles, brain, dural collections or bone (Table 24.2).

Plagiocephaly

Asymmetric head shape or plagiocephaly is common after birth and is a consequence of moulding during

delivery. Persistence of asymmetry may occur due to head positioning. Usually the asymmetry becomes less prominent as the child grows older and assumes a more upright posture. Babies born preterm may develop long heads with flattened sides (scaphocephaly). Some conditions have associated head shape abnormalities, e.g. flattened occiput (brachycephaly) in Down's syndrome.

Abnormal head shape may also occur due to partial craniosynostosis. In this condition there is fusion of one or more of the skull sutures. If all sutures are involved, microcephaly results, with inadequate space for brain growth and consequent raised ICP. Clinically palpable ridges are felt over the fused suture lines and there may be signs of raised ICP such as papilloedema. Skull X-ray will identify premature fusion of one or more sutures. The child requires referral to a craniofacial team.

Microcephaly and macrocephaly

The causes are listed in Table 24.2. These children are approached by:
- Full developmental history and examination.
- Neurological examination, including fundoscopy.
- Measuring the head size using a non-expanding tape across the forehead, above the eyebrows and over the most prominent parietal and occipital areas. The largest of three measurements is taken as the true reading.
- Measuring parental head circumference and plotting the results on an appropriate chart.

- Assessing for:
  - Dysmorphic features
  - Congenital abnormalities
  - Palpable sutures.

Isolated postural, familial or idiopathic abnormalities of head shape without any neurodevelopmental features do not require specialist referral.

Hydrocephalus

Hydrocephalus is an important cause of large head and is discussed fully in Chapter 28. Hydrocephalus occurs when there is an imbalance between cerebrospinal fluid (CSF) production and absorption, leading to an increase in pressure and fluid volume within the ventricles. This may be due to obstructive hydrocephalus where CSF flow is obstructed within the ventricular systems, e.g. aqueduct stenosis, posterior fossa tumours. Alternatively, in non-obstructive hydrocephalus, it may be due to lack of free flow of CSF within the sub-arachnoid space, affecting CSF absorption. This is seen in premature babies following intraventricular haemorrhage. Rarely communicating hydrocephalus can occur due to increased CSF production.

Apart from a large head size, clinical signs include sunsetting eyes, a bulging anterior fontanelle, prominent scalp veins, and papilloedema progressing to optic atrophy. Where ICP is high, there may be a history of headache, vomiting, decreased conscious level or tonic seizures. Ominous signs are bradycardia, hypertension, VI nerve palsy, changing upper motor neuron signs and decerebrate or decorticate posturing. These suggest imminent coning. It is important to check for signs of raised ICP in children presenting with tonic seizures, as management of these seizures without addressing the primary cause can be fatal.

Investigation by CT or MRI scan usually establishes the diagnosis and identifies the specific cause. Management of hydrocephalus is usually with a ventriculoperitoneal shunt, together with appropriate treatment of any underlying cause.

Faints and funny turns

This condition is also discussed from the acute paediatric perspective in Chapter 28.

Problem-orientated topic:

a child who is blacking out

Carol, a 12-year-old girl, presents with a history of three episodes of loss of consciousness followed by twitching. On the first two occasions she was in school: once while standing in school assembly and the second in the toilet. The third episode was while standing in the supermarket with her mother. Her mother describes Carol as going limp and slumping to the floor. She was unresponsive and had jerking of her arms, but recovered within 5 minutes. Carol describes the episode as feeling lightheaded followed by blacking out. The next thing she remembers is finding herself on the floor. There was no associated incontinence of urine on any occasion. Carol felt tired after the episodes and slept for a short time. Carol's mother gives a history of seizures as a teenager, but says she grew out of them. She is worried that Carol may be epileptic.

Q1. What is the likely cause of Carol's paroxysmal events?

Q2. What other conditions should be considered?

Q3. What should you look for in your clinical evaluation?

Q4. When is referral indicated?

Q1. What is the likely cause of Carol's paroxysmal events?

The setting of the episodes, with the description of preceding lightheadedness and visual loss, is characteristic of syncope. Syncope occurs quite frequently in school, places of worship and hairdressers. Other triggers include minor injuries, immunization and venepuncture.

Syncope is caused by hypotension and bradycardia, resulting in cerebral anoxia. The twitching seen is of short duration, of decreasing amplitude and non-epileptic in origin.

Q2. What other conditions should be considered?

Reflex anoxic seizures

Reflex anoxic seizures are common in childhood. They are typically triggered by unpleasant events, e.g. emotional trauma, and result in vagal induced asystole of short duration with resulting cerebral anoxia. The onset is rapid and there is no preceding history of light-headedness or visual loss. The child normally looks pale, loses consciousness and may have brief tonic or tonic–clonic seizures. These can be associated with

Table 24.3 Characteristics of epileptic seizures and psychogenic seizures

Feature	Seizure	Psychogenic seizure
Timing	Any — less frequent during activity	When many people around
Onset	Physiological spread Rhythmic movements	Non-physiological spread, non-rhythmic movement Movements in both limbs but conscious
Sound	Expiratory grunt on initiation Silent during tonic–clonic phase	Shout/groan throughout episode
Episodes	Each seizure type similar in different episodes Eyes — nystagmus Cyanosis may occur Incontinence may occur	Vary Bizarre eye movements may occur No cyanosis No incontinence
Recovery	Slow but orientated	Rapid, disorientated, amnesia

incontinence and tongue biting. Recognition that the attacks are triggered by an unpleasant event allows the correct diagnosis to be made. Management is by explanation and reassuring the family.

Beta-blockers or atropine may be helpful in recurrent and troublesome cases.

Psychogenic seizures/pseudoseizures

Psychogenic seizures are uncommon in children but increase during adolescence. The episodes occur more commonly in young people with true seizures but these episodes have different patterns, as detailed in Table 24.3. A detailed description of the episode and other behaviours, e.g. anxiety or panic attacks, or episodes of hyperventilation, is helpful in reaching a diagnosis. Emotional or sexual abuse can be a precipitant.

The features in Table 24.3 are only a guide. It is important to remember that not all of the features are present on every occasion.

Q3. What should you look for in your clinical evaluation?

Obtaining a detailed history with a careful clinical examination is time well spent. The diagnosis of paroxysmal events, whether epileptic or non-epileptic, is based on clinical assessment. Your diagnosis will be as good as your history. Video recordings of events, if available, are particularly useful and it is worth asking the families to obtain them in a child with frequent episodes.

History

Your history needs to focus on the exact sequence of events from before the episode up until complete recovery. History should be obtained both from observers and from the child, and should cover preceding events, where the event occurred, what the child was doing and whether the event was actually observed by the parents or the account is secondhand. It is common for parents to give a history of 'seizure' or 'fits' where a careful history can establish that the events are non-epileptic in origin. As mentioned earlier, even the occurrence of clonic movements does not automatically make the event epileptic. Asking the parent to mimic the episode can be helpful in diagnosis.

Symptoms suggesting an underlying condition, such as intracranial pathology, cardiac conditions, gastro-oesophageal reflux or chronic blood loss, should be obtained. A family history of similar episodes, along with an exploration of family dynamics, is important. The possibility of substance misuse, particularly in teenagers, needs to be considered.

Examination

A full physical examination, with a detailed cardiac and neurological examination including fundus examination and tests of coordination, is required. Remember to measure the head circumference.

Q4. When is referral indicated?

Non-epileptic disorders such as syncope and reflex anoxic seizures should be investigated with a 12-lead ECG for QTc measurement. An orthostatic test may be performed in older children. History of collapse during exercise or swimming, family history of sudden death, an abnormal cardiac examination or an abnormal ECG requires further cardiac evaluation. Referral is indicated for disorders thought to be epileptic in nature, and in children with neurological, cardiac or psychological difficulties.

Other non-epileptic paroxysmal disorders

Blue breath-holding spells

These occur in 4% of infants and toddlers and are precipitated by physical or emotional trauma. The child starts crying and holds the breath in a prolonged expiration, resulting in cyanosis. The resulting cerebral anoxia causes limpness and loss of consciousness for a short period of time. This may be followed by a small number of tonic–clonic jerks. The attacks last a few minutes and the child always recovers spontaneously. There is no need for any intervention, except reassuring the parents that the child will grow out of the episodes, usually by the age of 5 years.

Sleep phenomena

Night terrors
Night terrors occur in preschool children, usually in the early stages of sleep. Children are usually found sitting up in bed screaming and looking terrified. They do not recognize their parents and cannot be comforted. They have no memory of the episode.

Nightmares
Nightmares occur later in sleep. Children remain asleep but are distressed and, on wakening, have a good recall of the episode. They can be comforted by their parents.

Sleep myoclonus
Myoclonic jerking of the limbs or head is a common phenomenon and occurs most commonly in early phases of sleep in both neonates and children. It is important to check that it only occurs in sleep and it does not wake the child or cause any distress.

Daytime paroxysmal disorders

Day dreaming
Day dreaming involves episodes of vacant staring without any impairment of consciousness and is common in school-age children. It is a differential diagnosis of absence epilepsy and the key to differentiation is whether interacting with the child can interrupt the episodes.

Narcolepsy
Narcolepsy is the sudden onset of daytime sleep and is an uncommon disorder.

Cataplexy
Cataplexy is the sudden onset of loss of tone, associated with laughter or excitement. It may occur with narcolepsy or alone.

Shuddering
Shuddering is common in infancy and is characterized by rapid shivering movements without loss of consciousness. This is a benign disorder, which resolves as the baby matures.

Benign paroxysmal vertigo
In benign paroxysmal vertigo the child stops suddenly and looks frightened for a few minutes, perhaps in association with nausea, vomiting and nystagmus.

Masturbation/self-gratification
This usually occurs when the child is tired or bored and is associated with tonic posturing and staring. Masturbation can start from early infancy and is common in preschool children. It is managed by distracting the child and ignoring the behaviour. Masturbation with other sexualized behaviour raises concerns about sexual abuse.

Febrile convulsions

Problem-orientated topic:

a child with febrile convulsions

Two-year-old James presents with a history of episode of stiffness, followed by rhythmic jerking of all four limbs lasting 3 minutes, associated with a high fever. His parents feel that he was slightly drowsy after the seizure but is back to his normal self now, except for the fever.

Q1. What is the likely cause of James's symptoms?
Q2. What other conditions should be considered?
Q3. What should you look for in your clinical evaluation?
Q4. What investigations are appropriate?
Q5. When is referral indicated?
Q6. How should you counsel James's parents?

Q1. What is the likely cause of James's symptoms?

James has had a short generalized tonic–clonic seizure associated with fever, and has now made a full recovery apart from the underlying fever. The likely cause of his symptoms is a typical febrile convulsion.

A typical febrile convulsion is characterized by:
- Age 6 months to 5 years
- Generalized tonic–clonic seizure lasting less than 15 minutes
- Rapid and full neurological recovery
- Normal neurological examination including head circumference.

Q2. What other conditions should be considered?

- Central nervous system infections: meningitis, encephalitis or cerebral abscess
- Rigors and delirium associated with fever can mimic febrile convulsion
- True epileptic seizure: precipitated by fever, although within the typical age range this is rare.

Q3. What should you look for in your clinical evaluation?

History

A detailed history should be obtained from a witness of the event, and should cover:

- Child's health prior to onset of seizure
- Nature of onset of seizure, its progression and duration, whether any focal features were present at the start of the seizure
- How long it took for the child to recover after the seizure
- Enquiry into other symptoms that may explain the cause of the fever
- Family history of febrile convulsions
- History of developmental problems
- Immunization status.

Examination

Examination of the child at presentation should cover:

- Recording of body temperature
- Assessment of cardiorespiratory function
- Assessment of conscious level (*a*lert, responds to *v*oice, responds to *p*ain, *u*nresponsive — AVPU)
- Rashes, in particular petechial rash of meningococcal disease
- Signs of meningitis: neck stiffness, Kernig's sign
- Neurological examination, including fundoscopy and measurement of head circumference
- Ear, nose and throat examination.

A period of observation after a dose of antipyretics is helpful in assessment. With control of the fever the child often perks up and returns to his normal self, reassuring the parents and the doctor!

Q4. What investigations are appropriate?

A search for a focus of infection informs the choice of investigations to be performed. In the absence of any identified focus, urine should be collected for urinalysis, including nitrites and leucocytes as markers of infection. If any abnormality is shown, then the urine needs to be sent for microscopy and culture. If the child looks unwell or is under 18 months, then referral to hospital is indicated for septic screen, which could include full blood count, C-reactive protein, blood cultures and possibly chest X-ray and/or lumbar puncture.

An electroencephalogram (EEG) is not indicated for typical febrile convulsion. Neuroimaging is indicated for a focal seizure or if there are abnormalities on neurological examination. Neuroimaging may also be considered in children with previous developmental or neurological difficulties.

Q5. When is referral indicated?

Referral is indicated in the presence of any of the following:

- Focal seizure
- Prolonged seizure (urgent)
- Child with cardiorespiratory compromise (urgent)
- Presence of petechial rash (urgent)
- Presence of meningeal signs (urgent)
- Persistent altered consciousness (urgent)
- Abnormal neurological signs
- Child is under 18 months (urgent)
- Significant parental anxiety or inability to cope.

Parents find febrile fits terrifying, and most parents assume their child is dying during the seizure. It is often necessary to admit children with a first febrile convulsion for parental reassurance. Parents become more confident if the child has had a previous convulsion.

Q6. How should you counsel James's parents?

- What is a febrile convulsion?
  - Convulsion brought on by fever in a child aged 6 months to 5 years.
- What starts a febrile convulsion?
  - Any illness that causes high temperature, commonly cold viruses.
- Will it happen again?
  - Three out of 10 children who have a febrile convulsion will have a further convulsion.
- What should you do if it happens again?
  - If a child has a further seizure stay calm; you know what is happening.
  - Note the time so you know how long the seizure is lasting.
  - Only move the child if he or she is in a dangerous place.
  - Do not try to restrict the jerking movements.
  - Do not put anything into the child's mouth.
  - Call an ambulance if the seizure continues beyond 5 minutes.
  - As soon as the seizure ends, roll the child on to his or her side.

- – Arrange for a doctor to see your child to look for a cause for the fever.
- Is this epilepsy?
  - – No, this is not epilepsy.
- Will this lead to epilepsy?
  - – Most children who have febrile convulsions do not go on to develop epilepsy.
- Do febrile convulsions cause brain damage?
  - – Almost never, and only in children who have seizures lasting more than 30 minutes.

Epilepsy in primary care

(Hospital-based care of epilepsy is described in Chapter 25.)

Consider the following questions:

1. What is epilepsy?
2. Why do children develop epilepsy?
3. How is epilepsy classified?
4. What different seizure types are recognized?
5. How is epilepsy diagnosed?
6. How are paroxysmal episodes investigated?
7. What is an epileptic syndrome and why is it important?
8. How is epilepsy managed?
9. When is referral indicated?
10. What is the key information in counselling parents and children?

1. What is epilepsy?

An epileptic seizure is a transient clinical event that results from abnormal and excessive activity of a more or less extensive collection of neurons. If a person has more than one such seizure, he or she has epilepsy.

2. Why do children develop epilepsy?

Children develop epilepsy for different reasons:
- *Symptomatic epilepsy* occurs in children who have had their brain injured in some way, perhaps as the result of a severe head injury, perinatal hypoxic insult or meningitis.
- *Idiopathic epilepsy* has no demonstrable cause. This is the most common form of epilepsy.
- *Cryptogenic epilepsy* is where no cause can be found, although one is suspected: for example, in children with severe learning difficulties.

3. How is epilepsy classified?

Epilepsy is broadly classified into generalized and focal. Generalized seizures are caused by electrical disorder of both hemispheres of the brain and are associated with impaired consciousness. Focal seizures are caused by electrical discharges from one part of the brain and the person remains conscious. The electrical activity can spread to affect both sides of the brain and cause impairment of consciousness (secondary generalization).

The internationally accepted classification of epilepsy has been evolved by the International League Against Epilepsy.

 www.ilae-epilepsy.org

Follow the links to epilepsy classification and terminology

4. What different seizure types are recognized?

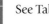 See Table 24.4.

5. How is epilepsy diagnosed?

Your diagnosis is as good as your clinical assessment. Principals of diagnosis include:
- Determining whether the episode is epileptic or non-epileptic from the history of witness and child. Getting the witness to mimic the event can be helpful. Video recordings are also useful.
- Identifying different seizure types.
- Looking for a history of neurological, developmental and possible genetic difficulties.
- Taking a family history.

6. How are paroxysmal episodes investigated?

All acute seizures should be investigated with measurement of blood sugar. In infants other biochemical abnormalities, e.g. hypocalcaemia, should be checked.

An interictal EEG can be helpful if a specific pattern is recognized. A normal interictal EEG does not rule out epilepsy. Abnormal EEG findings are found in 5% of the normal population. EEG recording during a seizure is helpful in differentiating epileptic from non-epileptic paroxysmal disorders. It is also useful in identifying the origin of the seizure. Sleep deprivation, sleep itself, photic stimulation or hyperventilation can be used during an EEG in an attempt to induce a seizure or abnormal electrical brain activity. Where the nature of the attacks is unclear, a video EEG can be useful.

A CT scan, or preferably an MRI scan, of the brain can be useful in identifying structural lesions and is valuable in children with focal seizures or complex difficulties. Neuroimaging is not routinely indicated

Table 24.4 Seizure types and features

Seizure type	Features
Generalized	
Tonic–clonic	During the tonic phase there is loss of consciousness and the child will fall, which may be associated with an expiratory noise. The eyes roll back and the muscles undergo tonic contraction. There is sudden onset of cyanosis. During the following clonic phase there is rhythmic jerking in all limbs. Loss of sphincter control is common
Tonic	The muscles of the whole body become stiff and the child falls if standing. Recovery is usually rapid
Atonic, drop attacks	The muscles of the whole body lose their tone and the child falls to the ground
Typical absence	Abrupt onset of impaired conscious level with cessation of motor activity or speech, a blank facial expression and flickering of eyelids, which last less than 10 seconds. The child continues with previous activity after the seizure. The child never falls to the ground
Atypical absence	Abrupt or gradual onset of impaired conscious level with cessation of motor activity or speech. More complex automatism, including lip smacking and fumbling. May be associated autonomic features such as flushing or micturition. Absences are longer and can cause the child to fall down
Myoclonic jerk	Brief, often symmetrical muscle contracture. Myoclonic jerks often occur shortly after wakening
Spasm	Lightning flexion of trunk, arms extended, abducted or flexed. Often occur in runs and are followed by child crying. Spasms occur more commonly on falling to sleep and wakening
Focal	
Temporal lobe	Child complains of unpleasant smells, abdominal sensations or déjà vu
Parietal lobe	Regular jerking (clonic movements) in one muscle group
Frontal lobe	Bizarre motor movements, e.g. thrashing, scratching genitals, vocalizations, dystonic movement. These may occur frequently
Occipital lobe	Crude visual distortions

in generalized seizures. Functional imaging with a positron emission tomography (PET) scan is only undertaken if epilepsy surgery is a possibility.

7. What is an epileptic syndrome and why is it important?

Children diagnosed with epilepsy syndromes have clinical and seizure characteristics that occur together. Seizures classified within a syndrome have a typical pattern and age when they start, and may produce specific EEG findings. The syndrome may follow a definite pattern of progression. Syndromes are important to recognize as they help the doctor to choose the most appropriate treatment and to be able to counsel the family accurately about the course of the condition, e.g. typical juvenile absence epilepsy, infantile spasms.

8. How is epilepsy managed?

Acute episode
- Note the time so you know how long the seizure is lasting.
- Only move the child if he or she is in a dangerous place.
- Do not try to restrict the jerking movements.
- Do not put anything into the child's mouth.
- Give oxygen if available.
- Check temperature and perform a blood sugar stick test.
- Give rectal diazepam if the seizure continues beyond 5 minutes and call an ambulance.

Table 24.5 Medications used for different seizure types

Seizure type	First-line agent	Second-line drug
Idiopathic generalized epilepsy	Sodium valproate	Lamotrigine
Focal epilepsy	Carbamazepine	Sodium valproate
Absence epilepsy	Sodium valproate	Ethosuxamide
Infantile spasm	Vigabatrin	Prednisolone

- As soon as the seizure ends, place the child in the recovery position.

Ongoing management
Long-term management of primary epilepsy is with anti-epileptic medication. The use of medication is based around the risk of recurrent seizures, the seizure type and recognized seizure patterns or syndromes, together with the wishes of the child and family (Table 24.5). Monotherapy is aimed for in all cases and the duration of treatment varies with response and recognized seizure patterns. The majority of anti-epileptic agents are started at a low dose, which is titrated up over the course of 2 months. The minimum dose that controls the seizures is used. Withdrawal of treatment is considered for most children who have been seizure-free for 2 years, except for lifelong epilepsy syndromes.

9. When is referral indicated?

All children with suspected epilepsy based on a detailed history should be referred to a paediatrician with an interest in epilepsy. For children with long-term epilepsy, care is usually shared between a general paediatrician and a paediatric neurologist (Ch. 28).

10. What is the key information in counselling parents and children?

- What epilepsy is
- Information regarding any underlying cause
- Benefits and side-effects of treatments
- Avoidance of precipitants where appropriate: sleep deprivation, drugs, alcohol, bright flashing lights
- How to manage a seizure episode
- Precautions; supervised bathing and swimming (in older children showering is safe), avoidance of climbing heights and cycling on busy roads
- Need for school to be informed and appropriate staff training in seizure management
- Allowing the child to live an otherwise normal life.

Absence epilepsy

Problem-orientated topic:

a child with episodes of blankness

Eight-year-old Lucy presents with a 3-month history of episodes when she becomes blank for a period of a few seconds. During these episodes she stands still, stares and flutters her eyelids.

Q1. What is the likely diagnosis?

Q2. What other conditions should be considered?

Q3. How will you clinically evaluate this child?

Q4. What investigations are indicated?

Q5. When is referral indicated?

Q6. What is the key information in counselling parents?

Q1. What is the likely diagnosis?

Staring episodes lasting for a few seconds with altered consciousness but no loss of postural tone constitute absence epilepsy. There may be associated fluttering of the eyelids, mouthing or minor twitching of the fingers. Episodes lasting more than 30 seconds are unlikely to be absence episodes.

Q2. What other conditions should be considered?

Day dreaming is common and is not associated with altered consciousness. Children can be made to 'snap out of it' if their attention is gained.

Complex partial seizures normally last longer and the child is drowsy afterwards. These seizures can have a premonition or aura and may involve automatisms (simple repetitive motor movements).

Atypical absence episodes are uncommon and mostly occur along with other seizure types. The onset and offset may be gradual, the duration is usually longer and changes in body tone are more pronounced, leading to a fall.

Q3. How will you clinically evaluate this child?

History

- A detailed description of the episodes from a witness and the child is key to the diagnosis. Asking the witness to act out the episode may be useful.
- Are there other types of seizure, especially myoclonic?
- Any history of neurological disorders?
- Any history of developmental difficulties? Has there been any recent loss of skills (regression)?

Examination

- Dysmorphic features
- Signs of neurocutaneous syndromes: unusual birth marks or rashes
- Abnormalities on neurological examination
- A timed 2-minute period of hyperventilation to evoke an absence seizure (ask the child to blow a piece of paper).

Q4. What investigations are indicated?

An EEG would be helpful in defining the epilepsy syndrome that is causing the absence seizures in Lucy. The EEG classically shows 3 per second spike and wave discharges during a seizure in children with typical absence epilepsy of childhood.

Q5. When is referral indicated?

If a diagnosis of absence seizures is made, with or without other seizure types, a referral to a consultant paediatrician is indicated.

Q6. What is the key information in counselling parents?

- Absence epilepsy is a form of epilepsy, which does not cause children harm beyond losing part of their day.
- There is no underlying cause — not a tumour.
- Absence epilepsy usually responds well to treatment.
- The child will usually grow out of the absence seizures. Out of 10 children, two will go on to have generalized tonic–clonic seizures in adult life.

Limp

Problem-orientated topic:

a child who is limping

Malcolm is a 5-year-old boy who is brought to see you by his Mum, as he has been miserable for 2 days and walking with a limp.

Q1. What conditions should be considered?

Q2. Which questions will be most helpful in determining the underlying cause?

Q3. What signs are helpful in determining the underlying cause?

Q4. What is the most likely cause of Malcolm's limp?

Q5. Which investigations would be useful and why?

Q6. What are the other common causes of an acute painful limp?

Q7. What are the common causes of chronic gait abnormalities?

Q1. What conditions should be considered? (Fig. 24.4)

54–57

A limp can be painful or painless. With a painful limp the child spends a smaller proportion of time weight-bearing on the painful limb. In painless limp children will spend an equal time on both limbs, but may shift their centre of gravity over the affected limb to help with their balance.

Q2. Which questions will be most helpful in determining the underlying cause?

Ask yourself if there is any evidence of:
- Local trauma or painful condition
- Infection

- Joint disease
- Systemic illness
- Weakness and/or altered muscle tone
- Leg length discrepancy.

History
- Is there any history of trauma?
- Is it painful or painless to walk?
- Are the difficulties acute, intermittent or chronic?
- Is there a history of fever?
- Does the child have any other condition or receive any medication?

Q3. What signs are helpful in determining the underlying cause?

See Table 24.6.

Q4. What is the most likely cause of Malcolm's limp?

Your history and examination reveal that Malcolm has complained of sudden onset of pain in his right hip on walking for the last 2 days. The pain and walking improve with paracetamol. He has never had this problem before. He had a cold 5 days ago but has otherwise been well. On examination he is afebrile and has no signs of a systemic disorder. There is no local deformity or swelling and he has decreased abduction and internal rotation. Neurological examination is normal. With encouragement he walks with an antalgic (painful) gait. These features would suggest a transient synovitis, which is managed by rest and analgesia. Recovery would be expected within a week.

Q5. Which investigations are useful and why?

See Table 24.7.

Q6. What are the other common causes of an acute painful limp?

These include minor trauma, ill-fitting shoes or ingrowing toenail.

Septic arthritis
Septic arthritis must be considered in all children who have a history of fever, look unwell and have a painful joint. Local signs are only seen in superficial joints. Leucocytosis, raised CRP and joint ultrasound with aspiration will confirm the diagnosis. Management is with analgesia and antibiotics, initially intravenously and later as a 3–4-week oral course.

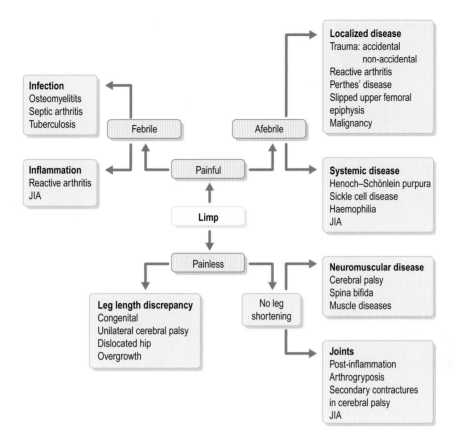

Fig. 24.4 **The child with a limp.**
  (JIA = juvenile idiopathic arthritis.)

Table 24.6 **Signs and diagnosis in children who limp**

Approach	What to look for	Diagnostic relevance
General	Temperature	Evidence of infection
	Does the child look unwell?	
	Pallor, lymphadenopathy, splenomegaly	Disseminated malignancy: leukaemia, neuroblastoma
Look		
Gait	Antalgic	Painful hip
	Hemiplegic	Cerebral palsy — hemiplegia
	Scissor gait	Cerebral palsy — diplegia
Skin	Petechial/urticarial rash	Henoch–Schönlein purpura
	Signs of trauma	
	Blisters on feet	Poorly fitting shoes
	Widespread bruising	Non-accidental injury, coagulopathy
	Local painful conditions	Ingrowing toenail
Leg length	See page 301	See page 301
Feel		
Joint	Temperature, tenderness, effusion	Infected or inflamed joint
	Deformity	Chronic inflammatory changes
		Malignant bone disease
Move	Range of movement	Evidence of pain, contractures
Neurological examination	Weakness with increased tone	Upper motor neuron disorder, e.g. cerebral palsy
	Weakness with decreased tone	Lower motor neuron or muscle disorder, e.g. spina bifida, muscular dystrophy

Table 24.7 Investigations used in children who limp

Investigation	Significance
X-ray of painful bone or joint	Identify bone and joint causes May be normal initially
FBC and film	Leucocytosis may indicate infection Sickle cell disease, leukaemia
ESR, CRP, plasma viscosity	Elevated in both local and systemic infective and inflammatory conditions
Clotting studies	Haemophilia Exclude other causes of purpura in Henoch–Schönlein purpura
Ultrasound of joint	Demonstrate effusion
Joint aspiration and culture	Septic arthritis
Technetium bone scan	Hot spots with infection, inflammation and malignancy

Perthes' disease

Perthes' disease is an avascular necrosis of the femoral head. It affects mostly boys between 3 and 10 years. The children are usually well and present with gradual onset of pain and limp. In 20% of cases Perthes' is bilateral. Plain X-ray shows increase density within the femoral head but may be normal initially. Management is bed rest, pain relief and traction. Most children recover well.

Slipped upper femoral epiphysis

This is displacement of the femoral head. It occurs most commonly in overweight boys at the start of their pubertal growth spurt. They present with a limp and hip or knee pain, which may have been precipitated by minor trauma. In 20% the process is bilateral. On examination the leg may be 1–2 cm shorter and externally rotated. Internal rotation and abduction may be limited. The diagnosis is confirmed by X-ray of the affected joint. Management is surgical, usually with pin placement in situ and weight reduction.

Q7. What are the common causes of chronic gait abnormalities?

Intoeing

In-toe gait can be due to:

- *Metatarsus varus*: in-turning of the forefoot in babies. Provided this can be passively corrected with ease, no further action is required.
- *Medial tibial torsion*: the tibia is rotated inwards compared to the femur. This is seen in toddlers, often with bow legs, and corrects spontaneously.
- *Femoral anteversion*: the femoral neck is twisted forwards more than normal. This presents in children who 'W sit'. It usually corrects spontaneously by 8 years.

Flat feet

All toddlers have flat feet, and most children develop a medial longitudinal arch. This can be demonstrated by standing the child on tiptoe. Very flat feet may result from lax ligaments and rarely from a connective tissue disorder, e.g. Ehlers–Danlos syndrome. Most children with flat feet have no problems and management is with reassurance. If the child complains of painful feet, an arch support may help.

Knock knees

Knock-kneed preschool children are common and a normal variant. They usually correct spontaneously by 10 years, and persistence beyond this age warrants referral. In children with pigmented skin look for other signs of rickets: enlargement of costochondral junctions and wrists. This can be confirmed by plain X-ray showing 'splaying and fraying' of the metaphyses and by bone biochemistry with decreased serum calcium, increased alkaline phosphatase and low vitamin D levels.

Toe walking

Toe walking is very common in 1–3-year-olds. It may persist beyond this age, usually from habit. Spastic hemiplegia or diplegia and Duchenne muscular dystrophy can present with toe walking. It is important when examining these children to look at their tone and power as well as the range of ankle movement. A normal creatine kinase excludes Duchenne muscular dystrophy.

Cerebral palsy

 Cerebral palsy (see also Ch. 29) is a cause of impaired motor function in children and can present with chronic abnormalities of gait as well as delayed gross motor development. Cerebral palsy is a persistent but not necessarily unchanging disorder of posture and/or movement due to a non-progressive defect or lesion in the brain in early life. Even though the condition affecting the brain is non-progressive, the clinical presentation can evolve and change. Children with cerebral palsy may have isolated motor difficulties or may have a number of comorbidities such as learning difficulties and epilepsy. The description of cerebral palsy can be based on distribution (unilateral, bilateral, either lower limb or whole body) or muscle tone (hypertonic, ataxic, dyskinetic).

Cerebral palsy is a clinical diagnosis with a number of different underlying causes. These may be:

- *Antenatal*, such as congenital malformations, antenatal stroke or congenital infection
- *Perinatal*, such as birth asphyxia, although this is a relatively unusual cause of cerebral palsy
- *Postnatal*, such as intraventricular haemorrhage in premature neonates or meningitis in the first year of life.

Cerebral palsy is discussed in detail in Chapter 29.

There will be a history of gross motor difficulties and on examination the child usually has altered tone and brisk reflexes. There may be tendon shortening, contractures, hip dislocation or leg length shortening, contributing to gait difficulties.

Talipes

- *Positional*. This is common and due to compression in utero. The foot is of normal size with a mild deformity, which can easily be corrected with passive manipulation. It resolves spontaneously over time and can be aided by corrective manipulation by parents.
- *Equinovarus*. This congenital malformation causes the foot to be inverted, supinated and adducted. The position of the foot is fixed and cannot be corrected by passive manipulation; the condition is frequently bilateral. It may occur spontaneously but is associated with neurological and muscle disorders. The treatment is commenced at birth with stretches, strapping and plaster casts. Surgery is necessary for significant abnormalities.
- *Calcaneovalgus*. This causes the foot to be dorsiflexed and everted. If the foot position can be passively corrected, then it usually corrects spontaneously with time.

Inequality of limb length

Causes may be:

- *Post-traumatic*: due to growth plate disturbance
- *Congenital*: developmental dysplasia of hip
- *Neurological*: unilateral cerebral palsy, poliomyelitis
- *Overgrowth*: arteriovenous malformation, syndromic.

History. Ask about a history of trauma or neurological disease.

Examination. Asymmetry can be judged by comparing the position of the patella when both hips and knees are flexed to 45 degrees. It is possible to identify

---

> **BOX 24.3 Causes of limb pain**
>
> **Bone**
> - Trauma:
>   - Accidental
>   - Non-accidental
> - Infection:
>   - Osteomyelitis
> - Tumours:
>   - Local, e.g. osteosarcoma
>   - Disseminated, e.g. leukaemia
> - Metabolic:
>   - Rickets
> - Growing pains
>
> **Joints**
> - Hypermobile joints
> - Infection
> - Systemic disorders:
>   - Vasculitis
>   - Inflammatory bowel disease
>   - Juvenile idiopathic arthritis
>   - Systemic lupus erythematosus
>
> **Neuromuscular**
> - Referred pain
> - Reflex sympathetic dystrophy: over-protection following minor injury

---

whether the femur or tibial component is short. It is also possible to measure leg length using the anterior superior iliac spine to medial malleolus as markers. Thigh length is measured from anterior superior iliac spine to tibial plateau. Look for skin abnormalities, e.g. haemangiomas. Assess for tone, moving the spine and lower limb joints through their full range of movement. Complete a neurological examination.

Management. Address the underlying cause and provide an orthosis where indicated, e.g. heel raise to shoe.

Limb pain

Limb pain in childhood is most commonly attributed to growing pains, where the aetiology of the pain is little understood. In the first instance it is important to exclude organic pathology, as listed in Box 24.3. The approach is the same as that for a child with a limp. A history compatible with growing pains, together with an examination failing to reveal any abnormality, is an adequate assessment in the first instance. Referral for investigation is indicated if there are any abnormal signs or the pain is always at one site or is severe or persistent.

Growing pains

These are episodes of pain in the lower limbs, which classically wake the pre-adolescent child at night. The

Spinal causes — central pain
- Discitis
- Tumour (benign tumours more common):
  - Bone, e.g. osteoid osteoma
  - Spinal cord, e.g. neurofibroma
  - Disseminated, e.g. leukaemia
- Diastematomyelia
- Epidural abscess
- Scheuermann disease
- Spondylolysis, spondylolisthesis

Muscular — localized to side pain ± scoliosis
- Poor posture:
  - Heavy school bags
- Trauma:
  - Muscle spasm
- Myalgia:
  - Secondary to viral or bacterial infection
- Urinary tract infection
- Stress-related

- Neurological symptoms or signs, including bladder or bowel dysfunction
- Persistent or increasing pain
- Systemic symptoms, particularly fever or weight loss

child is otherwise well and there are no abnormal findings on examination. The pain settles with massage, comforting or simple analgesia. Psychological factors have an association with limb pain and therefore it is important to enquire about possible predisposing, precipitating or perpetuating social factors.

Back problems

Back pain

Back pain is unusual in childhood and a cause needs to be sought (Box 24.4).

A careful history will help identify clues to the underlying cause. This includes the onset, duration of symptoms, the nature and site of the pain and any radiation (nerve root pain) or neurological symptoms such as weakness, or alteration of bladder or bowel function. Enquiry should be made into antecedent factors, general health and family history. Physical examination should cover spinal alignment, mobility, muscle spasm and areas of tenderness, together with a full neurological examination (Box 24.5).

Scoliosis

Scoliosis is lateral curvature of the spine, with resulting prominence of the posterior ribs. This is more obvious when children are asked to touch their toes. The most common cause is idiopathic scoliosis, but it is important to exclude other causes by clinical assessment (Table 24.8).

Clinical assessment includes a history of the age of onset and any associated pain or neurological symptoms, including difficulties with continence. This is followed by an enquiry into past history or family history of neuromuscular disorders or congenital malformations. Physical examination should start by excluding leg shortening as a cause of scoliosis; examine the child's spine sitting down and scoliosis due to leg shortening will resolve. Examination of the spine should record the site of the scoliosis, as well as any café au lait patches (neurofibromatosis), sacral dimpling or midline hairy patches associated with a spina bifida occulta. The forward bend test will reveal raised ribs on the convex side of the scoliosis. If no abnormalities are detected on this test, this suggests a positional scoliosis, which requires follow-up but no additional management apart from postural advice. Conclude with a neurological examination to exclude neuromuscular causes.

If an apparent scoliosis is identified due to leg length shortening, then this requires further evaluation along with a suitable orthosis such as a shoe raise. The remainder require X-ray to assess the scoliosis and exclude any underlying bony abnormality. The degree of scoliosis is assessed by Cobb's angle. This is formed by two perpendicular lines to the end plates of the superior and inferior ends of the vertebrae of the major curve on PA radiography.

If the Cobb's angle is:
- *Less than 20 degrees*, then observe 6–12-monthly, particularly during the adolescent growth spurt. Many mild idiopathic scolioses do not progress or resolve.
- *20–40 degrees or progressing rapidly*, consider bracing or a plaster jacket.
- *Greater than 40 degrees*, consider surgery to avoid respiratory compromise.

Torticollis

Torticollis is the term used for a twisted neck. It is a clinical sign that has a number of different causes (Box 24.6).

A clear history can help to elucidate the cause. For example, onset from birth would suggest a congenital abnormality or sternomastoid tumour. In later childhood the mode of onset, the presence of any

Table 24.8 Causes of scoliosis

Classification/subgroup	Features
Idiopathic	
Early onset	< 5 years, usually resolve
Later onset	Adolescent, mostly girls. Most common cause
Neuromuscular	
Neurological	E.g. cerebral palsy, neurofibromatosis
Muscular	E.g. Duchenne muscular dystrophy
Bony	
Congenital/infectious/malignant	Single vertebral anomaly or part of syndrome, e.g. VATER (*v*ertebral, *a*nal, *t*racheo-oesophageal, *r*enal)
Ligamentous	E.g. Marfan's syndrome
Apparent	Compensatory, e.g. due to leg length discrepancy

BOX 24.6 Causes of torticollis

Acute

- Inflammation:
  - Cervical lymphadenitis
  - Abscess: retropharyngeal, neck
  - Polyarticular juvenile arthritis
- Trauma:
  - Injury C1–C2 (associated with Down's)
- Atlanto-axial subluxation/dislocation
- Oculogyric crises, e.g.phenothiazines
- Posterior fossa tumour

Chronic

- Congenital:
  - Sternomastoid tumour
  - Bony abnormality
- Compensatory due to ocular cause:
  - VI nerve palsy/squint
- Neurological:
  - Posterior fossa tumour
- Bony/ligamentous:
  - Vertebral anomalies, e.g. Klippel–Feil

neurological symptoms, general health and any history of recent trauma, together with the past medical history and any medication, help to identify the underlying cause. Physical examination includes an assessment of the child's systemic wellbeing, the presence of a sternomastoid swelling, and lymph glands, as well as any ear, nose and throat, eye or other neurological signs.

The most common cause of torticollis in a baby is a sternocleidomastoid tumour (congenital muscular torticollis) due to birth trauma to the sternocleidomastoid. It presents with restriction of head movement in the first months of life, with a palpable swelling within the sternocleidomastoid. Management involves passive stretches taught by physiotherapists.

Further reading

Royal College of Paediatrics and Child Health 1997 Prevention and control of pain in children: a manual for health care professionals. RCPCH, London

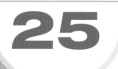

Nigel Kennedy

Abdominal disorders

LEARNING OUTCOMES

By the end of this chapter you should:
- Know how to diagnose the common and important conditions responsible for symptoms and signs in young children
- Know the causes of these conditions and details of the important conditions
- Know the appropriate management at primary care level
- Know when to refer for further hospital investigation
- Know how to take a full clinical history and examine the child to formulate a management plan.

Introduction

Symptoms related to the child's abdominal system present commonly to doctors in primary care. Many of these disorders are self-limiting and require no treatment, but less frequently, serious disease may be present and urgent referral to hospital is required. This chapter discusses an approach to these common symptoms.

Constipation

Problem-orientated topic:

a constipated child

Matthew is a 3-year-old who is brought to see you, his GP, because his mother is

Continued overleaf

MODULE FIVE

concerned that he is constipated. She tells you that he only has his bowels open every 4–5 days, and when he does, his stools are hard, small and pellet-like, and he often complains that passing the stool is painful. She has occasionally noticed red, streaky blood on the outside of the motion associated with some mucus. She is aware that he is constipated but wants help and advice to correct the problem.

Q1. What is constipation?

Q2. What are the common causes of this condition?

Q3. What would you look for in your clinical evaluation?

Q4. What investigations would be required?

Q5. How would you manage the situation at a primary care level?

Q6. When would you refer for specialist advice?

Infants
- Common:
  - Inadequate fluid or food intake
- Rare:
  - Hirschsprung's disease

Toddlers and children
- Common:
  - Secondary to minor illness
  - Anal fissure
  - Functional/psychological
  - No obvious cause
- Rare:
  - Anal stenosis
  - Hirschsprung's disease
  - Hypothyroidism
  - Hypercalcaemia
  - Neurological problems/hypotonia

- What does the child eat?
- Is the child thriving?

Examination

The examination will need to focus on recording the child's growth, with height and weight plotted on a centile chart. Signs of anaemia should also be sought, with palpation of the abdomen for abdominal masses, and a gentle but careful rectal examination can be helpful to confirm a loaded rectum.

Matthew has a history of infrequent bowel motions occurring every 4–5 days, which are hard and associated with some blood. It is likely that he has developed an anal fissure as a consequence of the hard stools, and the pain associated with defaecation is likely to encourage him to suppress the urge to defaecate, in order to avoid a painful experience. This will compound the overall problem, causing him to become more constipated and exacerbating the original problem.

Other causes, such as Hirschsprung's disease or hypothyroidism, are unlikely in this case but must be considered if the problem is ongoing.

Q1. What is constipation?

Constipation is defined as pain, difficulty or delay in defaecation. Parents have very different ideas about what constitutes constipation and some normal children may only have their bowels open 2–3 times a week. It is important to recognize that breastfed babies may only have a bowel motion every 7–10 days and this can be quite normal for them.

Q2. What are the common causes of this condition?

See Box 25.1.

Q3. What would you look for in your clinical evaluation?

History

In order to evaluate the problem, it is important to seek answers to certain questions. These include:

- Did the problem begin at birth, and if not, at what age? (Was there a delay in the passage of meconium at birth?)
- What does the parent/carer mean by constipation?
- Does the infant or child pass hard stools causing bleeding?

Q4. What investigations would be required?

As a rule, investigations are not required in the majority of children presenting with constipation. However, a plain abdominal X-ray may show excess faeces in the colon and help to confirm the diagnosis. Rare causes, such as hypothyroidism and hypercalcaemia, will require thyroid function and serum calcium levels to be measured.

Q5. How would you manage the situation at a primary care level?

- Give dietary advice to ensure that the child has an appropriate diet of cereals, fruit and vegetables, leading to a normal stool.
- Advise the use of stool softeners such as lactulose.
- Laxatives such as senna to stimulate the bowel may also be required.

There should be regular follow-up of the child, both by the GP and the health visitor, to ensure the restoration of a normal bowel habit and normal motions once the problem has been addressed. A sympathetic and reassuring approach to the problem by the healthcare team is essential in gaining and maintaining the confidence of the parents and child.

Early explanation of the problem to Matthew's parents, fluid and dietary advice, with increased cereal and fibre, may help to solve the problem. Left untreated, this may develop into a chronic situation requiring hospital paediatric care, enemas to empty the rectum and, in more severe cases, hospital admission.

Q6. When would you refer for specialist advice?

Hospital referral will be necessary for those children who do not respond to simple dietary measures or the introduction of faecal softeners and laxatives. For those children with gross constipation and impacted faeces, a short admission for rectal enemas to clear the rectum may be required; rarely, manual evacuation under anaesthetic may also be needed. For those children in whom an alternative diagnosis for the constipation, such as Hirschsprung's, may be considered, referral to the local paediatric department or designated clinic will be required for further investigation.

Causes of constipation in children

Common causes

Inadequate fluid
Young children may become fluid-depleted during a febrile illness, particularly if this is associated with vomiting. The constipation may resolve by the simple increase of fluids, but may also lead to later chronic constipation.

Anal fissure
A small tear in the anal mucosa can lead to painful defaecation associated with fresh rectal bleeding and may cause the child to suppress the desire to defaecate to avoid the painful experience. This itself may then lead on to the development of chronic constipation. Anal fissures heal spontaneously but symptomatic treatment to include faecal softeners and local anaesthetic jelly can be useful.

Functional constipation
This is by far the most common cause of constipation seen by GPs and health visitors. There may be an obvious precipitating cause in the history, such as an anal fissure or a febrile illness. The stools become hard, pellet-like and difficult to pass, and because of the pain the child is reluctant to attempt to pass them. Fresh blood may be present on the surface of the stools. The rectum becomes distended and loaded with faeces. It is particularly common in children with disability/immobility.

Rare causes

Hirschsprung's disease (Ch. 49)
Whilst this is a rare condition, with an incidence of 1 in 5000 live births, it must always be borne in mind in a child presenting to the GP with constipation. It is caused by an aganglionic segment of bowel and, while severe cases present in the neonatal period with delay in the passage of meconium or delay in the changing stool, less severe cases occur in infancy. Recurrent abdominal distension with infrequent passage of stools in the first month of life requires a full investigation and referral for a paediatric opinion. It must also be borne in mind that older children may still have the condition in a milder form with short-segment Hirschsprung's, and if the constipation does not respond to normal measures, Hirschsprung's must still be considered and referral to a paediatrician made.

Anal stenosis
One other condition to consider is anal stenosis, which can be diagnosed by a rectal examination. The problem usually responds to anal dilatation.

Endocrine causes
These include hypothyroidism and hypercalcaemia (Ch. 35).

Neurological causes/hypotonia
These include cerebral palsy and spina bifida (Chs 28 and 29).

Soiling and encopresis

Soiling

This term is usually used to describe the situation when there is leakage of liquid stool around impacted faeces in a child with chronic constipation, leading to staining of the pants. Treatment is to correct the underlying problem of chronic constipation and faecal impaction.

It can also be used to describe the situation when a child has not developed bowel continence by an appropriate age (usually 4 years). Management of this situation requires a regular toilet training plan along with a sympathetic and positive approach from GP and health visitor.

Encopresis

This describes a situation where a child who is not constipated passes stools in an inappropriate place. It indicates the presence of behavioural problems, sometimes severe. Referral to a child psychiatrist is usually necessary to explore the reasons behind the behaviour and to introduce behavioural management, along with providing a supportive attitude to overcome the problem.

Recurrent abdominal pain

Problem-orientated topic:

a child with recurrent abdominal pain

Tracey is an 11-year-old girl who presents to her GP with a 6-month history of recurrent abdominal pain. The pain originally began following an episode of chickenpox and has continued since then. She has only attended school intermittently since because of the pain, and the parents are becoming concerned about her. She describes the pain as being situated in the centre of her abdomen, around the umbilicus. There is no history of diarrhoea or vomiting but there is a family history of migraine.

Q1. What are the causes of recurrent abdominal pain?

Q2. What would you look for in your clinical evaluation?

Q3. When should you consider referral for hospital tests?

Q1. What are the causes of recurrent abdominal pain?

This is a common condition affecting 10–15% of schoolchildren, but only 1 in 10 has an organic problem. In

Table 25.1 Inorganic versus organic causes of abdominal pain

Non-organic pain (functional)	Organic pain
Periodicity	No periodicity
No constitutional upset	Associated with constitutional upset, e.g. weight loss, anorexia, fever
Periumbilical pain	Pain distant from umbilicus
Normal growth	Growth failure
Relationship to possible stress/domestic/school factors	Organ-specific symptoms, e.g. diarrhoea, polyuria, gastrointestinal bleeding

BOX 25.2 Causes of recurrent abdominal pain

- Idiopathic
- Psychogenic } (90%)
- Gastrointestinal:
  - Irritable bowel syndrome
  - Constipation
  - Oesophagitis
  - Peptic ulcer
  - Inflammatory bowel disease
  - Malabsorption
- Renal:
  - Urinary tract infection (UTI)
  - Renal calculus
- Hepatic:
  - Hepatitis
- Pancreatic:
  - Pancreatitis
- Gynaecological:
  - Dysmenorrhoea
  - Pelvic inflammatory disease
  - Ovarian cysts
  - Haematocolpos
- Others:
  - Lead poisoning
  - Sickle cell disease
  - Abdominal migraine

these children, the skill is to distinguish those with an organic problem from those with a non-organic (functional) problem (Table 25.1).

Recurrent abdominal pain represents pain of 3 or more months' duration.

The causes of recurrent abdominal pain are shown in Box 25.2.

Q2. What would you look for in your clinical evaluation?

History

It is important in these cases to take a detailed history from the child and parents to determine the precise

- Full blood count (FBC) and erythrocyte sedimentation rate (ESR)/C-reactive protein (CRP), to exclude anaemia or chronic infection
- Liver function tests (+ hepatitis serology), to exclude hepatitis
- Urea and electrolytes, to exclude renal disease
- Serum amylase, to exclude pancreatitis
- A midstream urine sample (MSU), to check for urinary infection
- A stool sample, for microscopy, culture and sensitivity, to exclude parasites, e.g. *Giardia*
- Occult blood × 3, to exclude gastrointestinal bleeding from inflammatory bowel disease or peptic disease
- Abdominal and pelvic ultrasound
- Abdominal X-ray for constipation, lead poisoning, renal calculi

nature of the pain, its frequency, its site and whether or not it affects their daily activities. Constitutional symptoms such as weight loss, anorexia or fever should be asked for and organ-specific symptoms likewise, e.g. renal — dysuria, frequency, haematuria regarding UTI/renal calculus. Gentle exploration into any domestic, school or family stress factors should also be made.

Examination

A full physical examination should be undertaken, both to elicit any abdominal signs and also, more importantly, to reassure the child and parents that the symptom is being taken seriously (Box 25.3). Growth measurements (height and weight) should be recorded and plotted on a centile chart. On general examination signs of anaemia and jaundice should be looked for. On abdominal examination evidence of organomegaly should be considered.

Q3. When should you consider referral for hospital tests?

Referral to hospital should be made if the child shows the following signs/symptoms:
- Constitutional symptoms/signs, e.g. poor appetite, weight loss
- Growth failure
- Gastrointestinal bleeding
- Organ-specific symptoms/signs, e.g. dysuria/haematuria (urinary tract).

Causes of recurrent abdominal pain

Non-organic/functional causes

Idiopathic recurrent abdominal pain

These are children who present with recurrent abdominal pain, usually in the periumbilical T10 distribution, associated with periods free from abdominal pain and with good health between episodes. They are often children who are high achievers with a history of colic as a baby.

General examination shows no abnormality, and growth and routine investigations are normal.

Management of the condition is one of strong reassurance, both to the child and the parents, that there is no specific cause for this condition, whilst accepting that the child is suffering attacks of pain. These cases are best followed up on a regular basis for a variable period of time, depending on the symptoms, and it often helps for children to keep a diary of their symptoms, graded by severity.

Abdominal migraine

Abdominal migraine is the name given to a condition from which some children suffer that involves recurrent episodes of abdominal pain, often associated with nausea and vomiting. The term cyclical vomiting used to be used for this condition and often patients required admission for intravenous fluids to be given and for the vomiting to settle. As well as periumbilical abdominal pain, some also suffer from headaches or develop classical migraine later on in adolescence or as an adult. There is often a strong family history of migraine. The condition described as abdominal migraine can sometimes be treated with pizotifen or a trial of food exclusion.

Irritable bowel syndrome

Some children with recurrent abdominal pain have a pattern of symptoms associated with some minor gastrointestinal upsets such as short-lasting diarrhoea alternating with constipation. There is usually no psychological stress identifiable. There may be a history of bloating and a past history of colic as an infant. It is thought that dysfunction of the autonomic nervous system to the gut may be responsible. Reassurance is the order of the day and the symptoms resolve spontaneously over time.

Organic causes of pain

- Gastrointestinal (Ch. 39):
  - Peptic ulcer
  - Gastro-oesophageal reflux disease
  - Inflammatory bowel disease
  - Constipation

- Urinary (Ch. 40):
  - Infection
  - Obstruction
  - Calculus
- Gynaecological:
  - Dysmenorrhoea
  - Ovarian cyst
- Others:
  - Lead poisoning.

In Tracey's case, provided that the history and physical examination are in keeping with a non-organic (functional) cause, strong reassurance from the GP/health visitor is satisfactory. In order to exclude the rarer causes of the condition, some investigations (Box 25.3) may be required, particularly if the pain is situated elsewhere in the abdomen or there are constitutional upsets.

Whilst the vast majority of these cases are functional in aetiology, organic causes must not be forgotten; in those cases that do not settle with reassurance, hospital referral after GP investigations is then appropriate.

Acute abdominal pain

Problem-orientated topic:

a child with acute lower abdominal pain

Mark, a 13-year-old boy, is brought to his GP by his parents with a 3-day history of lower abdominal pain associated with mild diarrhoea. He has a mild fever and has been off school. General examination shows some lower abdominal tenderness.

Q1. What are the causes of Mark's acute abdominal pain?

Q2 What would you look for in your clinical evaluation?

Q3. What investigations would be required?

Q4. When should you consider hospital referral?

Q1. What are the causes of Mark's acute abdominal pain?

Causes of acute abdominal pain in children are many and varied, and do not all lie within the abdomen (Boxes 25.4 and 25.5).

BOX 25.4 Causes of acute abdominal pain in children

Surgical intra-abdominal
- Acute appendicitis
- Intestinal obstruction
- Intussusception
- Inguinal hernia
- Peritonitis
- Meckel's diverticulum
- Pancreatitis
- Mesenteric adenitis
- Trauma

Medical
- Gastroenteritis (viral or bacterial, e.g. *Campylobacter*)
- Renal (UTI, renal stones, hydronephrosis)
- Henoch–Schönlein purpura
- Diabetic ketoacidosis
- Sickle cell disease
- Hepatitis
- Irritable bowel disease
- Recurrent abdominal pain
- Gynaecological causes (dysmenorrhoea, pelvic inflammatory disease, haematocolpos)
- Constipation
- Psychological
- Lead poisoning
- Porphyria

Extra-abdominal
- Lower lobe pneumonia
- URTI
- Testicular torsion
- Referred pain from hip/spine
- Shingles

Q2. What would you look for in your clinical evaluation?

The assessment of a child with acute abdominal pain requires a detailed history, a full examination by the GP and a decision as to whether the child requires further tests, usually carried out in hospital, or whether he or she can be monitored at home, with a review should the symptoms change or not improve.

A high index of suspicion of organic disease should be the rule with any child presenting with acute abdominal pain. A low threshold for either regular review by the GP or hospital admission must be used.

The history given in Mark's case should suggest the possibility of acute appendicitis, particularly associated

BOX 25.5 Common causes of abdominal pain according to age

Infant
- Colic
- Gastroenteritis
- Constipation
- Intestinal obstruction (intussusception, volvulus, incarcerated hernia, Hirschsprung's disease)

Preschool child
- Gastroenteritis
- Constipation
- Mesenteric adenitis
- UTI
- Trauma
- Sickle cell crisis
- Henoch–Schönlein purpura (HSP)

Schoolchild
- Gastroenteritis
- Appendicitis
- Constipation
- Functional abdominal pain syndromes
- UTI
- Mesenteric adenitis
- Pneumonia
- Sickle cell crisis
- HSP
- Inflammatory bowel disease

Adolescent
- Gastroenteritis
- Appendicitis
- Constipation
- Functional abdominal pain syndromes
- Inflammatory bowel disease
- Testicular torsion
- Ovarian torsion
- Threatened abortion
- Ectopic pregnancy
- Dysmenorrhoea

with localized lower abdominal tenderness/pain and fever. A history of mild diarrhoea is not unusual. The pain is also situated in the lower abdomen and should raise suspicion of an organic cause.

Other causes to consider in his case would be urinary tract infection/renal calculus and referred pain, e.g. scrotum, hip and spine. The overriding decision in such a case is whether a surgical opinion is required, and if so, referral to the appropriate paediatric surgical department will be necessary.

History

The type of pain, its duration and its position are very important features to ascertain from the history. However, in very young children this is not possible. A significant feature associated with pain is intermittent bouts of screaming, particularly associated with pallor. This is an important feature of an intussusception. Older children are more able to give a history and may relate a pain initially to the periumbilical area, only later moving to the lower abdomen and the right iliac fossa: for instance, in appendicitis. In general, children are poor localizers and generally point to the whole of the abdomen when asked to describe where the pain is maximal.

A history of blood in the stool may occur with intussusception (redcurrant jelly stools) but may also be associated with an acute gastroenteritis (e.g. *Campylobacter* infection, with abdominal pain and blood as strong features).

Other features such as a skin rash or arthralgia should be enquired for in relation to Henoch–Schönlein purpura.

Examination

On physical examination the position of the child is important. The child who lies still and is not keen to move may well have peritonism.

Localized tenderness is an important sign, as is tachycardia and/or fever. Examination of the throat or neck for signs of URTI may be relevant (mesenteric adenitis). Signs of peritonism, namely guarding and rigidity, will require a surgical follow-up and admission of the child to hospital. Rectal examination is an area of debate. In acute appendicitis it may be helpful in making a diagnosis of a pelvic appendix but it should not be a routine investigation.

Q3. What investigations would be required?

Investigations at primary care level may include an FBC for leucocytosis, ESR and a urine culture to exclude a UTI, but generally investigations are not undertaken by the GP but rather by the hospital paediatricians on referral of the child to hospital.

Q4. When should you consider hospital referral?

The most important question for the GP to answer in a child with an acute abdomen is whether he or she will require a surgical opinion, and hospital admission is essential if this question is raised. Conditions such as lower lobe pneumonia and diabetic ketoacidosis as extra-abdominal causes of acute abdominal pain must be borne in mind. Again, they usually occur with an ill child who will require investigation and referral to the local paediatric department.

Causes of acute abdominal pain in children

Infantile colic

This commonly occurs around the age of 3 months in full-term infants. The incidence is equal for bottle-fed and breastfed babies. Parents are aware of the infant having paroxysmal episodes of crying, often later in the day. During these episodes infants draw up their legs, exhibit fisting and sometimes are puce in the face. Sometimes the problem is relieved by the passage of flatus or faeces. Possible theories as to causation suggest that certain infants are susceptible to colic and it may be associated with hunger, aerophagy and abdominal distension, and overfeeding.

Differential diagnoses include intussusception, a strangulated inguinal hernia and also minor infections such as otitis media or UTI, which can present in a similar way.

The management consists of a full history and examination of the child to exclude any obvious cause and then strong reassurance to the parents that there is no abnormality and that the problem will resolve. Additional sucrose has been suggested as a treatment. For some mothers who are breastfeeding, the exclusion of cows' milk sometimes improves the problem, but if these mothers are on a diet free of cows' milk, it is important for them to take additional calcium and vitamins A and D. It is known that prolonged colic can be one of the precipitating factors in non-accidental injury.

Acute appendicitis

This is the most common cause of acute abdominal pain that a GP will see. The frequency is 3 per 1000 children. It may occur in very young infants up to teenagers and beyond. It is more difficult to diagnose in very young children. The old adage of 'grumbling appendix' is no longer tenable.

The classical presentation is of initially mild periumbilical abdominal pain, often associated with a mild fever, one or two episodes of diarrhoea, and then movement of the pain to the right iliac fossa and an increase in severity; in the presence of peritoneal irritation, the pain causes the child to lie still, since movement will aggravate it.

Clinical signs will include localized tenderness in the right iliac fossa, guarding and rebound tenderness. Should perforation have occurred and peritonitis ensued, a rigid board-like abdomen may be found.

The child requires to be referred to hospital as soon as possible, having been seen by the GP. Investigations in hospital are discussed in Chapter 39.

Treatment is appendicectomy.

Mesenteric adenitis

Children often present to their GP following a recent history of URTI with abdominal pain sometimes localized to the right iliac fossa. On examination there may be signs of residual infection in the throat or ears, possibly with cervical lymphadenopathy, but abdominal examination is entirely normal. It is thought that the condition is caused by acute enlargement of the abdominal lymph nodes that leads to the pain. Management is expectant and the condition resolves spontaneously.

Intussusception

This is a condition that commonly occurs between the ages of 3 months and 2 years, and is caused by invagination of one part of the bowel into another (see also Ch. 39). The most common site is the ileocaecal junction. It may follow an URTI or gastroenteritis. It is thought that enlarged Peyer's patches may form the leading edge of the intussusception.

The child is often brought to the GP by the parents because of episodic screaming. This is characteristically associated with pallor. In between bouts of pain, the child may appear quite well. Passage of diarrhoea with blood ('redcurrant jelly') is an important but often late sign of intussusception and requires the child to be immediately referred to hospital.

This is a diagnosis that should always be borne in mind with a child in this age group (3 months to 2 years), who has a history of episodic crying and associated pallor.

Management is discussed in Chapter 39.

Other causes

Other causes of acute abdominal pain that should be considered are shown in Box 25.6.

> **BOX 25.6 Other causes of acute abdominal pain to consider**
>
> - Diabetic ketoacidosis
> - Lower lobe pneumonia
> - Henoch–Schönlein purpura
> - UTI
> - Gynaecological causes, e.g. dysmenorrhoea

Vomiting in children

Problem-orientated topic:

a vomiting baby

Ruth is a 9-month-old baby who has a history of vomiting after feeds over the last 3–4 months. Mother describes Ruth as vomiting large quantities of food and is concerned that she is not getting adequate nourishment. She describes occasional small amounts of blood in the vomit. The child's weight chart appears to show static weight gain over the preceding 6 weeks. Vomiting appears to occur after both solid and liquid feeds. Up until recently Mother has not been concerned, but the onset of blood in the vomit and Ruth's static weight have brought her to your attention.

Q1. What are the common causes of vomiting in infants?

Q2. What should you look for in your clinical evaluation?

Q3. What, if any, investigations would be appropriate and when is hospital referral indicated?

BOX 25.7 Causes of vomiting in children

Newborn and infants
- Common causes:
  - Possetting
  - Gastro-oesophageal reflux
  - Gastroenteritis
  - Overfeeding
- Less common causes:
  - Pyloric stenosis
  - Intussusception (Ch. 39)
  - Occult infection, e.g. UTI
  - Raised intracranial pressure (Ch. 28)

Young children
- Common causes:
  - Gastroenteritis
  - Systemic infection
- Less common causes:
  - Toxic ingestion

Adolescents
- Common causes:
  - Gastroenteritis
  - Systemic infection
- Less common causes:
  - Migraine
  - Pregnancy
  - Bulimia
  - Raised intracranial pressure

Q1. What are the common causes of vomiting in infants?

See Box 25.7.

Regurgitation and possetting

In the first 6 months of life it is normal for children to regurgitate/posset small amounts of feed and this does not lead to any long-term problems. The condition usually rectifies itself once the child is sitting upright and particularly when he or she starts to walk. Sitting the child upright after a feed and not winding immediately after a feed can reduce the incidence of possetting. This is a common condition seen by GPs and health visitors alike, and requires only reassurance of the parents.

Gastro-oesophageal reflux

This condition (see also Ch. 39), an exaggerated form of regurgitation and possetting, is common in babies, in particular those with developmental disabilities such as severe cerebral palsy. It is caused by a lax gastro-oesophageal sphincter, which allows reflux of the stomach contents into the oesophagus. There are many degrees of the condition, from simple possetting to significant aspiration leading to oesophagitis, apnoea and recurrent chest infection. It is a possible cause of sudden unexplained death in infancy (SUDI, SIDS). It is thought that up to 50% of newborns will suffer from some degree of reflux, almost all resolving within the first year. It may be associated with abnormal neck movement (Sandifer's syndrome) and may lead to a number of complications, including bleeding/stricture from oesophagitis, failure to thrive, apnoea and Barrett's ulcer. There is a possible association with apparent life-threatening events (ALTEs) and SUDI but these are controversial.

In its mildest form the condition can be managed in primary care with advice on thickening feeds for bottle-fed infants, using thickeners such as Carabel and Nestagel. The use of posture, i.e. sitting infants upright after feeds rather than laying them supine, and the use of Gaviscon with the feeds, often improve the condition. Careful growth monitoring to ensure that the infants thrive is also important.

If these measures are not successful, referral to the paediatric department for further investigation should be undertaken. Further investigations include barium swallow, oesophageal pH monitoring and endoscopy. Drug therapy, including prokinetic agents and protein pump inhibitors, may be indicated. Should these not be effective, there is still a very small place for surgery with fundoplication.

Pyloric stenosis

This occurs in 7 per 1000 live births and has a 6:1 male:female preponderance. It is due to hypertrophy of the circular muscle of the pylorus and usually occurs between the ages of 3 and 6 weeks, presenting with increasingly progressive forceful vomiting of non-bile-stained fluid. Following the vomit, the child is hungry and anxious to feed again, but over a short period of time may lose a considerable amount of weight and become dehydrated, with visible peristalsis seen in the left hypochondrium and associated pyloric tumour palpable between the umbilicus and the right costal margin. A history of projectile vomiting should alert the GP to this possible diagnosis. Even if a pyloric tumour is not palpable, a child should be referred to hospital for further investigations, which may include a test feed, ultrasound scan or barium studies to confirm the diagnosis.

Treatment is surgical (Ramstedt's operation, pyloromyotomy). The surgery must be delayed until the child is biochemically normal, with correction of the metabolic alkalosis that can occur with this condition. Postoperatively children do very well, resuming normal feeds within a few hours, and continue to thrive. There is thought to be a connection between pyloric stenosis and athleticism.

Bowel obstruction

There are four features of intestinal obstruction, which include:

- Bile-stained vomiting
- Failure to pass stool
- Abdominal distension
- Visible peristalsis.

  Causes include:
- Hirschsprung's disease
- Volvulus secondary to a malrotation
- An incarcerated inguinal hernia.

Referral for a paediatric surgical opinion is essential in order to delineate cause and specific treatment.

Q2. What should you look for in your clinical evaluation?

History

A history of vomiting in a child of any age must be taken seriously and a full history and examination undertaken to ascertain the cause. Whilst the majority of these causes are minor and often self-limiting, there are major and serious causes that require hospital treatment and which need to be identified early to prevent any complications, e.g. meningitis, pyelonephritis and pyloric stenosis.

From the history the GP should ascertain the duration of the vomiting, the state of health of the child and whether the vomiting is associated with loss of weight, fever or diarrhoea to suggest an infective cause. The type of vomit should be enquired about, first to differentiate possetting from true vomiting, and then to establish the presence of blood-stained vomit, which may suggest oesophagitis. Bile-stained vomit suggests intestinal obstruction. Projectile vomiting may suggest pyloric stenosis.

Examination

A physical examination will include a full examination of the abdomen and scrotum. A high suspicion of causes outside the abdomen must be borne in mind, e.g. meningitis or pyelonephritis, both of which may present with vomiting. Otitis media is commonly associated with vomiting. Examination of the throat and ears will be required as well.

Vomiting is a common complaint of children who are brought by their parents, particularly in those under 1 year of age. As can be seen from Box 25.7, many causes must be considered. Ruth's vomiting suggests gastro-oesophageal reflux; in particular, traces of blood in the vomit suggest the development of oesophagitis. A static weight over the preceding 6 weeks poses the need for referral, investigation and possibly treatment, while the majority of cases at this age can be dealt with by health visitors and GPs, who should give reassurance after a full examination and weight check, with advice on thickeners and posture after feeds.

Q3. What, if any, investigations would be appropriate and when is hospital referral indicated?

Regurgitation and possetting

Although this condition usually just requires reassurance from the GP and health visitors, it is helpful to keep a record of the child's growth to check this is proceeding along satisfactory lines. Growth failure would indicate a need for hospital referral for further investigations.

Gastro-oesophageal reflux

Initial management (see also p. 312) is centred around posture after feeds, feed thickeners and use of Gaviscon. If these measures are not satisfactory, a hospital referral would be indicated for further investigations such as barium swallow, ultrasound and 24-hour pH intra-oesophageal monitoring.

Pyloric stenosis

A history of projectile vomiting requires hospital referral for further investigations by the paediatric department and probable referral to the surgeons for pyloromyotomy or Ramsted's procedure.

Bowel obstruction

If bowel obstruction is suspected, immediate referral to a paediatric surgeon is necessary in order for the problem to be further evaluated and, if necessary, for corrective measures to be undertaken surgically.

In Ruth's case, referral to a paediatrician would be appropriate, where a full history and examination will be undertaken and further investigations considered, to include ultrasound, barium studies and possibly oesophageal pH monitoring. The use of proton pump inhibitors and prokinetic agents should also be considered when the child is not thriving. Surgery has a very small place in the overall management.

Acute diarrhoea

> **Problem-orientated topic:**
>
> **a child with diarrhoea**
>
> Mohammed is a 10-month-old child who returned to the UK 2 days ago following a 4-week stay in Pakistan with his family. On the flight home he developed acute vomiting and diarrhoea. The diarrhoea has persisted on his return home, and his parents have brought him to the surgery because he is now reluctant to take his feeds and is drowsy.
>
> Q1. What are the common causes of diarrhoea?
> Q2. How would you assess the child in the surgery?
> Q3. How would you manage this situation at home?
> Q4. When would hospital referral be indicated?

Q1. What are the common causes of diarrhoea?

Acute diarrhoea is a common world-wide illness in young children under 5 and still has a significant morbidity and mortality. Whilst mortality has dropped significantly in the West, there is still significant morbidity and mortality

---

> **BOX 25.8 Causes of acute diarrhoea**
>
> - Viral gastroenteritis, e.g. rotavirus (common), echo and adenoviruses
> - Bacterial gastroenteritis, e.g. *Campylobacter*, *Shigella*, *Salmonella*, cholera, *Escherichia coli*
> - Protozoal, e.g. *Giardia*, *Cryptosporidium*
> - Others, e.g. otitis media, URTI, UTI, antibiotic-induced
> - Non-infectious gastrointestinal causes, e.g. intussusception ('redcurrant jelly diarrhoea')

in developing countries such as those in Africa, Asia and the Far East (Ch. 38). The majority of cases are caused by infectious agents but causes outside of the gastrointestinal tract must not be forgotten (Box 25.8).

Viral gastroenteritis

The most common viral agent is the rotavirus, which tends to cause outbreaks and epidemics in the winter months. It begins with a low-grade fever for 1–2 days, followed by the onset of vomiting and watery diarrhoea, which usually lasts from 1 to 5 days. Other viral causes include the echo- and adenoviruses, which can produce a similar picture but are less common than rotavirus.

Bacterial gastroenteritis

The picture here is similar to viral cases but a history of overseas travel is important if present. In addition, *Campylobacter*, *Shigella* and *Salmonella* are associated with blood-stained stools and abdominal pain is particularly a feature of *Campylobacter*. *E. coli* strain O157 may lead to haemolytic uraemic syndrome and acute renal failure.

Protozoal gastroenteritis

This is caused by *Giardia lamblia*, *Cryptosporidium* and *Entamoeba histolytica*.

Other conditions to consider

- Otitis media
- URTI
- UTI
- Antibiotic-induced diarrhoea, e.g. with amoxicillin.

Intussusception associated with blood-stained diarrhoea ('redcurrant jelly') is a late feature of this condition.

Q2. How would you assess the child in the surgery?

History

It is important to take a full history from the parents to determine the duration of the diarrhoea, frequency of stools and type of stool, i.e. soft, liquid and/or blood-stained. Recent overseas travel clearly is an important part of the history to determine.

Examination

On examination the abdomen is checked for tenderness or masses and the presence of bowel sounds. It is also important to consider systems outside of the abdomen. Examination of the ears, throat, chest and urine should be considered.

The history given for Mohammed is suggestive of acute gastroenteritis that began on his journey home, suggesting that the causative agent may have been acquired abroad. It is important to take a full history and perform a full examination, looking particularly for signs of dehydration and, if this is present, to assess the degree. Less than 5% dehydration may be managed at home, but 5–10% and certainly over 10% dehydration will require hospital referral. It is important to enquire about other family members to see if anyone else has been affected. A stool culture (Box 25.10 below) should be sent to the local laboratory and the child should be treated with oral rehydration fluid for 24 hours initially.

Important features of the history will include the presence of vomiting associated with the diarrhoea, and blood in the stool, both of which will raise the likelihood that the child may require paediatric hospital opinion.

Q3. How would you manage this situation at home?

The majority of these cases can be managed at home and will have negative stool cultures; they should be able to resume normal fluids and solids within 2 or 3 days of coming home. However, should they continue to have diarrhoea and vomiting, a hospital admission will become necessary and, depending on stool cultures and investigations such as blood tests, further treatment may be indicated.

The most important complication of acute diarrhoea is dehydration (Box 25.9). This is caused by the excess loss of water and sodium in the liquid stools, the loss not being compensated by oral intake. The presence of vomiting compounds the problem, but with acute diarrhoea and sickness, as a rule, the vomiting only lasts about 12 hours. Dehydration is assessed in three degrees by estimating the percentage of fluid loss: mild (less than 5%), moderate (5–10%) and severe (>10%). It is important to make an accurate assessment of the level of dehydration, as water makes up 80% of the body weight of infants.

Fluid deficit varies from 50 ml/kg (mild) in acute diarrhoea up to >100 ml/kg (severe) and can lead to dehydration ranging from mild to moderate/severe.

BOX 25.9 Degrees of dehydration

Less than 5% (mild)
- Dry mouth and lips

5–10% (moderate)
- Dry tongue
- Sunken eyes and fontanelle
- Loss of skin turgor
- Reduced urine output
- Tachycardia

10% and above (severe)
- Poor peripheral perfusion
- Drowsy
- Urine output nil for 12 hours
- Sunken eyes and fontanelle
- Tachycardia and reduced blood pressure

It is important, if possible, to measure body weight when the child is first seen and to compare this with the most recent weight from the parent-held records in order to obtain an estimate of the volume of body water lost. (1 kg body weight is equivalent to 1 litre of fluid.) However, this is not always possible and a clinical estimate of fluid loss has to be made (<5%, 5–10% and >10% — Box 25.9).

Mild dehydration (< 5%)

This can be managed at home. Cows' milk is stopped and clear fluids are given for 24 hours. Toddlers may be offered a flat cola drink or juices but young babies should be given oral rehydration fluids, which contain electrolytes and calories in the appropriate amounts: Na (60 mmol/l), K$^+$ (20 mmol/l), glucose (100 mmol/l). Breastfeeding should be continued throughout the illness.

Reintroduction of milk and solids can be started after 1–2 days of clear fluids because there is no longer any evidence for regrading milk feeds. Milk and solids can be reintroduced at an earlier age than was previously advised. A small minority of infants may relapse with diarrhoea because of a temporary lactose intolerance or cows' milk protein intolerance and may take longer to resume normal feeds with normal stools. The majority of children will be able to tolerate cows' milk and solids within a few days of the onset of diarrhoea.

There is no place for antidiarrhoeal or antiemetic agents in the management of acute gastroenteritis in children. Antibiotics, however, may be considered in specific situations, e.g.:
- *Campylobacter* — erythromycin
- Dysentery — ciprofloxacin
- *Giardia lamblia* — metronidazole.

- Blood-stained diarrhoea
- Diarrhoea for greater than 1 week
- History of overseas travel ⎱ Consider
- Ill child during epidemic ⎰ hospitalization

Stool cultures will need to be taken in order to confirm these bacterial causes (Box 25.10).

Q4. When would hospital referral be indicated?

Moderate (5–10%) to severe (> 10%) dehydration

If clinical assessment indicates that the child has a degree of dehydration of 5–10% or greater than 10%, the child should be admitted to hospital for further assessment and investigation. Treatment will include intravenous fluids, assessment of urea and electrolytes, stool culture and other investigations such as abdominal X-rays, blood cultures and MSUs as indicated.

Prolonged diarrhoea

This is discussed in more detail in Chapter 39.

Diarrhoea lasting for more than 14 days is defined as chronic and requires further investigation by the paediatric department.

Lactose intolerance (Ch. 39)

This is usually a secondary phenomenon following an episode of gastroenteritis. A primary form of lactose intolerance does exist and causes diarrhoea after the first milk feed. In non-Caucasian children it is normal for there to be no lactose in the brush border of the small intestine. The absence of the disaccharide lactase leads to watery stools due to osmotic diarrhoea. The stools have a low pH and positive reducing substances may be detected by using Clinitest tablets. Faecal sugars can be detected by stool chromatography.

Management

Management involves stopping lactose-containing milk and substituting with soya milk for a period of time until in secondary cases the brush border lactase is reformed, following which the infant will again be able to tolerate lactose in the diet. In the primary form, lifelong avoidance of lactose may be required.

Cow's milk protein intolerance (Ch. 44)

This occurs in between 2 and 7.5% of infants. It tends to occur in the first 3 months of life in babies fed on formula milk. Breastfed babies may develop it if their mothers are drinking cows' milk. The symptoms that the infants exhibit are varied and may include vomiting, which is common, usually about an hour after ingestion of the milk, loose stools, which may sometimes be blood-stained with mucus, abdominal pain, discomfort, crying and irritability. In addition, some children develop wheezing, cough or rhinitis and those with an atopic background may develop eczema and urticaria on areas of skin with which the milk has been in contact. Angioedema, producing acute stridor, and anaphylaxis are rare but can be delayed phenomena. Around 50% of children with cows' milk protein intolerance have other food intolerances and between 8 and 14% of them are intolerant to soya protein.

Diagnosis

Skin prick and radioallergosorbence testing (RAST) is unreliable, as is jejunal biopsy. Elimination diets and later milk challenge are the best ways to determine diagnosis. Natural history suggests that the condition will last a few months and has usually resolved by the age of 1 year. However, it may last up to the age of 3. To assist mothers in maintaining a cows' milk-free diet, the help of the paediatric dietician is very useful. There are several substitute milks that can be used, including soya milk and Pregestemil.

Toddler diarrhoea (chronic non-specific diarrhoea — CNSD)

This condition, which occurs in infants from the age of 6 months to around 5 years, is sometimes described as irritable bowel syndrome of infancy. It is essentially diarrhoea without failure to thrive, and is associated with rapid gastrocolic transit time. It comes under the umbrella of the functional bowel disorders and is one of the spectrum of motility disorders of the gastrointestinal tract. An alternative name is 'peas and carrots diarrhoea' since the diarrhoea often contains undigested food particles. The incidence is greater in male infants.

It is known that the diarrhoea is made worse by a high-roughage diet, a diet with additional fruit and sugary drinks. An important factor on examination is that there is no failure to thrive. Growth charts must be checked and plotted in order to ensure that this is the case.

Management

Removal of excess fruit juices may help, and exploration of a possible food allergy can sometimes be useful. There is sometimes a history of atopy. Diets low in fat are known to reduce intestinal transit time, and stress in the family or personal stress may be a factor. However, the prime feature of these infants is that they are healthy and thriving but have loose stools. Management is strong reassurance that the condition will improve spontaneously. Increasing the fat intake in the diet sometimes helps in increasing the transit time. A trial excluding cows' milk and eggs may sometimes be effective. Loperamide may be used symptomatically. Stress management strategies have been employed. The condition resolves spontaneously by the age of 5.

Blood in the stool

Problem-orientated topic:

a child with blood in the stool

Sam is a 3-year-old with a history of constipation. His mother reports that he only passes a motion once or twice a week and the stools are hard when passed. She has noticed some bright red bleeding on the outside of the stool recently when he has been straining for long periods. She also mentions that he cries with the passage of the stool.

Q1. What are the causes of blood in the stool?

Q2. What important features in the history and examination should you look for?

Q3. What is your management of this problem?

Q1. What are the causes of blood in the stool?

See Box 25.11.

Sam's history is very typical of a child with constipation (infrequent stools that are hard when passed). The bright red blood is present as a result of straining and the development of an anal fissure, which also causes him to cry when passing the stool.

Q2. What important features in the history and examination should you look for?

History

A history of constipation is important and helpful, also the colour of the blood and whether the blood is on the outside of the stool or mixed with it. Red blood suggests

---

BOX 25.11 Causes of blood in stool

Neonates
- Swallowed maternal blood
- Necrotizing enterocolitis
- Haemorrhagic disease of newborn
- Midgut volvulus
- Anal fissure

Well child
- Bright red blood:
  - Anal fissure, polyp or rectal prolapse
  - Milk allergy
- Large amount of blood:
  - Meckel's diverticulum
  - Peptic ulcer
  - Oesophageal varices

Sick child
- Gastroenteritis (*Campylobacter/Shigella/Salmonella*)
- Intussusception
- Henoch–Schönlein purpura
- Crohn's disease
- Ulcerative colitis

---

bleeding from the lower bowel, a black stool (melaena) suggests bleeding from the upper gastrointestinal tract, and with an intussusception the associated diarrhoea is described as 'redcurrant jelly' with blood mixed with the motion.

A history of pain associated with constipation suggests an anal fissure. Inspection of the anus is important to identify this cause.

A history of bleeding from other sites, e.g. epistaxis/urine, would suggest a generalized bleeding disorder rather than a local cause and would require further investigation.

Examination

On examination a history of diarrhoea, bleeding and associated fever suggests gastroenteritis. Henoch–Schönlein purpura — a combination of abdominal pain, arthralgia and characteristic rash on extensor surfaces — should be looked for (Ch. 33). Sexual abuse should also be considered (Ch. 37).

Q3. What is your management of this problem?

With constipation and anal fissure, investigations are not necessary at primary care level but advice is necessary about the management of the constipation with softeners and bowel stimulants.

With anal fissure stool softeners and anaesthetic jelly may relieve the symptoms while the fissure heals.

Hospital referral

- Intussusception requires surgical referral for further investigation.
- Recurrent red rectal bleeding requires surgical follow-up to exclude conditions such as a rectal polyp.
- Swallowed maternal blood can be differentiated using the APT test.

Scrotal swelling

Problem-orientated topic:

a child with a swollen scrotum

John is a 5-year-old boy who is brought to see you with a 6-hour history of increasingly severe pain in the scrotum. His mother has noticed that the scrotum is swollen and is anxious to seek your advice.

Q1. What are the causes of scrotal swelling?

Q2. How do you manage these conditions?

Q3. What complications may arise?

Q4. When is hospital referral indicated?

Q1. What are the causes of scrotal swelling?

In evaluating the cause of a scrotal swelling (Box 25.12) there are important features in both the history and physical examination that will help to determine the diagnosis and the course of management.

Scrotal pain must always be considered seriously in a child of any age, as the possibility of a testicular torsion must not be missed. In John's case, he should be seen as soon as possible by the GP and as far as possible the cause of the testicular pain and swelling should be ascertained. Conditions such as a hydrocele, which are painless, and an inguinal hernia, likewise painless unless it becomes incarcerated, are usually not difficult to establish. The differential diagnosis between testicular torsion and epididymo-orchitis may be difficult at times, and should not be made without a second opinion, which will require a hospital surgical referral to the paediatric team. With testicular torsion, time is paramount, and if delay occurs, the affected testis will become ischaemic and atrophy, and function will be lost.

BOX 25.12 Causes of scrotal swellings

Painful
- Testicular torsion
- Epididymo-orchitis

Usually painless
- Hydrocele
- Inguinal hernia (pain if incarcerated)

Q2. How do you manage these conditions?

Hydrocele

A hydrocele is a collection of fluid in the tunica vaginalis. It may communicate with the peritoneal cavity via a patent processus vaginalis, in which case it may vary in size. Most, however, do not fluctuate in size and are separate from the peritoneal cavity. They usually resolve by the age of 18 months but occasionally require surgical treatment. The development of a hydrocele in an older boy should raise the suspicion of testicular malignancy. Clinically, hydroceles are often present at birth. They do not extend into the groin unless there is a communication into the peritoneal cavity. The testis cannot be palpated through the fluid and they can be transilluminated. Treatment is surgical if the condition has not resolved by the age of 18 months.

Inguinal hernia

An inguinal hernia characteristically causes intermittent swelling in the scrotum and is particularly noted when the child is crying or straining. The swelling can be massaged out of the scrotum back into the abdomen through the inguinal ring. Inguinal hernias in childhood are indirect (associated with a patent processus vaginalis). Premature infants are more at risk of an inguinal hernia.

Management of an inguinal hernia is surgical, and referral to a paediatric surgeon is the preferred choice. The hernia may become incarcerated and irreducible. This is an acute surgical situation requiring immediate referral. Pressure on the testicular vessels produced by the incarcerated bowel within the confined inguinal canal may also lead to testicular necrosis and subsequent atrophy. An irreducible hernia may lead to abdominal distension resulting from bowel obstruction.

Testicular torsion

This occurs usually before the age of 6 years. The torsion occurs suddenly and is extremely painful. The testis and epididymis twist on the spermatic cord, usually within the tunica vaginalis. This is commonly associated with an abnormal attachment of the tunica (clapperbell testis) or an undescended testis.

Urgent surgical treatment is required to prevent ischaemic damage to the testis. At operation both the affected testis and the contralateral normal testis should be fixed in the scrotum (orchidopexy) to prevent recurrence of the torsion.

Torsion of a testicular appendage (hydatid of Morgani) can present with acute scrotal pain, usually on the upper pole of the testis, and may mimic testicular torsion. Treatment is surgical.

Epididymo-orchitis

Epididymo-orchitis in the absence of urinary tract abnormalities, e.g. a neuropathic bladder or reflux, is uncommon in young boys and a swollen tender testis and hemiscrotum must be assumed to be due to torsion until proved otherwise. The child must be referred for an immediate surgical opinion. Orchitis may occur with mumps. Epididymo-orchitis requires antibiotic treatment; the symptoms and signs may mimic testicular torsion and frequently require a surgical opinion first.

Q3. What complications may arise?

The hernia may become incarcerated and irreducible. This is an acute surgical situation requiring immediate referral. Pressure on the testicular vessels produced by the incarcerated bowel within the confined inguinal canal may also lead to testicular necrosis and subsequent atrophy. An irreducible hernia may lead to abdominal distension resulting from bowel obstruction.

Q4. When is hospital referral indicated?

The management of an inguinal hernia is surgical, and all patients with this condition should be referred to a paediatric surgeon.

Food allergy (see also Ch. 44)

Food allergy occurs in between 5 and 30% of infants. The common foods involved include milk, egg, fish and peanuts. It is usually an IgE-mediated response. Histamine may also be involved in reactions to strawberries, egg white and cheese. Atopic individuals are more prone to food allergies. They are generally of a temporary nature, although allergy to wheat gluten (coeliac disease) is usually lifelong.

Egg intolerance

This occurs in 1.6% of infants. It first appears around 6 months of age. Within 1 hour of ingestion of egg, a rash (erythema) appears around the mouth, associated with urticaria of the oral mucosa. Angioedema of the face may occur, with stridor and wheezing. Anaphylaxis is rare. Skin prick and RAST testing is unreliable. The treatment is to exclude egg. The prognosis is good. By the age of 3 years most children have lost the egg allergy and are able to eat egg without problems. A few cases have a lifelong allergy and are required to exclude egg permanently.

Peanut allergy

The prevalence of peanut allergy in the Western world is about 0.5%. Atopic children are more prone to this condition. Commonly, ingestion of peanuts causes urticaria and may cause angioedema leading to wheeze, tightness of the chest, cough and breathlessness. Acute anaphylaxis is not uncommon. A lifelong allergy is common. Treatment consists of exclusion of peanuts, the use of antihistamines and subcutaneous injection of 1:1000 adrenaline (epinephrine) using Epipen. Skin testing under controlled conditions may also be appropriate to determine whether the allergy is present or not.

Food additives

Allergies occur to tartrazine (an azodye or yellow colouring agent), which can lead to urticaria, asthma and rhinitis. Sulfites are another food additive that can lead to wheezing, particularly in children with pre-existing asthma.

Iron deficiency anaemia

This is a very common problem seen by GPs in babies and toddlers and is due to a combination of rapid growth requiring extra iron, a diet deplete of iron-rich foods and, in some children, chronic blood loss. It is usually asymptomatic initially, but with falling haemoglobin levels the child may then suffer from lethargy and anorexia, and low levels of iron may affect intellectual function. Apart from pallor of mucous membranes, splenomegaly may be detectable in 10% of cases and systolic flow murmurs are frequently heard. Blood loss should always be considered a possibility, although dietary causes predominate.

Secondary causes (blood loss) include:
- Nose bleeds
- Meckel's diverticulum
- Gastrointestinal polyps
- Peptic ulceration due to *Helicobacter pylori*.

Pica and breath-holding have also been shown to relate to low haemoglobin values.

The prevalence of iron deficiency anaemia ranges from 12 to 40% of 1–2-year-olds if deprived populations are included.

Investigation

The initial investigations at primary care level are haemoglobin, blood film and serum ferritin. In iron deficiency anaemia the haemoglobin is low (< 10 g/l). The blood film shows microcytic hypochromic red blood cells and the serum ferritin is low, indicating iron deficiency.

Management

Treatment is with iron supplements orally (ferrous sulphate/fumarate/gluconate) and measurement of the haemoglobin periodically. Parents should be encouraged to give a diet to the child containing iron-rich foods. On oral iron treatment haemoglobin should improve by approximately 1 g/dl per week. If the haemoglobin does not improve on iron therapy, consider the reasons shown in Box 25.13.

Failure of the haemoglobin to respond to iron therapy will require referral to a paediatric or haematology department for further investigation.

Prevention

Breastfeeding protects against iron deficiency anaemia, as the iron is absorbed more effectively. Cow's milk should not be given to infants under 1 year, as this may cause blood loss from the gastrointestinal tract.

Bruising

Apart from bruising on the legs of toddlers, which is a common finding, and cough purpura on the face, which can occur with coughing and vomiting, bruising must always be taken seriously. A full assessment should be made, with referral for further investigations if appropriate (see also Ch. 43). Box 25.14 lists the common causes of bruising in the different ages but these will all require hospital referral for haematological and other paediatric investigations to ascertain the precise cause and management plan.

Neonatal jaundice

Problem-orientated topic:

a jaundiced baby

Sarah is an 8-week-old breastfed baby born at term, who was noted to be jaundiced in the first week of life and remains jaundiced now. She is feeding well but the parents are concerned because the jaundice does not appear to be clearing, as it has in other babies at the clinic. She is brought to see you for your advice.

Q1. What causes of jaundice must be considered at this age?

Q2. What is your clinical approach to this problem?

Q3. When is hospital referral indicated?

BOX 25.13 Failure of iron therapy

- Non-compliance
- Wrong diagnosis, e.g. haemoglobinopathies, thalassaemia, chronic renal failure, chronic infection, myeloproliferative disorders
- Lead poisoning
- Chronic blood loss, e.g. cow's milk protein allergy, Meckel's diverticulum, epistaxis

---

BOX 25.14 Causes of bruising in children

Neonates
- Birth trauma, e.g. cephalohaematoma and subconjunctival haemorrhage
- Coagulation disorders, e.g. haemorrhagic disease of the newborn (vitamin K-dependent factors), haemophilia, liver disease
- Thrombocytopenia: maternal autoimmune thrombocytopenia
- Congenital infection, e.g. cytomegalovirus and rubella
- Thrombocytopenia with absent radius (TAR syndrome)

Infants
- Coagulation disorder:
  - Haemophilia
  - Late-onset haemorrhagic disease
  - Liver disease
- Thrombocytopenia:
  - TAR syndrome
  - Congenital infection
  - Idiopathic thrombocytopenic purpura (ITP)
  - Malignancy
  - Wiscott–Aldrich syndrome
- Trauma:
  - Accidental
  - Non-accidental injury (NAI, child abuse)

Older children
- Trauma, both accidental and NAI
- Bleeding disorders: ITP, haemophilia and von Willebrand's disease
- Liver disease
- Bone marrow failure, e.g. leukaemia
- Infections, e.g. meningococcal sepsis
- Haemolytic uraemic syndrome
- Vasculitis, e.g. Henoch–Schönlein purpura
- Systemic lupus erythematosus (SLE)

Q1. What causes of jaundice must be considered at this age?

Jaundice (see also Ch. 48) in the neonatal period is a common problem presenting to GPs. Around 60% of normal infants will show signs of jaundice in the first week but the majority will have resolved by the end of the second week. Persistence of the jaundice beyond this time must be considered to be pathological until proved otherwise and requires a very thorough assessment. There are several reasons why children are clinically jaundiced in the first week or so (Box 25.15) and these include:
- Haemolysis in the first days as the haemoglobin concentration falls
- Reduced lifespan initially of the red blood cells (70 days as opposed to 120)
- Liver immaturity with reduced glucuronyl transferase activity, leading to reduction in conjugation of bilirubin initially.

Unconjugated bilirubin is fat-soluble and bound to albumin. Unbound unconjugated bilirubin in excess may lead to the serious complication of kernicterus.

This may lead in turn to the development of cerebral palsy, choreoathetosis, nerve deafness and mental retardation.

Breast milk jaundice (unconjugated form)
This occurs in breastfed babies who are thriving but remain jaundiced for a period longer than 2 weeks. The cause is unknown but breastfeeding may be allowed to continue quite safely for as long as the mother wishes. On cessation of breastfeeding the jaundice will disappear and there are no complications of the condition.

Hypothyroidism (unconjugated form)
This condition is now screened for using the neonatal (Guthrie) screening test. If jaundice continues for more than 2 weeks, however, thyroid function testing should be undertaken and hypothyroidism excluded.

Sarah presents with a typical history for a breastfed term baby. She is well and the jaundice generally does not fluctuate very much. Tests will show that the bilirubin is unconjugated, generally < 200 μmol/l, and it is quite safe to advise the mother to continue breastfeeding until she decides to stop or her milk becomes insufficient. There is no associated risk of the jaundice to the baby.

It is, however, important to investigate the jaundice with a full history and examination of the child, and with investigations to ascertain the level of serum bilirubin and the amount of conjugated and unconjugated bilirubin, in order to exclude the other conditions listed in Box 25.15. These will require hospital referral as appropriate and further investigations as outlined in the chapter.

Q2. What is your clinical approach to this problem?

The GP must take a careful history to ascertain when the jaundice started and the state of wellbeing of the infant. The colour of the stools and urine must be asked for. Pale stools and dark urine suggest an obstructive cause and require prompt early referral for further investigation.

Measurement of total and unconjugated levels of bilirubin must be made to determine the type of jaundice present. A level of bilirubin > 200 μmol/l requires hospital referral.

The common situation of physiological and breast milk jaundice, both of which are associated with an unconjugated hyperbilirubinaemia, are self-limiting, but raised levels of conjugated bilirubin suggest the possibility of either a hepatic or a post-hepatic cause for the jaundice and hospital referral is essential.

Prolonged jaundice lasting more than 2 weeks (Box 25.15) requires full explanation, in particular to rule out an infective cause such as a UTI or neonatal hepatitis and, most importantly, obstruction to biliary outflow from biliary atresia, which requires prompt surgical treatment to prevent complications. Potential complications include biliary cirrhosis and portal hypertension (Ch. 49).

Q3. When is hospital referral indicated?

Hospital referral is indicated in the following situations, to which the GP must be alert:
- Early onset of jaundice within the first 24 hours
- A serum bilirubin > 200 μmol/l
- Conjugated hyperbilirubinaemia (plus pale stools/dark urine)
- An ill baby who is jaundiced in whom the immediate cause is not apparent.

Lumps in the neck

> **Problem-orientated topic:**
>
> ## a child with swellings in the neck
>
> Anna is a 2½-year-old who is brought to see you because her parents have noticed swellings on either side of the neck following a series of upper respiratory infections that she has been experiencing over the last 2 months or so. They tell you that she is generally well, with a good appetite and full of energy, but appears to be prone to these recurrent infections. They are concerned that she has an underlying problem and seek your advice.
>
> Q1. What are the important causes of cervical lymphadenopathy?
> Q2. When should hospital referral be considered?

Q1. What are the important causes of cervical lymphadenopathy?

This is a common presentation to GPs and requires a careful assessment to determine the cause and reassure the parents and child. The most common neck swellings that a GP will see are cervical lymph glands, usually in the anterior cervical chain, but posterior triangle cervical lymph nodes also occur (rubella).

> **BOX 25.16 Causes of cervical lymphadenopathy**
>
> **More common**
> - Cervical adenitis, e.g. URTI, tonsillitis, otitis media, rubella
> - Glandular fever, parotid enlargement, e.g. mumps
> - Mastoid enlargement, e.g. mastoiditis
> - Cervical abscess
>
> **Less common**
> - Thyroglossal cyst
> - Branchial fistula remnant
> - Thyroid enlargement (goitre)
> - Tuberculosis (Ch. 44)
> - Lymphoma (Ch. 51)
> - Leukaemia (Ch. 51)

See Box 25.16 for causes of cervical lymphadenopathy.

Cervical adenitis

Enlargement of the cervical glands in the anterior cervical chain commonly occurs with infections such as tonsillitis, pharyngitis and otitis media. The glands enlarge but remain discrete and are tender on palpation. Viral infections predominate as the cause of enlarged cervical lymph nodes but bacterial causes can occur and may require antibiotics. Spontaneous resolution of the underlying enlarged lymph nodes is the normal course of events, but in many children glands do not totally resolve and remain as a persisting cervical lymphadenopathy. This triggers attendance at the surgery and a request for the GP to examine the child.

A full history is obtained from the parent and child to determine the length of history, any preceding symptoms or signs to suggest viral infection, and whether antibiotics have been given already. Examination of the throat and ears is undertaken, along with examination of the neck to determine the site of the cervical swelling/lymphadenopathy. It is also important to examine other lymphatic areas such as the axillae and groin and to exclude enlargement of the liver and spleen. Specific clinical signs such as palatal petechial haemorrhages in glandular fever may be found, and in myeloproliferative disorders a bleeding tendency may also be found due to low platelets leading to purpuric rash.

Infectious mononucleosis (glandular fever) can lead to a severe exudative tonsillitis associated with generalized lymphadenopathy and splenomegaly and, in particular, large painful cervical lymph nodes. Palatal petechiae also occur. It is important to suspect this on clinical grounds and to arrange a specific test (Monospot/Paul–Bunnell) to confirm the diagnosis, as antibiotics play no part in the management; indeed, if these children are given amoxicillin they may develop a florid and extensive maculopapular rash.

Malignancy

A more serious cause of persistent cervical lymphadenopathy may be myeloproliferative disorders including leukaemia and lymphoma (Ch. 51). In these situations the nodes tend to be fixed — matted together and non-tender, and the child has constitutional symptoms including fever, night sweats, weight loss and malaise. There may also be hepatosplenomegaly and lymphadenopathy at other sites. These children require urgent referral to the hospital paediatric department for further assessment.

Thyroid swelling (goitre)

Here the swelling is anterior in the midline of the neck. A smooth diffuse swelling on both sides of the neck may be due to hypo- or hyperthyroidism. In addition, a pubertal goitre can occur, particularly in girls who have normal thyroid function tests.

Mastoid swelling

This is a tender swelling over the mastoid process behind the ear, with the ear displaced anteriorly, associated with the presence of otitis media; this requires immediate hospital referral for ENT assessment, intravenous antibiotics and possible surgery to drain the mastoid.

Midline swellings of the neck

These may be caused by:
- Submental lymph node.
- Dermoid cyst.
- Thyroglossal cyst. These cysts arise from the thyroglossal duct, which develops at the base of the tongue and migrates into the neck in the development of the thyroid gland. Cysts may become infected and cause a swelling in the anterior part of the neck. They characteristically move with the tongue and on swallowing. They require surgical excision following referral to a paediatric surgeon.
- Ectopic thyroid or goitre at the site of the normal thyroid.

Branchial fistulae/remnants

Persistence of the second branchial cleft may give rise to a blind-ending sinus or fistula between the tonsillar fossa and the skin overlying the anterior border of the sternomastoid muscle at the junction of its lower third and middle third. A mucous discharge may occur and occasionally the fistulae become infected. Treatment is by surgical excision after the first 6 months of life.

Table 25.2 Investigations for neck swellings

Test	Reason
FBC/film	To exclude anaemia and myeloproliferative disorder
White blood count (WBC)	Raised in bacterial infections
Atypical lymphocytes	Present in glandular fever
Paul–Bunnell/Monospot	Positive in glandular fever
Cytomegalovirus/ Toxodye test	To exclude CMV infection and toxoplasmosis
Throat swab	Group A haemolytic *Streptococcus*

Investigations

See Table 25.2.

Anna presents with a typical story of a child suffering from upper respiratory viral infections associated with cervical adenopathy. In between the episodes of infection she is well and thriving but continues to have bouts of infection that tend to make her unwell and produce concern in the parents. A full history and examination are essential for the aetiology, and rare causes such as tuberculosis, lymphoma and leukaemia must not be forgotten. Investigations as listed will be necessary in order to establish the precise diagnosis.

Following investigation Anna is found to have a normal blood count and a negative Monospot, CMV and toxoplasmosis dye test; the most likely cause of her cervical lymphadenopathy is recurrent URTI, which will have no long-term detrimental effect. Parents are reassured and advised that no further investigation is necessary.

Q2. When should hospital referral be considered?

Hospital referral should be considered for all children in whom the cause of the cervical swelling is not apparent. In particular, initial investigations such as full blood count may lead to a diagnosis, e.g. myeloproliferative disorder, that requires immediate hospital referral. It may be possible for the GP to manage conditions in primary care such as throat and ear infections, glandular fever and other viral infections. Thyroid goitre requires investigation with thyroid function tests, ultrasound and hospital referral. Parotid enlargements may occur with mumps and be managed by the GP. Mastoid enlargements generally require assistance from the ENT department. Cervical abscess, thyroglossal cysts and branchial fistulae will all require the assistance of the paediatric surgeons in order to treat these problems.

26

Disorders of the urinary tract

LEARNING OUTCOMES

By the end of this chapter you should:
- Know the basic anatomy and physiology of the urinary tract
- Recognize common and less common patterns of urinary incontinence in children and be able to offer appropriate treatments for enuresis
- Know the appropriate investigations for children with suspected and proven urinary tract infections
- Recognize normal and abnormal frequency of micturition, and know how to assess the child who appears to be passing excessive amounts of urine
- Be able to describe in detail the appropriate treatments for children with uncomfortable urination
- Know the likely causes of macroscopic and microscopic haematuria in children and the indications for referral
- Be able to discuss the psychosocial aspects of urinary dysfunction in children, and have an informed understanding of the relevance of possible sexual abuse to urogenital problems.

You should also take this opportunity to ensure that:
- You can take a proper history of voiding
- You know how to test urine accurately with commonly available dipsticks
- You can undertake simple microscopy of urine
- You can give detailed advice and support on the use of enuresis alarms
- You can examine the scrotum and external genitalia.

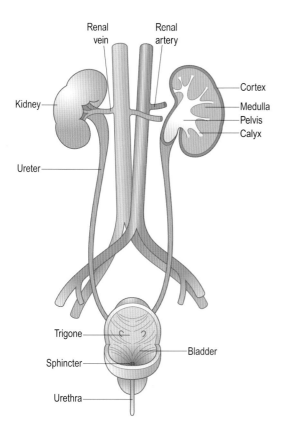

Fig. 26.1 The anatomy of the urinary tract.
(Adapted with permission from the Virtual Autopsy site of the Clinical Division of Pathology, University of Leicester.)

Basic science: the anatomy of the urinary tract

The renal system (Fig. 26.1)

The kidneys are essentially regulatory organs that maintain the volume and composition of body fluid by filtration of the blood and selective reabsorption or secretion of filtered solutes.

The kidneys are retroperitoneal organs (i.e. they are located behind the peritoneum) situated on the posterior wall of the abdomen on each side of the vertebral column, at about the level of the 12th rib. The left kidney is slightly higher in the abdomen than the right, due to the presence of the liver, which pushes the right kidney down.

The kidneys take their blood supply directly from the aorta via the renal arteries; blood is returned to the inferior vena cava via the renal veins. Urine excreted from the kidneys passes down the fibromuscular ureters and collects in the bladder. The bladder muscle (the detrusor muscle) is capable of distending to accept urine without increasing the pressure inside; this means that large volumes can be collected (700–1000 ml) without high-pressure damage to the renal system occurring.

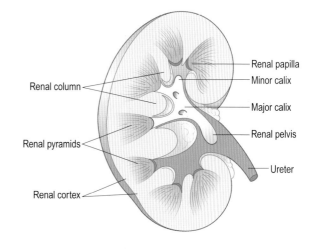

Fig. 26.2 Structure of the kidney

When urine is passed, the urethral sphincter at the base of the bladder relaxes, the detrusor contracts, and urine is voided via the urethra.

The structure of the kidney (Fig. 26.2)

On sectioning, the kidney has a pale outer region — the cortex — and a darker inner region — the medulla. The medulla is divided into 8–18 conical regions, called the renal pyramids; the base of each pyramid starts at the corticomedullary border, and the apex ends in the renal papilla, which merges to form the renal pelvis and continues to form the ureter. In humans, the renal pelvis is divided into two or three spaces — the major calyces — which in turn divide into further minor calyces. The walls of the calyces, pelvis and ureters are lined with smooth muscle that can contract to force urine towards the bladder by peristalsis.

The cortex and the medulla are made up of nephrons — the functional units of the kidney — and each kidney contains about 1.3 million of these. Each nephron is made up of:

- *A filtering unit: the glomerulus*. As blood is filtered through this sieve-like structure, 125 ml/min of filtrate is formed by the kidneys. This filtration is uncontrolled.
- *The proximal convoluted tubule*. Controlled absorption of glucose, sodium and other solutes goes on in this region.
- *The loop of Henle*. This region is responsible for concentration and dilution of urine by utilizing a counter-current multiplying mechanism; basically, it is water-impermeable but can pump sodium out, which in turn affects the osmolarity of the surrounding tissues and will affect the subsequent movement of water in or out of the water-permeable collecting duct.

325

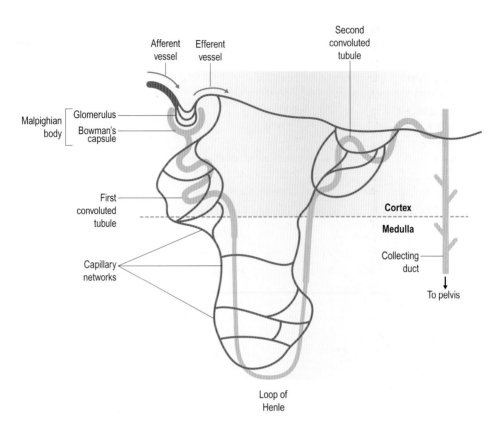

Fig. 26.3 **Structure of the nephron**

Labels in figure:
Afferent vessel — Efferent vessel — Second convoluted tubule — Malpighian body [Glomerulus / Bowman's capsule] — First convoluted tubule — Capillary networks — Loop of Henle — **Cortex** — **Medulla** — Collecting duct — To pelvis

- *The distal convoluted tubule.* This region is responsible, along with the collecting duct that it joins, for absorbing water back into the body. Simple maths will tell you that the kidney does not produce 125 ml of urine every minute. Around 99% of the water is normally reabsorbed, leaving highly concentrated urine to flow into the collecting duct and then into the renal pelvis.

The structure of the nephron is shown in Figure 26.3.

Enuresis

Basic science of enuresis

Control of micturition

The human bladder has to manage the two associated functions of storing and emptying. To achieve dryness, children need a compliant bladder capable of expanding to adequate volume, and working detrusor and sphincter muscles. In addition, the autonomic control must be such as to manage appropriately coordinated contraction and relaxation.

The sympathetic nervous system releases noradrenaline (norepinephrine) to stimulate contraction of the bladder neck and posterior urethral sphincters, and simultaneously relax the detrusor muscle, so that urine storage

may take place. When it is time to empty the bladder, this is achieved by acetylcholine release from the preganglionic nerves (S2–S4) of the parasympathetic nervous system, stimulating detrusor contraction.

Any detrusor contraction in babies is accompanied by simultaneous sphincter relaxation, so that wetting results immediately. The process of potty training is thought to be one of recruiting supraspinal polysynaptic reflexes to bring the processes of inhibition and stimulation of detrusor contractions, as well as contraction and relaxation of the sphincters, under voluntary control.

Social and behavioural science

The stages of social development that underpin childhood emotions involve a progression from the realization of object permanence in the infant (required for trust in a parent's return, for example), through the egocentric stages of magical thinking in the toddler to the stages of logical thinking, conception of time and differentiation of self from others, which progress through childhood, leading to the establishment of independence and abstract thinking that characterize adolescence (Ch. 3).

Psychological distress, which can manifest as enuresis, can be interpreted against this developmental background.

Anxiety is a normal behavioural response to an event that is perceived as threatening or dangerous. Separation anxiety occurs when children are separated from their parents and is a normal reaction, which in some circumstances can become excessive. The majority of children rapidly reduce the onset and frequency of distress as they develop new social relationships and become confident that parents will reliably and predictably return.

Bullying and sexual abuse are examples of threats to the child's wellbeing that can result in disturbed behaviour patterns, including enuresis, regression, aggression or sexualized behaviour. Masturbation is a normal childhood behaviour from infancy onwards, and is usually devoid of ulterior significance. Healthy children may also experience sexual behaviour with their peers from the onset of puberty, but appropriate social support within the family, school and neighbourhood can help the child to avoid adverse consequences of exploratory behaviour. Sexual abuse happens to children of all ages and to both sexes, in all social classes.

Developmentally appropriate environmental challenges, such as change of school or teacher, may lead to transient emotional disturbances, including enuresis, as may the loss reactions that occur with family breakdown or bereavement.

Control of micturition requires attentional skills, which are closely dependent upon successful biological development. Difficulty with attention is a common impairment in many childhood developmental conditions. Attention is the process of focusing on relevant information and inhibiting responses to irrelevant stimuli — for example, prioritizing the bladder over playtime!

Problem-orientated topic:

a child with daytime and night-time wetting

Neil, who is 7 years old, attends the village primary school where he is doing well academically. He enjoys football and cub scouts, and has several good friends, but he avoids sleepovers because he is nervous about his bed-wetting. Several times a week he will also have slightly wet pants in the daytime, and this happens on holidays as well as at weekends. He says he does not know anything about it until he feels the dampness. Mum, who works in a supermarket, and Dad, who works for the council, are both supportive of Neil, and his older sister does not tease him about it.

Q1. When should one become concerned about wetting?

Q2. What is the likely cause of Neil's daytime wetting and bed-wetting?

Q3. What other conditions should be considered?

Q4. What should you look for in your clinical evaluation?

Q5. What investigations might be appropriate?

Q6. When is referral indicated?

Q1. When should one become concerned about wetting?

See Box 26.1.

BOX 26.1 Enuresis: guidelines for concern

- Daytime urinary symptoms accompanying bed-wetting in children older than 3 or 4 years suggest there may be an underlying bladder dysfunction
- Between 2 and 4% of children are still enuretic at puberty, and although some will resolve in adolescence, others will turn out to have hereditary enuresis with a high chance of this persisting into adult life
- Secondary bed-wetting after the child has been dry should prompt enquiry about emotional upset; in particular, bullying or sexual abuse should be considered as possibilities
- Bed-wetting may be a sign of urinary tract infection (UTI), particularly if accompanied by frequency or dysuria

Q2. What is the likely cause of Neil's daytime wetting and bed-wetting?

Primary enuresis would be the most likely cause of bed-wetting, but the daytime wetting is a greater cause of concern.

Bladder dysfunction needs to be considered, particularly the urge syndrome, as well as simple inattention to the need to void. In urge syndrome, the volume of urine lost is usually very small, only enough to cause damp patches on the child's underwear.

Rarely, incontinence may be due to structural abnormalities of the urinary tract, such as posterior urethral valves, or abnormalities of the nervous system.

Q3. What other conditions should be considered?

See Box 26.2.

Physiological causes

• Maturation — primary enuresis
• Inattention to the need to void (much more common in boys)
• Giggle incontinence
• Constipation

Pathological causes

• Neurological:
  – Detrusor hyperreflexia
• Bladder dysfunction:
  – Primary detrusor instability
  – Secondary detrusor instability (can result from over-frequent voiding in an attempt to avoid incontinence)
  – Urge syndrome
  – Urge incontinence
• Congenital malformation:
  – Spinal dysraphism
  – Posterior urethral valves
• Genetic:
  – Hereditary enuresis persists into adulthood in 1–2% of cases
• Psychosocial:
  – Anxiety
  – Bullying
  – Sexual abuse

Q4. What should you look for in your clinical evaluation?

Key points

• A good history and physical examination will help to distinguish children with neurological or bladder dysfunction from those with simple enuresis.
• It is also important to assess the psychosocial dimensions of the problem.
• It is vital to ascertain the child's and parents' views on desired approaches to the problem.

History

• Medical history:
  – Establish whether wetting is nocturnal or happens in the day.
  – Check bowel control.
  – How much wetness? How often? (In urge syndrome, the volume of urine lost is usually very small, causing only dampness on the underwear.)
  – What circumstances? Does this suggest inattention or a relation to stress?
  – Is there ever any pain? (Pain can be a feature of detrusor instability.)
  – Is the child aware when wetting?
  – Is there associated urgency? If so, is this primary or secondary to frequent micturition in an attempt to avoid incontinence?
  – Has the child ever been dry (primary or secondary enuresis)?
  – Potty-training attempts?
  – Previous treatment?
  – Other medical conditions, especially diabetes mellitus or insipidus?
  – Drinking habits?
• Family history:
  – Who has had bed-wetting problems?
• Birth history:
  – Congenital malformations?
  – Good stream observed as neonate?
• Psychosocial history:
  – Personality — happy, easygoing, recent change?
  – Affect?
  – Family relationships?
  – Interests, sports, pastimes?
  – School performance? Any reluctance to attend, school refusal or truancy?
  – Peer relationships? Bullying?
  – Any sexualized behaviour?

Examination

Physical examination should include general inspection, looking particularly at the back for evidence of occult sacral and spinal anomalies (Ch. 28), such as unusual hairy patches, vascular malformations, asymmetry or dermal pits.

In the abdomen, inspect, palpate and percuss for a full bladder, and check for the faecal loading of constipation.

In appropriately chaperoned conditions, check the genitalia, looking for epispadias and any evidence of sexual abuse (p. 231). Ballooning of the foreskin is rarely of concern. Anal tone and sensation should be checked where there is any possibility of bladder dysfunction.

Neurological examination includes power, tone, and sensation in the lower limbs.

Q5. What investigations might be appropriate?

Your clinical evaluation should guide any investigations (Table 26.1).

Q6. When is referral indicated?

• To access incontinence services (e.g. enuresis nurse or buzzer provision)

Table 26.1 Investigations in a child with wetting

Investigation	Relevance
Blood count, haematocrit	Polyuria to assess plasma hydration
Urea, creatinine and electrolytes	Renal impairment or hyponatraemia
Urine dipstick for glucose	Mandatory to exclude diabetes in all cases of polyuria or secondary urinary incontinence Follow up positive tests with blood glucose test
Urine dipstick for blood and protein	If renal impairment suspected
Urine dipstick for protein, white cells and nitrite	To exclude urinary tract infection
Mid-stream urine culture and microscopy	If nitrites or pyuria
Urine concentration test	Polyuria to exclude diabetes insipidus N.B. Early morning specific gravity is not reliable
Urine acidification test	Polyuria in context of renal impairment
Urine plasma osmolality	Polyuria to exclude nephrogenic diabetes insipidus
Urodynamic studies	A bladder is defined as unstable if urodynamic investigation shows detrusor contractions during the filling phase while the patient is attempting to inhibit voiding

- Urological assessment for persistent primary daytime enuresis where a voiding problem is suggested by the voiding chart
- May need cystoscopy or imaging if primary urethral valves are suspected
- May need urodynamic studies if proven neurological disorder or if history suggests detrusor instability.

Polyuria

Basic science of urine formation

The process of urine formation has three distinct parts: filtration, reabsorption and tubular excretion. During glomerular filtration, blood pressure forces all small molecular components of blood into the lumen of the nephron through the pores in the walls of the glomerular capillaries and pores in the wall of the Bowman's capsule. As the filtrate passes through the tubules of the nephron, up to 99% of the water is reabsorbed into the bloodstream, together with many solutes. A process of active tubular excretion supplements the initial glomerular filtration, and allows for some larger molecules to be excreted in urine.

In the younger child it may be difficult to distinguish polyuria from enuresis, as incontinence (the cardinal feature of enuresis) may accompany the frequent micturition that defines polyuria. The distinguishing feature is that polyuria involves the passage of abnormally large daily quantities of urine (over 50 ml/kg/24 hrs as a rough guide in the school-age child).

In the absence of dehydration, polyuria has to be accompanied by polydipsia — the drinking of excessively large or frequent amounts of fluid — and it is important to tease out whether the drinking is the primary phenomenon or is a response to involuntary polydipsia.

> **Problem-orientated topic:**
>
> **a child with frequent urination**
>
> Fatima is 7 and came to the UK from Somalia when she was 2. The school nurse has referred her because teachers have noticed over the past 6 months that she cannot last through a double class period (1 hour 20 minutes) without needing to go to the toilet. She is starting to get teased by the other children for this. She is always drinking large amounts of water, but appears to be embarrassed by her thirst rather than seeking to draw attention to herself. Her mother cannot recall a time in recent months when Fatima has had less than about 15–20 drinks in a day. So long as she is allowed to go to the toilet on request and to get up as frequently as she needs to at night, Fatima does not wet herself.
>
> Q1. When should one become concerned about children who urinate often?
>
> Q2. What is the likely cause of Fatima's polyuria?
>
> Q3. What other conditions should be considered?
>
> Q4. What should you look for in your clinical evaluation?
>
> Q5. What investigations might be appropriate?
>
> Q6. When is referral indicated?

- Children who regularly pass over 50 ml urine per kg of their body weight in 24 hrs should be referred for investigation
- It will sometimes be apparent that excessive water drinking has become a habit for the child, from which he or she is easily distracted, and in such children a policy of encouraging distraction and gently restricting to more normal drinking is all that is needed
- In the absence of evidence that the child can manage happily on a lower fluid intake, it is probably safest to refer for assessment before attempting water deprivation

Q1. When should one become concerned about children who urinate often?

See Box 26.3.

Q2. What is the likely cause of Fatima's polyuria?

As far as can be assessed from the history, Fatima does not seem to have evidence of compulsive water drinking or to be attention-seeking.

There is a strong possibility that her thirst is secondary to excessive urine production, and the two likely causes are diabetes insipidus — a lack of antidiuretic hormone (ADH) — or a failure of the kidneys to respond to ADH. Such primary renal concentration defects are known as nephrogenic diabetes insipidus (Ch. 40).

Q3. What other conditions should be considered?

See Box 26.4.

Q4. What should you look for in your clinical evaluation?

Key points
- A good history is crucially important in helping to decide whether psychogenic polydipsia or attention-seeking behaviour is likely.
- Examination should firstly exclude signs of dehydration, and it is then important to look for the stigmata of chronic disease, including growth stunting.
- Features of chronic renal disease may include palpable kidneys in polycystic disease, pallor and anaemia.
- In thinking about diabetes insipidus, look for signs or symptoms of head injury or brain disease.

Physiological causes
- Excessive fluid intake, particularly fluids containing caffeine (e.g. cola drinks)
- Excessive salt load (consider deliberate poisoning, p. 229)

Pathological causes
- Endocrine:
  - Diabetes mellitus (Ch. 35)
  - Diabetes insipidus (Ch. 35)
- Chronic illness:
  - Nephrogenic diabetes insipidus (Ch. 40)
  - General renal failure
  - Isolated defect of renal concentration
- Genetic:
  - Sickle cell anaemia (Ch. 43)
- Psychosocial:
  - Psychogenic (Ch. 30)
- Pharmacological:
  - Diuretic treatment

- Any child of Mediterranean or Afro-Caribbean origin should have sickle cell disease excluded (Ch. 43).

History
- Medical history:
  - When did the problem start?
  - Daily pattern of urination/drinking?
  - Any record of total input and output?
  - Fed well/grown well?
  - Brain injury or surgery?
  - Meningitis/encephalitis?
  - Tuberculosis/sarcoid?
- Family history:
  - Sickle cell trait/disease?
  - Polycystic kidneys?
  - Renal failure?
  - Diabetes mellitus or insipidus?
- Psychosocial history:
  - Family dynamics happy?
  - Other evidence of attention-seeking?

Examination
- Growth stunting?
- Pallor/anaemia?
- Signs of head injury?
- Palpable kidneys? Polycystic?

Q5. What investigations might be appropriate?

See Table 26.2.

Table 26.2 Investigations in a child with polyuria

Investigation	Relevance
Blood count, plasma viscosity or erythrocyte sedimentation rate	Excludes anaemia
Sickle cell screen	Sickle cell disease a common cause of nephrogenic diabetes insipidus in susceptible populations
Urea, creatinine and electrolytes	Chronic renal failure
Plasma glucose	Excludes diabetes mellitus
Formal water deprivation test (this should only be done in a hospital setting)	Osmolality of an early morning urine sample is often taken as a measure of urinary concentration in children with a history of polydipsia and polyuria, but studies have shown that only around 4 normal children out of 5 will have an osmolality of 600 mmol/kg or more in an early morning urine, making this test too non-specific for routine use
Magnetic resonance imaging (MRI)	Studies of posterior pituitary if diabetes insipidus suspected
Renal ultrasound	Polycystic disease and small shrunken kidneys of chronic renal failure

Q6. When is referral indicated?

All children with unexplained polyuria not responding to gently encouraged fluid restriction should be referred to hospital for further assessment.

Dysuria in girls

Problem-orientated topic:

a girl with painful urination

Shelley is 8. She has not started her periods yet. She tells her mother that it hurts her whenever she passes urine. Sometimes it hurts so much that she cries. Her mother says Shelley denies 'interfering with herself', yet it is getting to be so much of a problem that she is frightened of going to school. She is an only child and lives with her mother (a beauty therapist) and stepfather (a builder). She has no significant past illness. Shelley feels the urge to pass urine a lot of the time, but tends to 'hang on' because it is so sore. She has sometimes had a little buff-coloured staining on her pants but has not noticed any blood in her urine. Initially, she got some relief from cool baths but this has not lasted.

Q1. When should one become concerned about uncomfortable urination?
Q2. What is the likely cause of Shelley's dysuria?
Q3. What other conditions should be considered?
Q4. What should you look for in your clinical evaluation?

Q5. What investigations might be appropriate?
Q6. When is referral indicated?

Q5. What investigations might be appropriate?
Q6. When is referral indicated?

BOX 26.5 Dysuria: guidelines for concern

- Dysuria that is persistent and troublesome should always be fully assessed
- Most often this distressing symptom is relievable
- A further concern about dysuria is that sometimes it may represent a child's distress following sexual abuse, or may even be a symptom of sexually transmitted disease

Q1. When should one become concerned about uncomfortable urination?

See Box 26.5.

Q2. What is the likely cause of Shelley's dysuria?

Shelley is most likely to have simple vulvovaginitis of childhood.

Q3. What other conditions should be considered?

See Box 26.6.

Q4. What should you look for in your clinical evaluation?

Key points
- Vulvovaginitis in prepubertal girls is common and the challenge for clinicians is to diagnose and treat

BOX 26.6 Causes of dysuria

Physiological causes

- Tight or nylon underwear causing excessive local warmth
- Masturbation
- Inexperienced tampon use

Pathological causes

- Dermatological:
  - Dermatitis, including the perineal dermatitis of gluten enteropathy and Crohn's disease (Ch. 39)
  - Sensitivity to irritants like bubble bath or perfumed soap
  - Eczema (Ch. 37)
  - Psoriasis (Ch. 36)
- Infective:
  - Lower UTIs, most commonly due to faecal organisms
  - Candidal vulvovaginitis
  - Sexually transmitted disease, including *Chlamydia* and gonococcal disease
  - Threadworms
- Psychosocial:
  - Child sexual abuse (p. 231)

simple conditions with a minimum of fuss, whilst at the same time remaining vigilant about the possibility of sexual abuse and sexually transmitted disease.

- A good history and simple external physical examination, backed up by culture of a vulval swab and mid-stream urine (MSU), will generally be all that is needed to diagnose simple vulvovaginitis.
- Examination of external genitalia in children is a sensitive issue. Cultural norms must be respected and the examination must always be fully chaperoned by a nurse.

- Where there is any possibility of sexual abuse, the examination is best performed by someone with specialist expertise, and in all cases the appropriate swabs must be taken (Ch. 37).

History

- Medical history:
  - Clarify symptoms: genital pain, pruritus, dysuria/haematuria, frequency of micturition, vaginal discharge/vaginal bleeding?
  - Tampon use in the older child
  - When did symptoms start?
  - Were there any triggers to the symptoms?
  - Any history of a dermatological condition, e.g. eczema?
  - Bubble baths or perfumed soaps?
  - Enuresis or faecal soiling?
  - What type of underclothing is worn?
  - How does the child wipe to clean herself after using the toilet?
- Psychosocial history:
  - Sensitive enquiry around possibility of sexual abuse.
  - Enquire if caregiver has any concerns about sexual interference.
  - Ask directly about the possibility of a foreign body.
  - Normal masturbatory behaviour?

Examination

- Inflammation and excoriation of the labia majora, labia minora, clitoris and introitus
- Hymen intact?
- Vaginal discharge/stains on underwear.

Q5. What investigations might be appropriate?

Your clinical evaluation should guide any investigations (Table 26.3).

Table 26.3 Investigations in a child with dysuria

Investigation	Relevance
Mid-stream or clean-catch urine	Lower urinary tract infections commonly
Vulval swab (bacteriology and *Candida*)	If vaginal discharge detected
Full sexually transmitted infection (STI) screen, including swabs in specialist culture and transport media and rubbed on glass slides	Whenever STI is suspected, it is vital to avoid half-measures and ensure proper samples are taken. Positive results must be followed up by family screening
Full blood count	Chronic dermatitis (also consider checking serum zinc levels and excluding gluten enteropathy)
'Sellotape slide'	Threadworms are a common cause of vulvovaginitis in the younger child. More sensitive test than stool microscopy
Pelvic and renal ultrasound	Check for urinary tract abnormalities if UTI proven or any anomaly of external genitalia

Q6. When is referral indicated?

All children in whom sexual abuse is suspected should be referred for expert examination in accordance with local practice guidelines. Likewise, if there is a possibility of retained foreign body, children should be referred to a paediatric gynaecologist.

Prepubertal girls with simple vulvovaginitis can be satisfactorily treated in primary care. Simple clear advice to parents and child, backed up by leaflets, can be helpful. Children have a tendency to wipe their bottoms forwards, increasing the likelihood of faecal contamination of the vulva because of the proximity of the anus. Advice on wiping, improved hygiene practices, avoiding local irritants such as bubble baths, and possibly advising salt baths or showers after defaecation may be all that is needed

Some authors recommend the use of topical oestrogen creams for resistant cases, on the grounds that hypo-oestrogenization of childhood genitalia reduces introital protection against infection, as the mucosa is thin and alkaline and there is a paucity of the protective 'Doderlein's bacillus' (*Lactobacillus acidophilus*). However, this is not without hazard, as there is systemic absorption of topical oestrogens and repeated applications may lead to side-effects such as breast enlargement.

Another contentious point for primary care is the use of antifungal creams or steroid/antifungal combinations. Creams such as Canesten are best reserved for children in whom *Candida* has been isolated, and likewise Daktacort, although effective for mild dermatitis and some bacterial and fungal infection, risks masking other problems if used blindly.

Acute urinary tract infection

Problem-orientated topic:

a child with a urine infection

John is 4 and has been dry by day and by night since he was 2. Yesterday he was off-colour at the preschool playgroup, and was sick just before bedtime. He woke in the night having wet the bed, and Mum thought he was hot. He now complains of tummy ache and his urine has an offensive smell. John's parents are university teachers of Nigerian origin and he has two older brothers, both well. John was born by full-term normal delivery after an uneventful pregnancy and has thrived since. His urinary stream has always been good but he tends not to drink a lot of fluid. A dipstick shows no blood but +protein, +++ white blood cells and ++nitrite. His temperature is 38.2°C.

Q1. When should one become concerned about urine infections?

Q2. What is the likely cause of John's urine infection?

Q3. What other conditions should be considered?

Q4. What should you look for in your clinical evaluation?

Q5. What investigations might be appropriate?

Q6. When is referral indicated?

BOX 26.7 Acute urinary tract infection: guidelines for concern

- Earlier evidence about the risks of urine infections in the child under 5 years of age, causing scarring leading to chronic pyelonephritis has recently been challenged
- Nevertheless, it remains true that UTIs are under-diagnosed and it is particularly important to establish the diagnosis in infants and toddlers, in whom sample collection is the most difficult. Using syringes to collect fresh nappy urine where bags or clean-catch specimens are impractical is often possible in primary care. A fresh specimen should be sent for phase contrast microscopy or culture
- As in adults, the absence of proteinuria, and pyuria and nitrites on dipstick testing are strongly reassuring that infection is unlikely
- If infection is established, differentiate between lower UTIs in the child who is only mildly unwell, and acute pyelonephritis, which usually merits immediate intravenous therapy

Q1. When should one become concerned about urine infections?

See Box 26.7.

Upper urinary tract infections (acute pyelitis and pyelonephritis) are the more serious forms of UTI, both form the risk of septicaemia and on account of the complications of chronic pyelonephritis causing renal damage. Upper UTIs are rarely accompanied by dysuria. Sometimes there is loin pain, or more usually in children, vague abdominal pain. This condition is discussed in Chapter 40. The child is usually febrile and may have systemic symptoms, e.g. vomiting.

BOX 26.8 Causes of urinary tract infection

Physiological causes

- Perineal hygiene problems include wet nappies being left too long and causing balanoposthitis in boys, as well as forwards wiping after defaecation in girls
- Poor fluid intake is a predisposing factor for lower UTIs, as high urine throughput is an important protection against cystitis
- All ascending infection is much more common in girls than boys (5:1), as the direct short female urethra offers less protection than the male urethra
- Voiding dysfunction is a highly important contributing factor and raises the importance of avoiding constipation

Pathological causes

- Blood-borne:
  - The majority of acute renal infections are believed to be bacteraemic in origin. They are more common following acute gastroenteritis
- Genetic:
  - Structural anomalies of the urinary tract predispose to infection, and they are a particular problem for children with spina bifida
  - Vesico-ureteric reflux has a strong familial component
- Instrumentation:
  - Ascending UTIs are an ever-present risk in children who have to be catheterized

Lower UTIs frequently cause dysuria. The child can have vague abdominal pain or even systemic symptoms of diarrhoea or vomiting. Children with lower UTIs are often afebrile.

Q2. What is the likely cause of John's urine infection?

John could have either an upper or a lower UTI, and the difficult decision here is whether to admit him to hospital for systemic therapy. Unless there are excellent facilities for specimen collection and transport in the practice, it seems reasonable to ask the local paediatric unit to obtain a high-quality urine specimen for culture and to guide on treatment.

Q3. What other conditions should be considered?

See Box 26.8.

Q4. What should you look for in your clinical evaluation?

Key points

- UTIs are often missed because they are not considered. In all febrile or unwell children, in whom a positive diagnosis has not been established, UTIs must be excluded.

History

- Medical history:
  - Previous infections?
  - Any known renal or urological problems?
- Psychosocial history:
  - Nappy changing practices
  - Perineal hygiene
  - Drinking habits.

Examination

- Temperature
- Hydration
- Capillary refill
- Pulse and blood pressure
- Abdominal tenderness
- Renal enlargement or tenderness
- Perineal soreness.

Q5. What investigations might be appropriate?

Your clinical evaluation should guide any investigations (Table 26.4).

The further investigation of UTI in hospital is discussed in more detail in Chapter 40.

Q6. When is referral indicated?

Most children with UTIs have an excellent prognosis, with resolution of reflux by 4 years of age. The greatest risk of renal involvement in UTI is in newborn boys and pre-school-age girls.

Any child who is unwell, and most children under 6 months, should be admitted for intravenous antibiotics. The management of UTI in hospital is discussed in Chapter 40.

Haematuria

Haematuria is potentially a very serious symptom in children and urgent referral to hospital may be required (Ch. 40). The approach in primary care is described in this chapter.

Table 26.4 Investigations in a child with urinary tract infection

Investigation	Relevance
Dipstick urine tests	The presence of white cells and nitrites on dipstick testing is a strong pointer to UTI, and red cells or protein may also be found BUT absence of all of these does not exclude UTI in the unwell child, and other causes such as glomerulonephritis must be considered for haematuria and/or proteinuria
Blood count, with white cell differential	High neutrophilia a strong pointer to infection
Urea, creatinine and electrolytes	Renal function should be checked in any *unwell* child with UTI and in children with recurrent UTIs
Urine culture and phase contrast microscopy	Important in all children in whom UTI is suspected, as screening dipstick tests may miss important infection
Blood culture	Important for all potentially bacteraemic children, including infants under 1 year
Lumbar puncture	Should not be omitted in unwell infants just because a UTI has been diagnosed
Suprapubic aspiration	For children too young to obtain an MSU and with a high probability of UTI, or who are unwell and warrant more invasive investigation

Problem-orientated topic:

a boy with haematuria

Jason is 5 years old and in his first year at school. He drew his mother's attention to his dark urine ('coca-cola wee') and the sample that his mother brought to surgery tested +++blood and +protein on dipstick. He has never had any serious illness and there is no family history of haematuria or renal problems. Jason is well grown and energetic, and rarely misses school, though he did have a few days off recently with a cold. He has no pain on passing urine and has noticed no rashes or anything else out of the ordinary.

Q1. When should one become concerned about blood in urine?

Q2. What is the likely cause of Jason's haematuria?

Q3. What other conditions should be considered?

Q4. What should you look for in your clinical evaluation?

Q5. What investigations might be appropriate?

Q6. When is referral indicated?

Q1. When should one become concerned about blood in urine?

See Box 26.9.

Q2. What is the likely cause of Jason's haematuria?

Jason is likely to have post-infective acute glomerulo-nephritis (Ch. 40), possibly post-streptococcal. It

BOX 26.9 Haematuria: guidelines for concern

- Significant haematuria is determined by finding more than 5 red blood cells per high-power field on a slide of fresh spun urine
- A dipstick test will detect red blood cells but in addition will detect myoglobin and haemoglobin, which are also clinically important findings
- After a positive dipstick, it is imperative to do a urine analysis. Other causes of red urine include dietary ingestion of beetroot or blackberries, treatment with rifampicin or sedimentation of urate crystals, which may cause red discoloration on a nappy
- Deformed red cells on phase contrast microscopy or casts in the urine usually indicate glomerular involvement, but the absence of casts does not rule out glomerular pathology
- Proteinuria accompanying microscopic haematuria makes significant renal pathology more likely, but small amounts of protein are usually detected when haematuria is macroscopic and do not have ominous significance

is essential to check for oedema and hypertension, and to arrange for baseline blood and urine investigations.

This condition will need careful monitoring until it has fully resolved, but in the majority of cases there are no long-term sequalae.

Q3. What other conditions should be considered?

See Box 26.10.

BOX 26.10 Causes of haematuria

Physiological causes
- Idiopathic transient haematuria is not uncommon
- Exercise haematuria resolves within 48 hours
- Familial benign haematuria is usually asymptomatic

Pathological causes
- Infective:
  - UTIs (Ch. 40)
- Traumatic:
  - Blunt abdominal trauma
  - Perineal trauma
- Immunological:
  - One of the most frequent causes for persistent or intermittent gross or microscopic haematuria during childhood is Berger's disease (IgA/IgG nephropathy). It affects males:females (2:1). Progressive disease develops in 30% of patients. The development of hypertension, diminished renal function or proteinuria > 1 g/ 24 hr indicates a poor prognosis. There are many other rarer forms of glomerulonephritis
- Acute illness:
  - Renal vein thrombosis (Ch. 40)
  - Haemolytic uraemic syndrome (Ch. 40), though uncommon, is the most common cause of acute renal failure in young children and follows an acute gastroenteritis or upper respiratory tract infection (URTI)
  - Neonatal asphyxia
- Chronic illness:
  - Systemic lupus erythematosus (Ch. 33)
  - Chronic glomerulonephritis (Ch. 40)
  - Idiopathic hypercalciuria: excessive gastrointestinal absorption of normal dietary calcium intake or a defect in renal calcium reabsorption
- Haematological:
  - Bleeding diatheses and thrombocytopenias
- Genetic:
  - Alport's syndrome (familial nephritis)
- Congenital:
  - Rare vascular abnormalities: haemangiomas, arteriovenous malformations
- Neoplastic:
  - Nephroblastoma (Ch. 51) and other rare tumours
- Drugs:
  - Heparin, warfarin, aspirin, penicillins, sulphonamides, cyclophosphamide
- Psychosocial:
  - Factitious bleeding (interference by child or carer, p. 229)

Q4. What should you look for in your clinical evaluation?

Key points
- As so often in paediatrics, the key question is 'Is this child unwell?'
- Haematuria, whether microscopic or gross, carries very different implications if the child is unwell.
- Look carefully for evidence of fever, poor feeding, dehydration or oedema, and always check the blood pressure and for coexistent proteinuria.

History
- Medical history:
  - Any symptoms of a UTI, such as dysuria and frequency? Any suprapubic pain?
  - Any recent URTI or sore throat?
  - Any skin rashes or vesicles?
  - Are the stools loose or bloody?
  - Any recent trauma?
  - Any joint pains or swellings?
  - What medications does the child take?
- Family history:
  - Sickle cell disease or trait?
  - Renal disease, transplants or dialysis? Hearing deficits?
- Psychosocial history:
  - Any pointers to factitious illness?

Examination
- Anaemia or jaundice?
- Growth retardation?
- Oedema is a prominent finding in acute glomerulonephritis.
- Blood pressure recording is vital, as hypertension is a serious finding.
- Examine external genitalia for a local cause of bleeding (e.g. urethral caruncle).
- Look for any rashes, evidence of trauma and bruising, petechiae and purpura (look especially at feet, thighs and buttocks for Henoch–Schönlein purpura, Ch. 33).
- Examine all joints for signs of arthritis — red, warm or swollen.
- Abdominal masses or tenderness? Enlarged kidney(s)?

Q5. What investigations might be appropriate?

Your clinical evaluation should guide any investigations in primary care. Investigation of glomerulonephritis is discussed in Chapter 40.

Q6. When is referral indicated?

Until recently, all children with asymptomatic microscopic haematuria would have been referred for further investigation. It now seems that a reasonable policy in respect of the well child with no proteinuria, in whom an infection has been excluded, is to check and record the blood pressure and to monitor urine dipstick tests at intervals until blood is no longer detected, in order to check that proteinuria does not develop.

A reasonable policy for a well child reporting macroscopic (gross) haematuria is to recheck the urine in a few days if physical examination is normal and there is no family history of renal disease. Then, if the dipstick is still positive, obtain a fresh sample for phase contrast microscopy and to check the spun urine for blood, casts, protein, white blood cells and bacteria.

All infants and unwell children with haematuria should be referred for immediate investigation, as should any child with hypertension, oedema or reduced urine output.

The management of glomerulonephritis is discussed in Chapter 40.

Painless scrotal swelling and maldescent of testis

Basic science of testicular descent

During fetal development, the testis is formed within the peritoneal cavity. As it descends through the inguinal canal and into the scrotum, the testis brings with it an extension of peritoneum, known as processus vaginalis (PV). After the testis has completed descent, the PV closes off and becomes a fibrous cord with no lumen. Once the duct connecting scrotum to abdomen has closed off, neither abdominal contents nor peritoneal fluid should gain access to the scrotum or inguinal canal. If the PV does not close, it is referred to as a patent processus vaginalis (PPV).

A communicating hydrocele occurs if the PPV is only large enough to allow fluid to pass. Herniation of other abdominal contents can occur if the PPV is larger.

At any point along its descent, the testis may become arrested, resulting in maldescent, with either an impalpable testis or one that is palpable at the inguinal ring

Problem-orientated topic:

a baby with painless scrotal swelling

Yousef is 1 week old and is due to have a circumcision for religious reasons next week.

He is a healthy neonate, but his parents have noticed a unilateral painless swelling on the right side and are concerned.

Q1. When should one become concerned about painless scrotal swelling in infants?

Q2. What is the likely cause of Yousef's scrotal swelling?

Q3. What other conditions should be considered?

Q4. What should you look for in your clinical evaluation?

Q5. What investigations might be appropriate?

Q6. When is referral indicated?

Q1. When should one become concerned about painless scrotal swelling in infants?

See Box 26.11.

BOX 26.11 Painless scrotal swelling: guidelines for concern

- Infant hydroceles need no action, as the vast majority will have resolved within the first year of life as the patent processus vaginalis closes
- Inguinal hernias require surgical repair, and opinion differs as to how early this should be performed on infants. Seek local advice from a paediatric surgeon
- For older children and those awaiting routine surgery, parents should always be told to report any tenderness suggestive of incarceration
- In preterm babies, hernia is common and the timing of surgical repair is a matter of expert judgment, weighing risks of complication against those of intervention

---

Q2. What is the likely cause of Yousef's scrotal swelling?

He is likely to have an innocent infant hydrocele. You should examine him to ensure that he does not have an inguinal hernia and to check his testicular descent.

Q3. What other conditions should be considered?

See Box 26.12.

Physiological causes
- Neonatal hydrocele (80–90% of newborns have a patent processus vaginalis)
- Varicocele (uncommon in children)

Pathological causes
- Developmental:
  - Inguinal hernia
- Trauma:
  - Post-traumatic hydrocele
- Neoplastic:
  - Tumours of the testis (benign or malignant) should be considered in the older child

Q4. What should you look for in your clinical evaluation?

Key points
- Clinicians will usually be able to reassure parents on the basis of a thorough examination.

History
- Medical history:
  - Check if the child is unwell.
- Birth history:
  - Hernias in preterm babies require very careful evaluation because of the risk of complication.

Examination
- Transillumination is useful to characterize hydroceles, but beware the hernia that transilluminates.
- Checking testicular descent is part of routine paediatric surveillance in boys. Warm hands and a gentle technique are needed to perform adequate examination in a calm child. If conditions are not ideal, the examination should be repeated.
- Check for inguinal lymphadenopathy.

Q5. What investigations might be appropriate?

Investigations play little part (Table 26.5).

Scrotal pain

Problem-orientated topic:

a boy with scrotal pain

Sean is 12 and over the past 24 hours he has noticed intermittent discomfort 'in the balls'. His scrotum has now become very uncomfortable, particularly on the left side where it is noticeably swollen. The pain radiates up into his abdomen, and it is so sore that it is difficult for him to walk. He feels sick and his temperature is 38.0°C.

Q1. When should one become concerned about scrotal pain?

Q2. What is the likely cause of Sean's scrotal pain?

Q3. What other conditions should be considered?

Q4. What should you look for in your clinical evaluation?

Q5. What investigations might be appropriate?

Q6. When is referral indicated?

Q1. When should one become concerned about scrotal pain?

See Box 26.13.

- Any acute scrotal pain needs careful evaluation
- To miss an acute torsion of the testis is to risk total unilateral loss of gonadal function through infarction
- Strangulated inguinal hernia is another surgical emergency
- Likewise, epididymo-orchitis merits prompt antibiotic therapy

Q2. What is the likely cause of Sean's scrotal pain?

The dilemma here is that Sean's history does not permit reliable distinction between testicular torsion, strangulated hernia and epididymo-orchitis.

Table 26.5 **Investigations in a boy with painless scrotal swelling or undescended testis**

Investigation	Relevance
Routine blood count and urinalysis	Routine preoperative checks for children having surgery are all that is needed

Q3. What other conditions should be considered?

See Box 26.14.

Q4. What should you look for in your clinical evaluation?

Key points
- A good history and physical examination will establish the diagnosis in most cases.

History
- Medical history
- Family history
- Birth history
- Psychosocial history.

Examination
- Transillumination — classically hydroceles transilluminate but beware, so may hernias.
- Purpuric rash of Henoch–Schönlein purpura over scrotum (may have associated vasculitic rash of buttocks and lower limbs, arthritis, abdominal pain with gastrointestinal bleeding, and nephritis.
- Haematoma to indicate trauma?

Q5. What investigations might be appropriate?

Your clinical evaluation should guide any investigations (Table 26.6).

Q6. When is referral indicated?

Early surgical consultation is vital, as delay in scrotal exploration and relief of torsion of a testis will result in testicular infarction within 8–12 hours. Keep the child fasted pending surgical review.

Epididymo-orchitis should be managed with antibiotics once a suitable urine sample has been sent. Young infants or systemically unwell children should be admitted for intravenous antibiotics.

Most patients can be successfully managed as outpatients. Adolescents with epididymo-orchitis should have sexually transmitted infection excluded.

Circumcision

Basic science of penis development

At birth, the shaft of the penis and the glans forming the rounded end are separated by a sulcus. The bilaminar foreskin covering the glans penis is called the prepuce. Before birth, prepuce and glans have developed as one tissue, and before a boy's foreskin can retract, the prepuce must separate from the glans, a process that may take several years. The prepuce has a protective function, shielding the delicate glans from faecal and urinary irritation.

Circumcisions are done for religious as well as medical reasons (Box 26.15). There is a wealth of information on the Circumcision Information and Resource Pages (CIRP), including factual descriptions of the procedure. However, there is a strong detectable bias on this site against subjecting children to the procedure, which

Table 26.6 Investigations in a boy with scrotal pain

Investigation	Relevance
Blood count	More important to exclude anaemia than to base decisions on white cell count, which can be misleading
Urea and electrolytes	Check renal function
Urine culture and microscopy	Obligatory for all
Meatal swab for *Chlamydia* and gonococcus	Adolescents with epididymo-orchitis must have STI excluded
Ultrasound and radiology	Rarely helpful here, although some authorities recommend duplex ultrasound to check blood flow

BOX 26.15 Circumcision

- Religious circumcision is often practised by non-medically qualified practitioners. For this reason many paediatric surgeons prefer to offer the procedure in order to ensure that children receive the benefits of sterile procedures in clinical settings
- The procedure is often performed without anaesthesia, as some doctors prefer to avoid local anaesthesia, both on account of the local pain and transient swelling induced by the local anaesthetic, and because of the cardiovascular risks in small infants, risks that can also occur following systemic absorption of topical anaesthetic creams
- General anaesthesia is generally avoided in young babies and immobilization is crucial
- Circumcision involves removal of a considerable proportion of the preputial skin along with peripenic dartos muscle, the frenar band and part of the frenulum. This can make urethroplasty in later life more difficult for those men who are unfortunate enough to damage their urethra
- Cheesy smegma consists of the discarded epithelial layers of glans and inner foreskin. Adult smegma also contains a lubricating substance from Tyson's glands around the base of glans penis
- Hygiene in the infant involves cleaning around the meatus of the foreskin. It should not involve probing with cotton buds or attempts at retraction
- Retraction of the foreskin may not happen until school age in many boys. It is of no concern until the time the pubescent child starts to get erections, and then it is rare for non-retraction to be a problem. Retraction should never be forced
- Painless ballooning of the foreskin on micturition in children is not of concern, as it merely represents the separation of glans from prepuce in the prelude to the foreskin becoming retractile
- Penile cancer is a very rare cancer in adults, but used to be more common in uncircumcised men. However, since the present epidemic of human papillomavirus, causing penile warts (which are a risk factor for penile cancer), there is likely to be little protective advantage in circumcision
- STIs such as syphilis and herpes simplex may cause penile ulcers and are more common in uncircumcised men. Penile warts and gonococcal and non-gonococcal urethritis are, however, more common in circumcised men. Candidal balanitis may be asymptomatic in males and is equally common in circumcised and uncircumcised men, although those who are circumcised are more likely to notice visible signs of thrush
- Opinions differ on the effect of circumcision on the transmission of HIV infection and on cervical cancer. Any effect is now considered small, and unlikely to constitute an indication for circumcision
- Lower UTIs are up to ten times more common in uncircumcised male infants

many doctors perceive as cruel in the absence of strong medical indications. The religious and cultural drivers towards circumcision in some families are very strong, notwithstanding the secular and religious arguments reviewed on the CIRP website.

 www.cirp.org/

Phimosis

This occurs when the opening of the foreskin becomes narrowed, to the extent that problems develop, such as irritation or bleeding from the edge of the foreskin, dysuria, hesitancy or even urinary obstruction. It is most common in adolescence.

Balanoposthitis

This occurs when the phimotic foreskin becomes white, hard and scarred. Advanced changes in the prepuce are

BOX 26.16 Possible medical indications for circumcision in childhood

- Phimosis causing pain or urinary obstruction
- Painful erections due to non-retraction of foreskin in adolescence
- Irreducible paraphimosis

known as balanitis xerotica obliterans and can become cancerous if left untreated, which is why circumcision is usually advised for this condition.

Balanitis

This is irritation of the glans, and occurs under the same conditions as cause nappy rash, especially ammoniacal dermatitis. Rarely it can be a marker for diabetes if heavy glycosuria has stimulated candidiasis.

Paraphimosis

This occurs if the foreskin has been retracted past the sulcus and not replaced. If the retracted skin becomes swollen, it then forms a tight painful band around the penis. This surgical emergency can often be treated by skilled manipulation, but sometimes reduction under anaesthesia or emergency circumcision is needed (Box 26.16). The condition can always be avoided if the foreskin is never left retracted.

Skin disorders

LEARNING OUTCOMES

By the end of this chapter you should:
- Know the common causes of pruritus
- Know how to diagnose and manage mild to moderate eczema
- Know the causes of napkin rash and how to manage this condition.
- Be able to recognize common birthmarks and give appropriate advice to the parents
- Be able to recognize and manage common discrete skin lesions.

Itching (pruritus)

(See also Ch. 36.)

Problem-orientated topic:

a child with an itchy scalp

Susan is a 6-year-old girl whose mother has noticed that she has developed an itchy scalp over the last 2 weeks. Her 4-year-old sister has also started scratching in the last week.

Q1. What is the likely diagnosis?

Q2. What investigations are required?

Q3. How would you manage this condition?

Q4. When should a child with prolonged itchiness be referred to hospital?

Q1. What is the likely diagnosis?

A careful history and examination is essential in all cases. In particular, ask about the following:
- Is there a rash?
  - Eczema (examine flexures and face)
  - Psoriasis (flexor surfaces)
  - Scabies (palms and soles)
  - Pityriasis rosea (Ch. 33)
- Contacts?
  - Scabies
  - Head lice
  - Fungal infection (ringworm)

- Systemic upset?
  - Chickenpox
  - Infected eczema
  - Allergic reaction.

Further history indicates that other children at Susan's school also have itchy scalps and examination reveals the characteristic egg cases of the lice on several of her hair shafts (see below).

Q2. What investigations are required?

Investigations into the cause of itching in primary care are limited, but the following should be considered:

Skin scrapings should be sent for mycological examination for confirmation of a ringworm fungal infection.

If scalp ringworm is considered, a plucked hair sample should be sent for examination.

Scraping of a scabietic burrow can isolate the mite, its larvae, empty egg cases or faecal material.

Patch testing of the skin for allergens in childhood eczema has limited value.

Q3. How would you manage this condition?

The management of head lice and other differential diagnoses are described below.

Q4. When should a child with prolonged itchiness be referred to hospital?

The most common causes of itching should be diagnosed and managed in a primary care setting. In this case the vignette suggests head lice infestation; this should be diagnosed by examination of the hair for egg cases and appropriate treatment prescribed. Scabies is another diagnosis which, if thought of, should be readily diagnosed and treated. Many cases of mild atopic dermatitis and eczema can be managed at home, but children with more resistant cases should be referred to a dermatologist.

Head lice (*Pediculosis capitis*)

This is due to infestation by the human head louse (*Pediculosis humanus capitis*) and is very common in school-age children (4–11 years). The louse is contracted through close head contact, often in classrooms or amongst siblings. Parents may also be infested.

The louse is 1–3 mm long and lives off blood sucked from the host's scalp. Females lay eggs (nits) on hair shafts close to the scalp. These are light grey in colour and may be very extensive. The nymphs hatch in 7 days and mature in 10–14 days, when they mate and lay eggs.

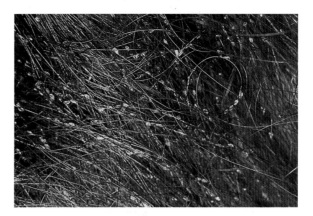

Fig. 27.1 Nits attached to hair shafts

BOX 27.1 Strategies for managing head lice

- Only treat if live lice are identified on fine combing to avoid drug resistance
- Apply an aqueous lotion to the whole scalp and leave for 12 hours
- The most effective evidence-based lotions are permethrin, synergized pyrethrin or malathion 0.5%
- Apply an aqueous lotion at night and wash out the following morning. Repeat application 7 days later
- Resistance may be a problem in some areas and local information on best choice is recommended

Children present with scalp pruritus and examination of the hair confirms the presence of live lice or egg cases (Fig. 27.1).

Management strategies are summarized in Box 27.1.

Eczema

Eczema (also referred to as atopic dermatitis) is a very common skin disorder of children. In the UK it is estimated that 1 in 5 school-age children suffer from this condition. It is a polygenic disorder with a strong family history of atopic disorders such as asthma and hay fever. Eczema may also be caused by contact with a variety of substances, including detergents and some metals (nickel jewellery is a common irritant). Exclusive breastfeeding for at least 6 months has been shown to reduce the risk in atopic families.

The most common presenting feature is an itchy rash over the face or limb flexures (antecubital fossa, backs of knees). In infants evidence of scratching or rubbing the skin must be sought. The skin appears dry, red and inflamed, particularly in the flexures, neck or face.

Lifestyle changes
- Use cotton clothes next to the child's skin.
- Avoid using scented soaps
- Avoid biological washing powders and fabric softeners
- Keep the child's nails short to avoid the trauma of scratching
- At night cotton mittens may be helpful

Exclusion diets
- These have not been shown to be helpful in mild and moderate cases

Reduce itching
- Emollients (moisturizing ointments or creams) reduce water loss from the skin, thereby preventing dryness
- Use emulsifying ointment instead of soap
- Give oral antihistamines
- Chlorphenamine maleate
- Hydroxyzine hydrochloride

Topical steroids
- These should be used sparingly and in low concentration (mild strength) during acute flare-ups of the eczema
- Apply thinly to the affected area

Infected eczema
- Antibiotic cream or oral medication if there are exudates or crusting of lesions

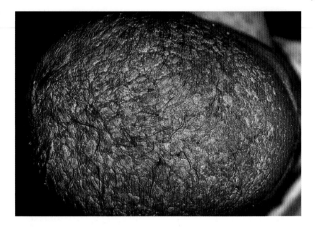

Fig. 27.2 **Severe cradle cap**

The management of more problematic eczema is discussed in Chapter 36.

Cradle cap

In infants in the first few months of life eczema may present as 'seborrhoeic dermatitis'. It is often referred to as 'cradle cap' when affecting the scalp and associated with thick flakes on the head and behind the ears, but is not sore or itchy (Fig. 27.2). It may also affect the nappy area (see below). It is usually self-limiting and disappears by the age of 1. Basic management is with moisturizing (emollient) creams and bath oils.

www.eczema.org

Scabies

This is due to infestation by the mite *Sarcoptes scabiei*, which causes intense itchiness. The mite is acquired by direct skin-to-skin contact and is highly contagious. The adult female mite burrows into the skin and lays its eggs. The larvae mature and mate, and the cycle is repeated every 2 weeks. Itchiness is due to an allergic reaction to the mites and their products. Symptoms occur after 6 weeks of primary infection, but within 48 hours of reinfestation.

The diagnosis is suggested by itching in several family members at the same time and the definitive diagnosis is made on identification of the subcutaneous burrow (Fig. 36.14). In older children the burrow is usually seen on the hands, but in younger children and babies scabies often affects the face, scalp, head, palms and soles. Longer-standing infestation can cause widespread eczematized lesions, particularly on the trunk. Very young babies do not scratch but appear miserable.

Management is summarized in Box 27.3.

Long-standing scratching of the affected lesions leads to splitting of the skin and thickening (lichenification) with increased pigmentation in dark-skinned children. Cracked skin may weep ('wet' eczema) and become secondarily infected.

Involvement of the face is common and particularly distressing for the child and family. The cheeks and forehead are frequently involved initially, with itching, dryness and inflammation. The eyelids may be involved (blepharitis) particularly, causing thickening of the lower eyelid in long-standing cases.

Eczema is a chronic condition that is likely to relapse and remit during childhood. There is no cure but in many cases simple remedies will control the unpleasant symptoms of the condition. Around 50% of children with eczema will clear by 12 years of age.

Management in primary care can be considered under several headings (Box 27.2).

Children with moderate or severe eczema or those not responding to basic management should be referred to a specialist paediatrician or paediatric dermatologist.

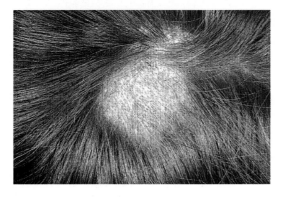

Fig. 27.3 Scalp ringworm with a patch of hair loss.
(Reproduced by permission from Blackwell Science.)

Scalp ringworm (tinea capitis)

This highly contagious condition is due to a fungal infection and particularly affects Afro-Caribbean children. It causes intense itchiness of the scalp and on examination there is usually patchy alopecia with scaling (Fig. 27.3). The scales may be confused with cradle cap. A kerion occurs rarely; this is a boggy mass with multiple pustules, often with lymphadenopathy of the neck.

Diagnosis is made by finding the fungus on a hair or scale sample. Treatment is with an oral antifungal agent such as griseofulvin until the fungus is eradicated.

Urticaria

This refers to itchy hives or wheals, usually lasting only a few hours. It may be due to contact with noxious plants (nettles) or be the result of allergy to some foods (e.g. strawberries). The lips may be affected as the result of food allergy and this is an IgE-mediated reaction. Rarely swelling of the tongue and glottis may occur, which may be life-threatening; this may result from nut allergy (Ch. 44). Insect bites may cause a very itchy papular urticaria.

Table 27.1 Clinical assessment of a nappy rash

Cause	Distinguishing features
Contact (ammoniacal)	The whole of the napkin area is affected, but the skin creases are spared
Thrush	The skin in the nappy area is bright red and the skin creases are involved. Satellite lesions may extend beyond the napkin area
Seborrhoeic dermatitis	Red rash with flakes and pustules. There are often eczematous patches elsewhere, particularly the scalp
Psoriasis	Rare. Red scaly rash often involving non-napkin areas

Nappy rash

Problem-orientated topic:

a baby with nappy rash

Shoaib is a 6-month-old baby who has developed a sore, red rash in the nappy area. He screams when he passes urine and his mother has noted that he has been febrile on occasions. Four weeks earlier he developed a less severe nappy rash, which improved spontaneously.

Q1. What is the differential diagnosis of this rash?
Q2. What is the management?

Q1. What is the differential diagnosis of this rash?

Nappy rash is a very common occurrence in babies and may be severe. Some babies develop repeated episodes of this condition.

Table 27.1 lists the causes and distinguishing features of nappy rash.

Q2. What is the management?

The major points in the management are summarized in Box 27.4.

Contact (ammoniacal) nappy rash

This is now a very uncommon condition with the widespread introduction of disposable absorbent nappies. The effect of bacteria on urine is to produce ammonia, which, if in contact with the skin for a prolonged time, leads to inflammation. Contact dermatitis in the nappy

- Keep the nappy area dry and clean by changing frequently
- Use disposable nappies, which absorb water, rather than towelling
- Leave the baby without a nappy whenever possible
- Use a barrier cream (e.g. zinc and castor oil, petroleum jelly, Sudocrem)
- If the skin is very inflamed, use a mild steroid cream (1% hydrocortisone) before applying the barrier cream
- If thrush is present, use an antifungal cream (see below)

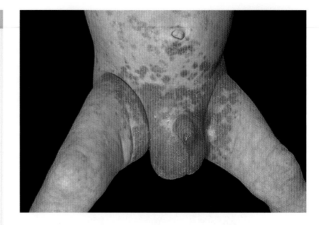

Fig. 27.4 *Candida* nappy rash.
(Reproduced with permission from Blackwell Science.)

area also occurs rarely as few mothers wash towelling nappies in sensitizing biological washing powders.

The characteristic feature of contact nappy rash is that the skin creases are usually not red, as the nappy does not come in contact with the creases except if secondary fungal or bacterial infection occurs. Treatment is based on prevention of the skin being exposed to urine and faeces for a long time and use of a barrier cream.

If recovery does not occur rapidly with this treatment, secondary infection should be considered and an antifungal cream with 1% hydrocortisone used. Rarely secondary bacterial infection occurs and this is usually staphylococcal. Severe infection is associated with a fever and an oral antibiotic (flucloxacillin) should be given.

Once the nappy area has recovered, the mother should be advised on basic hygiene measures to prevent recurrence.

Thrush (*Candida*) rash

Fungal infections cause a very red and sore nappy rash with involvement of the skin creases. Sometimes small satellite lesions develop on the abdominal wall or thighs outside of the nappy area (Fig. 27.4).

General treatment should be instituted, as outlined above, together with an antifungal cream or ointment (miconazole 2% or nystatin). If the skin is very sore, a combined antifungal and 1% hydrocortisone cream is recommended.

Birthmarks

Birthmarks may be divided into vascular and pigmented lesions (Box 27.5). Birthmarks are common and may affect 1 in 3 babies. The most common is the naevus flammeus. Apart from cosmetic concerns,

BOX 27.5 Types of birthmark

- Vascular
- Naevus flammeus
- Strawberry naevus
- Port-wine stain
- Pigmented
- Mongolian blue spot
- Café-au-lait spots
- Moles

birthmarks are usually benign. Pigmented birthmarks are less common than vascular marks, but if large may become malignant.

Naevus flammeus (stork's beak mark)

These relatively small vascular naevi are extremely common and become more obvious when the baby cries (Fig. 27.5). They are most frequently seen on the nasal bridge or forehead in the midline, over the nape of the neck or on the eyelids. They usually fade as the baby gets older.

Strawberry naevus (capillary haemangioma)

These naevi are often not present at birth but grow rapidly over the first few weeks and months to become raised red lobulated tumours (Fig. 27.6). They then remain fixed in size before regressing and completely resolving. Around 95% disappear by the time the child is 9 years old.

Strawberry naevi most commonly occur on the face, scalp, back or chest. They may cause mechanical problems

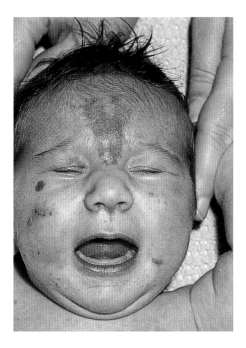

Fig. 27.5 Naevus flammeus.
(Reproduced with permission from Blackwell Science.)

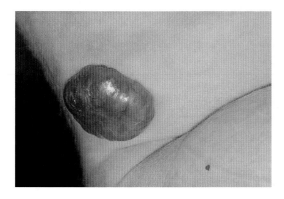

Fig. 27.6 Strawberry naevus in a 3-month-old baby

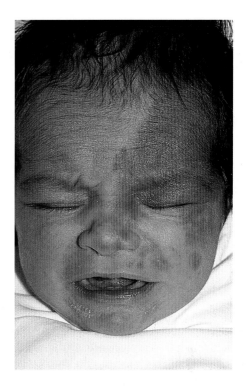

Fig. 27.7 Port-wine stain in the upper trigeminal area.
(Reproduced with permission from Blackwell Science.)

bution (Fig. 27.7). It has an incidence of 0.3% in newborn babies. It usually does not fade and may cause distressing facial disfigurement. There may be local tissue overgrowth in the region of the haemangioma. Port-wine stains around the eye may be associated with glaucoma.

The Sturge–Weber syndrome is a combination of port-wine naevus over the face with intracranial calcification and often convulsions.

Management is usually with cover-up cosmetics, but laser treatment may be effective in causing the lesion to fade. Best results are obtained when the laser treatment is started early in life.

Mongolian blue spot

This is a common pigmented macular lesion seen in pigmented babies (Fig. 27.8). It is blue or slate-grey in colour and occurs over the lower back and buttocks. It may be mistaken for a bruise and child abuse may be suspected. It usually fades as the child gets older, but is always benign and requires no treatment.

Café-au-lait spots

These are light-brown pigmented lesions that usually develop in childhood. Multiple lesions or large lesions greater than 2 cm diameter may be a feature of neurofibromatosis (Ch. 28).

if they compromise the eye, mouth or nose as they grow. Rarely capillary haemangioma may occur in the upper respiratory tract, leading to life-threatening obstruction of the airway.

They may ooze blood if subject to constant rubbing, but serious haemorrhage is very rare.

A cavernous haemangioma refers to a deep capillary haemangioma that causes a lump and often a blue discoloration of the skin.

Treatment is rarely required, as the natural history is for them to regress spontaneously.

Port-wine stain

This is a flat haemangioma, most commonly unilateral and found on the face in the trigeminal nerve distri-

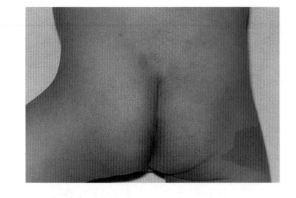

Fig. 27.8 Mongolian blue spot in gluteal cleft and café au lait lesion on thigh.
(Reproduced with permission from Blackwell Science.)

Pigmented naevi (moles)

These are very common; they are usually small but grow as the child grows. Rarely a large congenital pigmented naevi occurs and is very disfiguring. If larger than 10 cm in diameter, it has an increased risk of malignancy (melanoma). Careful follow-up observation of the lesion should be arranged.

Other common skin lesions seen in primary care

Contact dermatitis

This is due to an allergen causing a delayed hypersensitivity reaction. In children the most common sensitizing substance is nickel, used in cheap jewellery and studs. There is erythema and blistering at the contact site.

The localization of the lesion usually suggests the cause. The allergen should be avoided and the lesions, if severe, respond rapidly to hydrocortisone 1% cream.

Impetigo

This is a highly contagious skin lesion due to *Staphylococcus aureus* or *Streptococcus pyogenes*. It most commonly presents in young children (2–6 years) as multiple golden crusty lesions growing slowly in size and reaching 2 cm in diameter (Fig. 27.9). It is not usually painful or itchy and does not scar. In some cases the crusts develop following a bullous eruption (blistering). Impetigo may occur in already damaged skin, such as in eczema or scabies.

A swab from the lesions should be taken, as meticillin-resistant strains (MRSA) are common. Topical flucloxacillin cream is recommended in mild cases with few lesions, but topical antibiotics will not eradicate organisms on uninvolved skin. Oral flucloxacillin or erythromycin is

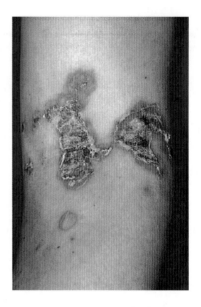

Fig. 27.9 Lesions of impetigo with satellite lesions.
(Reproduced with permission from Blackwell Science.)

recommended in more severe cases. Resistance is growing and microbiological sensitivities of the organism may guide the choice of antibiotics.

Warts

These are common and are caused by the human papillomavirus. They may occur as common warts (usually on hands and feet) or plantar warts (verrucae). In the vast majority of cases the wart resolves spontaneously after a number of years. Genital warts are discussed in Chapter 37.

If treatment is required, topical application of salicylic acid or cryotherapy is beneficial, but the latter is painful and not advised in young children.

Molluscum contagiosum

This is a common lesion in children 2–5 years old. It is contracted from affected children by direct contact and lesions are due to a human poxvirus. The lesions appear as multiple 1–10 mm dome-shaped papules with a central depression, usually occurring on the trunk or limb flexures (Fig. 27.10). The natural history is for the lesions to resolve spontaneously within 8–12 months, but new ones can occur by autoinoculation.

In view of their benign and self-limiting natural history, no treatment is recommended.

Cold sores

These are due to herpes simplex virus (HSV-1) infection and cold sores develop when the HSV is reactivated.

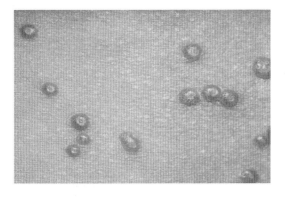

Fig. 27.10 Molluscum contagiosum lesions.
(Reproduced with permission from Blackwell Science.)

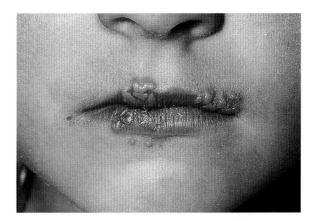

Fig. 27.11 Cold sores.
(Reproduced with permission from Blackwell Science.)

The lesions usually affect the lips, but may also involve the mouth, and start with tingling followed by multiple vesicles erupting in a group (Fig. 27.11). It is self-limiting but tends to recur. Children with eczema may develop a more severe form of HSV-1 infection (eczema herpeticum) with multiple lesions, fever and malaise.

Treatment of cold sores is by topical aciclovir cream until the lesion resolves.

Index

Myoclonus, 48
sleep, 293

N

Naevus
congenital melanocytic, *82*
flammeus (stork mark), *74*, *82*, 346,
347
pigmented, 348
strawberry, *82*, 346–347, *347*
Nail-biting, 220–221
Nails, examination, 51
Nappy rash, *345*, 345–346, *346*
candidal (thrush), *345*, *346*
contact (ammoniacal), *345*, 345–346
Narcolepsy, 293
Nasal polyps, 282
Nasogastric tube (NGT) feeding,
newborn infants, 84
Nasopharyngeal aspirate (NPA), 270
National Health Service (NHS)
data collection, 154–155
organizational structure, 155, *156*
responsibility for improving health, 178
National Institute for Clinical Excellence
(NICE), 112
clinical audit process, 134–136
National Screening Committee (NSC), 162
antenatal screening policy, 165, *165*
childhood screening policy, *168*
criteria for screening programmes, 162,
163
neonatal screening policy, *167*
National Service Framework (NSF),
Children's, 135, *156*, 157–158
implementation, 158
standards, 157
Neck
examination, 51, *51*
in newborn, 72–74, *74*
lumps, *322*, 322–323, *323*
midline swellings, 323
torticollis, 302–303, *303*
Needs assessment *see* Health needs
assessment
Negative predictive value (NPV), *56*,
161–162
Neglect *see* Child neglect
Neighbourhood, 143, *143*
Neisseria meningitidis infection *see*
Meningococcal disease
Neonatal deaths, major causes, *5*
Neonatal intensive care, ethical issues, 114
Neonatal screening, 84–85, *90*, 167–168
blood spot, 84–85, 167, *167*
hearing, 85, *160*, 168
policy, *167*
Neonates *see* Newborn infants
Nephrons, 325–326, *326*
Nephrotic syndrome, *45*
Nervous system
development, 8–10, *9*
examination *see* Neurological
examination
malformations, 9, *9*

Neural tube, closure, 9
Neural tube defects, 9
maternal serum screening, 91
Neuroimaging, 291, 294, 295–296
Neurological disease
constipation, 306
vaccination, *174*
Neurological examination, 46–50
cranial nerves, *48*, 48–49
eye and squints, 49–50
limbs and gait, 46–47, *47*
newborn infants, 79–81
tremors and movement disorders,
47–48
Neuropeptide Y (NPY), 255
Neuroplasticity, 19
Newborn infants
antimicrobial prescribing, 106
attachment *see* Attachment
breastfeeding, 25–28, 82–83
bruising, causes, *320*
drug metabolism, 103, *103*
drug toxicity, 103–104
ethical and legal issues, 113–114
evaluation, 71–85
feeding advice/problems, 28, 82–84
history, 71–72
jaundice *see* Jaundice, neonatal
pain assessment, 106
physical examination, 72–82, *73*,
167
physiological changes, *28*
Newborn Screening Programme Centre,
167
NHS *see* National Health Service
NHS Direct, *156*
NICE *see* National Institute for Clinical
Excellence
Nightmares, 293
Night terrors, 293
Ninth (IX) nerve, *48*, 49
Nits, 343, *343*
Nociceptors, 284
Non-judgmental attitude, 213
Non-steroidal anti-inflammatory drugs
(NSAIDs), 107
Non-verbal communication
development, 11
talking to patients/families, 64
Noradrenaline (norepinephrine), 326
Nose
bleeds, 282
examination, 52
NSC *see* National Screening
Committee
NSF *see* National Service Framework
Nuchal translucency (NT), 91, 166
Number needed to treat for benefit
(NNT$_B$), *131*
Numerators, 151
Nursery schools, 198
Nursing staff, role in communication
with families, 65, 66, 67
Nutrients
in infant and toddler foods, *30*
requirements, calculations, *31*

Nutrition, 24–33, *142*
assessment, 30–31, 42
childhood, 30
fetal, 24–25
in infancy, 25–32
in pregnancy, 24–25
role in growth, 237
strategies to tackle obesity, 185
see also Diet; Eating; Feeding; Food(s)

O

Obesity, *149*, 184–185, 255–261
causes, 256, *256*, 260–261
clinical assessment, 256–258, *257*,
258, *259–260*
complications, 184–185, 260, 261
facts and figures, *185*
investigations, 258, *258*
management, 260, 261
nutritional, *258*, 260–261
prevention, 185, 261
prognosis, 261
screening, 168
Objective pain scale (OPS), 284
Oculomotor (III) nerve, *48*, 49
Odds ratio, 130–131, *131*
Oestrogen cream, topical, 333
Olfactory nerve (I), *48*
Omission of treatment, 112
Opioids
analgesic (opiates), 107, 285
endogenous, 284
Optic nerve, *48*
Oral rehydration fluids, 315
Orchidometer, *52*
Orchitis, 319
Organ retention, 112–113
Organ transplant recipients,
immunization, 174
Ortolani's test, 78
Osmoregulation, newborn infants, *28*
Otitis media
acute (AOM), *268*, 268–269
chronic suppurative (CSOM), 269
neck swellings, 322, 323
Ottawa Charter for Health Promotion
(1986), 182, *183*, 184
Oucher Scale, 106
Outbreak control, 175–176
Outcomes
clinical audit, 133
monitoring by data collection, 134
Outpatients
major causes of attendance, *6*
writing GP letters, 68–69
Over-active child, 218–219
Over-the-counter medicines, 105
Oxygen saturation, measurement, 120
Oxytocin, *26*

P

Paediatricians, 157
attributes, 4
duties, *4*

DVD Player access instructions

- Place the DVD in the DVD player and press play. Use the Up, Down, Left and Right arrows on your remote control to navigate the menus. Press **Enter** or **Play** to make a selection.

DVD-ROM access instructions

Windows

- Locate the DVD icon in **My Computer** or select **'Start'**, **'Programs'** and the name of the DVD software
- Click the DVD icon or the name of the DVD software and the **Main Menu** will appear.

Mac

- The DVD will auto-start unless **auto-start** has been disabled in **System Preferences**.

System requirements

This is a Region 0 enabled DVD so is compatible with any DVD player.
A NTSC-compatible television/monitor is required to display the content correctly.

Windows PC

PC Based Pentium 450 MHZ
Windows 2000 or higher
256 MB RAM or higher
32 MB or higher Graphics Card
4x DVD-ROM drive
Display Resolution of 800 × 600 or greater
Sound Card and Speakers
Software which supports DVD-Video playback

Mac

Power PC G4 300 MHZ, I-Mac, I-Book
Macintosh OS 9.2 or higher
256 MB RAM or higher
32 MB or higher Graphics Card
4x DVD-ROM drive
Display Resolution of 800 × 600 or greater
Sound Card and Speakers
Software which supports DVD-Video playback

Technical support

Technical support for this product is available between 7.30 a.m. and 7.00 p.m. CST, Monday through Friday.
Before calling, be sure that your computer meets the minimum system requirements to run this software.
Inside the United States and Canada, call 1-800-692-9010.
Inside the United Kingdom, call 0-0800-6929-0100.
Rest of World, call +1-314-872-8370.
You may also fax your questions to +1-314-523-4932,
or contact Technical Support through e-mail: technical.support@elsevier.com.

Elsevier DVD-Video licence agreement